Intermittent Fasting For Women Over 50 & Autophagy Mastery (2 in 1): Detox Your Body, Improve Hormonal Health & Promote Extreme Energy+ 10 Weight Loss Hypnosis& Meditations

Intermittent Fasting For Women Over 50: Promote Longevity& Extreme Energy, Detox Your Body, Improve Hormonal Health& Reset Your Metabolism+ 5 Rapid Weight Loss Hypnosis& Meditations

The Wellness Hub

TABLE OF CONTENTS

INTRODUCTION

Today's fast-paced, nutrient-deficient world wreaks havoc on the human body. Pollutants weaken our immune systems, our cells can't properly engage in the process of autophagy, which recycles usable cellular materials while discarding toxins and unnecessary cellular waste. This has an affect on everything in the body and even in the mind, creating downward spirals that can take a person's entire future with it. But there are ways of combating and even reversing the corrosive effects of a toxic body and mind. It's widely known in the medical field that people who engage in regular physical exercise have:

- Roughly 30% lower risk of early death

- Roughly 50% lowered risk of type 2 diabetes

- Roughly 35% lowered risk of coronary disease

- Roughly 35% lowered risk of stroke

- Roughly 20% lowered risk of breast cancer

- Roughly 50% lowered risk of colon cancer

Fasting is a powerful weapon for weight loss and general good health. People who participate in intermittent fasting cut four to seven percent from their waistline over six months.

And women have special health considerations to take into account when combating illness, especially where fasting and diet are concerned. Before any woman fasts or begins a new regiment (after consulting with a doctor), she should be aware of the building-block general information as well as the particulars we'll present here.

And that information is sorely needed. Here are some frightening US statistics to make the point a bit clearer.

- Over 15% of women over 18 are in fair or poor health

- Less than half of women 18 years and over met the guidelines for physical activity

- 12.7% of women 18 years or over currently smoke cigarettes: 12.7%

- Over 41% of women 20 years or and over who are obese

- Over 45% of women 20 years or older have hypertension or are taking antihypertensive medication

- 11% of women under age 65 do not have health insurance

- Leading causes of death of women are (in order) heart disease, cancer, and stroke

Perhaps that makes the urgency for remedy even clearer. Women are facing a widespread health crisis which spans the globe. Don't become the next statistic. Take your life and your health into your own hands, into your own minds, and turn things around now, while you still can.

Because there are natural remedies for such lethal conditions. This book is your guide, to them and to other remedies for other conditions! This book provides the history as well as the best information. It offers you findings from cutting edge studies and experiments. Here, you can learn everything you need to know about autophagy, fasting, hormonal imbalances and more. You'll practice leading methods of weight loss and roads to general good health; detoxing and cleansing, diet, exercise, yoga, meditation, even hypnotism. You'll get a working knowledge of good health from the molecule to the entire body. You'll learn what and what not to eat and why. You'll learn how your body and mind work and how they can work together. You won't just learn, you will *do*; putting the concepts into action which will change your body, your mind, your life.

These exercises come from leading experts, programs chosen to address the subjects in this book. The data is from the world's most trusted sources (like The World Health Organization). This book, like all our books, makes complex scientific information easy to understand and making complicated concepts easy to ingest. We help countless readers improve their lives, more of them all the time, on subjects as diverse as leadership skills and mental disorders and more. Readers come to us to help them remedy the things which plague their lives and so many others.

This book addresses the discrepancy between body and soul, between temporary satisfaction and true happiness. The benefits go deeper than that. We'll walk you through the processes you'll come across. Wellness is the destination at the end of (this leg of) your journey, and we'll take that journey with you to see through every step.

Statistics prove these approaches work. Generations of longevity all over the world prove it. And new technology illuminates what was once misunderstood or unknown to modern science. Now they've finally caught up with the technologies creating electronic light, processed foods, a barrage of media.

In fact, there's so much diverse information here, just one lesson well-learned may very well change your life. The chapter on fats and cholesterol alone will teach you the difference between good cholesterol and bad. It's a difference which may be taking you by surprise even as you read this introduction). That alone could be the difference between life and death. Even understanding what autophagy is, how and why it works, is worth the price, since this alone will change how you look at yourself, your body, your life. It's your body, you should know how it works. It's your mind, you should know how to properly use it.

You know these things are true. And you know you haven't got a choice. Chances are, the problem has been going on for a while if you're seeking help now. As you read this, your bones may be becoming brittle, your blood may be thickening. You eating that things you want but you know you don't need. You may be living on the powder keg of an impending stroke or heart attack. Or you may be looking at the long, slow decline that may rob you of the perfect life you have worked hard for. Don't let your dreams or your body die. Your good health is in your own strong hands, figuratively and literally. If not now, when? It's easy to be jaded or to procrastinate, but it's crucial you take the next step. The first step was picking up this book, seeking help. The next step is to read the book and accept that help. The next steps are all in this book. Read them, understand them, question them.

Always consult with a physician before changing your diet or exercise programs. Don't strain your body or your mind. Drink plenty of fluids, especially water.

Remember when reading this book that all elements we come across will interact with others. You won't be able to master one without understanding the other. Also, the information here is presented in a very particular order, each section building on the section before it and preparing the reader for the section to come. So while this is definitely a reference book in part, meant to be looked at time and again, it is also mean to be followed. Try exercise before moving on yoga; try yoga before meditation. Each prepares you for the next.

We're also going to make clear that this is about you. You don't have to live for others, to impress others, nor can you save others. So even though the chances are you have friends or loved ones who share maladies illustrated here, you can only tell them so much.

You'll have to lead by example. Think about adopting some of these practices even if your muscular integrity and weight are in good shape. You can always be better. Stress always comes up, and that can causes inflammation and related conditions. Good health is about deliberate action and mindfulness. We can all always be more deliberate, more mindful. Anybody can always be in better physical or mental health. All we need information, inspiration, dedication.

So just do it. Read the book, do the exercises, engage in the practices, Share it all with your family and friends. They'll all want to know you're leaner and healthier and happier, with a vibrant glow and clear skin. They'll beg to know, and you'll be ready to share your secrets. You can lead them down the road to wellness which none of you may have realized existed. Now you hold the roadmap. You're already taking the first steps. Now take the rest; we'll take them together.

So, let's begin!

SECTION 1: AUTOPHAGY AND FASTING

CHAPTER ONE: Autophagy

Autophagy is the human body's method of flushing out damaged cells. It's the body's way of regenerating healthy, new cells. *Auto* refers to *self* and *phagy,* means *to eat.*

Autophagy removes dysfunctional cells and can recycle some parts of those cells for use in cellular cleaning and repair, which it does by way of organelles called *autophagosomes*, a process which binds unwanted cellular matter with other cellular components called *lysosomes*. A lysosome breaks the material down, allowing some materials to be reused and others discarded.

Benefits of Autophagy

Autophagy has innumerable benefits, the sum of which is longevity and overall good health are among the most noticeable. What goes on behind the scenes is even more intriguing. Autography is known to have protective or curative effects on:

- Alzheimer's and Parkinson's disease, as well as other neurodegenerative diseases.

- Cancer

- Alcohol- and drug-induced liver damage

- Wilson's disease

- Nonalcoholic fatty liver

Diet and Autophagy

Take a look at these horrifying statistics:
- Obesity affected 13% of adults globally in 2016

- Obesity often fosters metabolic syndrome (high blood pressure, type 2 diabetes, and low HDL cholesterol

- 700 million adults are obese

- Obesity if linked to roughly five million deaths each year around the world

- Obesity accounts for about 13% percent of adults worldwide

- 39% of adults are overweight

- One in every five children and adolescents globally are overweight

- 34 million people (over ten percent of the population of the United States, have diabetes

- Roughly 26.8 million people (10% of the population) have diagnosed diabetes

- Over 7 million people have undiagnosed diabetes

Seems pretty straight forward, doesn't it? It's a pretty simple natural process, one that's meant to happen all the time, but which has slowed to a crawl in a lot of our bodies in this modern and toxic age. Really, it's the key to longevity, practically the fountain of youth. And that only makes sense. When your cells are healthy, you are healthy. When your cellular metabolism is unhealthy, your whole body will be unhealthy.

Yet this is new and exciting information to a lot of people. It can and should bring new hope to everyone, particularly for women. Because women face issues of youthfulness and vitality which men do not necessarily face.

Because, autophagy or not, men and women age differently, in ways both social and biological. Men remain in their reproductive years far longer than women do, so their bodies may remain vital for longer. They may become more handsome with age. Women's bodies are no longer reproductive fairly early in life, with everybody's lifespans longer than in previous generations. Though life expectancy has waned slightly in the past few years, the average man in the US still lives to be over seventy years old, and the average woman close to eighty. Nature stops focusing on the post-partem female body, as it no longer has any innate, natural value. She may have sociological value, but not in the same way that an aging man has. Because, sociologically speaking, the rigorous standard of youth and beauty to which women are held simply doesn't apply to men. As men age, they often become wealthier, and men are held up to a different bar in this regard as women are in the other regard.

So knowing the value of autophagy may be of particular importance to women who would like to see their skin cells replacing themselves, the renewed vitality which comes from autophagy.

And one of the best ways to kickstart autophagy is fasting, which is where our study takes us next. But read carefully, as the rules for men and women may differ. As with the rest of the book, we'll review the books in general, as they apply to men and women both, then move into the territory where women need special guidance or information. The things which apply to men only are left for another book.

CHAPTER TWO: Fasting

Fasting is where body and mind will meet, as we'll see soon enough. It's also where the past and the future meet, and it's about to be squarely in the present of your life. Because, of all the things we're going to look at here, fasting is perhaps the oldest. Fasting occurred in man's earliest era, when he was still a part of the food chain. A million or so years ago, during the paleolithic era, our ancestors often had to go long periods without eating. That was when they hunted. Hunts were often long, prey was not always abundant or easy to kill. This is when the human body as it basically is today programmed itself to react to foods. It's how protein and carbohydrates and fats became prioritized in the human physiology.

But our lifestyles were different then, much more active to burn more calories. And the foods were more pure, whole foods and good fats and carbohydrates. Fat was helpful in the winter, when food was scarce and fasting necessary.

Our lives are barely recognizable from those of our ancestors, but our bodies have hardly changed at all. We're a bit taller now, leaner, we live longer. But our environment is more toxified, our lifestyles more sedentary. Involuntary fasting still occurs among the meal-insecure of our third-, second-, and even first-world countries.

But voluntary fasting has risen from the dark corners of political protest and religious dedication and into the mainstream, becoming something of a trend. And there are good reasons for that. It integrates with everything we'll look at in this book, from autophagy to yoga to meditation and beyond. It has a number of health benefits, and a few health risks as well, particularly for women. A lot of people fast, but few people do it wisely or well. And fasting incorrectly can do more harm than good, so read on and always consult with your doctor!

On the whole, fasting is one of the very best ways of instigating autophagy, which puts it next on our list. Some of the benefits of fasting include:

- Gut, heart, immunity, and brain health

- Body composition

- High energy

- Appetite management

- Anti-aging and longevity

- Willpower, self-control, and relationship with food

There are different types of fasts for different results.

Caloric liquid fasting (CLF) is best for general digestive health. These liquids-only fasts (low-sugar juices, bone broth, water, unsweetened coffee and tea) may last between one and five days.

Non-caloric liquid fasting (unsweetened tea, coffee, and water) are best for fast weight loss, and they can last between one and seven days. This cellular cleanse is ideal to instigate autophagy.

Intermittent fasting is probably best for body composition.

There are two fasting cycles; intermittent or short-term fasting, and long-term fasting.

Note: Always start a fast with a period of light eating equal to half the length of the expected fast.

Intermittent Fasting

Fasting has a lot of the same benefits of autophagy, including weight loss, muscle strength, improved metabolism, improved organ health, and overall longevity. Studies show that intermittent fasting may generate a weight loss of three to eight pounds over three to 24 weeks. Similar studies show the same thing, but to lesser degrees. Intermittent fasting can boost norepinephrine, which elevates the metabolic rate from roughly four percent to almost 14%.

Intermittent Fasting and Weight Loss

Intermittent fasting has a demonstrable effect on weight loss, as we've seen. And while intermittent fasting has many other benefits to the human body, weight loss is certainly one of them. Before we go much further, it's important to note that fasting of any sort is not recommended for women who are pregnant, sufferers of low blood pressure or diabetes, anyone under the age of 18, or anyone who has had or may have an eating disorder.

Losing weight is basically about burning more calories than you consume. But the body isn't that simple. There's a bit more to losing weight than caloric balance and there's also more to intermittent fasting than just losing weight.

It's important to understand what factors may affect weight loss. They include:

- Sleep

- Gender

- Age

- Stress

- Genetics

- Medication

- Hormones

- Microbiome

- Metabolic rate

- Health status

- Food quality

Intermittent fasting is more of an eating schedule than a diet. It's less about *what* you eat, but *when* you eat … and when you *don't,* as we'll see in greater detail shortly.

Benefits of intermittent fasting for weight loss include:

- Ease of use

- Flexibility

- Self-awareness

- Self-control

What about the drawbacks of intermittent fasting? Not everybody loses weight with intermittent fasting. Why is that?

- Premenopausal women may not lose weight with intermittent fasting, and the practice may even be detrimental. We don't recommend it for premenopausal women.

- Overeating during the eating windows is another reason some people fail to lose weight. Limiting alcohol intake is also crucial to weight loss with intermittent fasting.

- Insufficient exercise may limit weight loss during an intermittent fast.

Different Methods of Intermittent Fasting

One popular, simple way to do is known as *the 16/8 method*. It requires daily fasting for between 14 and 16 hours with an 8- to 10-hour eating window. The eating window allows for two or more healthy meals, low in carbohydrates. Water, coffee, and no-calorie drinks are allowed.

Variations on this approach include 13/11 (13 hours fasting with an 11-hour eating window), 18/16 (18 hours fasting with a 16-hour eating window) and 20/4 (20 hours fasting with a four-hour eating window). The 13-hour approach may begin at noon and end at one in the morning, basically a breakfast-and-early-lunch cycle. The 20/4 approach offers an eating window for any preferred meal; a long breakfast, lunch, or dinner. The 18/16 approach staggers the schedule, so you're eating breakfast one day, lunch the next, dinner the next.

Another method of short-term fasting is *the 5/2 diet*, which divides the week into two blocks; two days and five days. Dieters eat as they normally would for five days, but they restrict their caloric intake for the other two days. The two days can be staggered throughout the week or be sequential. Those two days might include two small meals of 250-300 calories each (men are recommended to intake 300-400).

There is also the *Eat Stop Eat* method, which entails fasting for 24 hours periodically. Dieters may eat at 6 pm on one day, then fast until dinner the next night. Coffee and water and zero-calorie beverages are allowed during fasting times.

Eating regularly and moderately during non-fasting days is important; don't double-up to compensate. Also, twenty-four hours can be a long time for a lot of novice dieters. Newcomers might try16 hours at first, then expand.

Alternate-day fasting requires one day of regular eating followed by one day of fasting (or very limited intake, 500-600 calories max). If done on a weekly cycle, it generates two eating days or two fasting days in a row.

The Warrior Diet offers small portions of raw fruits and vegetables during the day and one big meal at night.

Spontaneous meal-skipping is a forgiving and non-committal form of intermittent fasting. It involves the dieter occasionally skipping meals. It's a myth that the human being needs to eat every couple of hours. The body can certainly survive missing one meal every now and then. This is a good introduction to fasting.

Short-term fasting's drawbacks may include dizziness or lightheadedness, distractedness, cloudy thinking, and nausea.

Long-term Fasting

Short-term fasting includes a full day, but long-term fasting may go on for two days or more.

A *dry fast* is the most extreme type; no food or beverage of any kind, including water. It can have terrible effects on the body, including sin, kidney, and liver damage, heart problems, and tooth loss. Don't go longer than twenty-four hours without drinking something.

Water fasting is like dry fasting but with water, and only water. No calories are consumed. Juice fasting allows only whole fruit or vegetable juices. A broth fast is comparable, providing liquid and also minimal caloric intake. But neither juice, broth, or coffee fasting are true fasting.

Weight loss is among the most prominent effects of water fasting as the body works through the storage of glycogen and turns to protein and fat for fuel. Fasters may lose one to two pounds per day of water weight. This will slow as the body turns to the fats for fuel.

Long-term fasting promotes autophagy, which we know has crucial health benefits.

One study found benefits of long-term suffering to cancer patients undergoing chemotherapy (fasting for an average of five days), and sufferers of hypertension (an average of ten days of fasting).

Long-term fasting also allows a dieter to reset their relationship with their favorite foods. What was habitual may become repulsive, as it often is with ex-cigarette smokers.

The dangers and risks of long-term fasting include loss of heart muscle and even heart failure. Mineral deficiencies (magnesium and potassium) may only worsen the effects. Infectious diseases can also be a threat to long-term fasters, who may suffer weakened immune systems.

Mood swings, low energy, irritability, and an increase in cortisol and norepinephrine, stress hormones may occur. This creates a fasting high, encouraging more (and more dangerous) fasting. Fasting also releases toxins from fat quickly, reintroducing toxins into the blood before they're disposed of.

The long-term fast can end lifelong cycles of bad dieting and malnutrition and bad diet, eating disorders, and food-related conditions like type-2 diabetes and obesity. It can also lead to the faster confronting the emotional causes of eating disorders.

Keep in mind that like pregnant mothers, some people should forgo fasting. They include:

- Children

- Elderly

- Sufferers of kidney or liver problems

- Women who are trying to get pregnant (and obviously those who already are)

  Anyone who is going to fast long-term, here are some tips:

- Talk to your doctor

- Explain to your friends and family to help socialize

- Get a fasting coach or counselor

- Integrate meditation and/or yoga

- Integrate supplements (calcium, potassium, magnesium, sodium, phosphate)

- Forgo vigorous exercise

Fasting Apps

There are lots of fasting apps, and we don't have the time to run through them all. We're setting some which are designed specifically for women for our book on fasting for women, but there are plenty which are good for both men and women, and each has its benefits. All are free to download for Windows or IOs.

Zero is a popular app with a variety of valuable benefits:

- Fasting customization

- Fasting tracking of progress and goals

- Fasting journal entry

- Integration with smart devices and wearables

Fasting Tracker also has a number of handy benefits, including:

- Fasting adjustment

- Logging of weight, waist size, ketones and glucose

- In-app community for support

- Videos and articles

BodyFast offers some unique features, including:

- Fasting coach

- Fasting timer

- Statistics

- Weight tracker

- Notification alerts

- No advertisements

- Sharing progress

- Staying accountable to friends on various popular social platforms

Vora offers:

- Daily fast tracking

- Export information to CVS

- Tracking others' progress for inspiration

  Fastient offers:

- Visualization of fasting progress

- Journaling of fasting progress and experience

- Checking fasting history

- Import previous fasts from comparable apps

- Progress pictures

- Quick-tag

- Emojis

- Dark mode

FastHabit allows the users to:

- Stop, restart, or even to adjust fast

- Keep weight loss records

- Visualize progress in percentages

- Set fasting reminders and receive notifications

But whatever type of fasting you choose, you'll have to break that fast sometime, and that brings us to our next chapter; breaking a fast.

Women and Fasting

Women who fasted intermittently can have a decrease of glucose tolerance. Women's metabolisms can suffer from intermittent fasting.

Rodent studies found that alternate-day fasting had significant hormonal changes on female rats. Studies on humans found that non-obese females had metabolic responses which may be not as robust of men of their age, indicating that fasting could be antagonistic or even dangerous to your health.

Intermittent fasting can cause hormonal imbalances in females if done incorrectly. Females may be very sensitive to signals of starvation. If the body senses it is being starved, it will increase production of the hunger hormones ghrelin and leptin.

When females experience insatiable hunger after food deprivation, they may be experiencing the increased production of those hormones. it is the female body's way of protecting a potential fetus, even when a woman is not pregnant.

Females may ignore these hunger cues, which causes the signals to get even louder. Or they ignore them, fail, then binge and follow it up with more deprivation and starvation again. The cycle can throw your hormones off and even stop ovulation.

In animal studies, female rats' menstrual cycles stopped and their ovaries shrank and they experienced more insomnia than male counterparts after two weeks of fasting. Male rats experienced lower testosterone production).

Intermittent fasting for longer periods can disrupt the female hormonal balance, causing fertility problems and worsening eating disorders like anorexia, bulimia, and binge eating.

Intermittent fasting may be hard on the female body if you jump in too quickly. If you are a woman or fasting for the very first time, you may prefer modified (or crescendo) intermittent fasting.

Crescendo fasting requires fasting only a few days. Females may get more benefit without throwing their hormones into a frenzy. This is a gentler approach which helps the body adapt to fasting. And if women do it right, it may be an amazing way to lose body fat, reduce internal inflammation, and boost energy.

Not every woman needs crescendo fasting, but it will promote success in most. Crescendo fasting entails fasting for two to three nonconsecutive days a week (Tuesday, Thursday and Saturday). Here are some particulars:

- On fasting days, do light cardio or yoga

- Fast for 12 to 16 hours

- Eat normally on strength training/HIIT days

- Drink plenty of water (Tea and coffee with no sweetener or milk)

After two weeks, add one day of fasting.

Consider taking five to eight grams of BCAAs during a fast. A branched chain amino acid supplement gives fuel to the muscles and has few calories which can take some of the edge off of the fatigue and hunger.

Fasting for Women

Intermittent fasting may be of benefit many men, it can have a negative effect on women's metabolism and hormones. Females report serious problems, including metabolic disruption, binge eating, and lost menstrual periods. Early onset-menopause while intermittent fasting may occur in some women, even women in their early twenties.

Intermittent fasting can be disruptive of female hormones. Because hormones regulate key functions like metabolism, ovulation, and even mood, they are very sensitive to your energy intake. Changing how much and when you eat can negatively impact the reproductive hormones.

This can have a ripple effect, causing health issues.

One-way fasting affects the reproductive hormones of men and women. This is due to the hypothalamic-pituitary-gonadal (HPG) axis: The hypothalamus releases the gonadotropin releasing hormone (GnRH), telling the pituitary gland to secrete luteinizing hormone (LH) and also follicular stimulating hormone (FSH).

LH and FSH then turn and act upon the gonads. LH and FSH both stimulate production of progesterone and estrogen, necessary for ovulation and to support pregnancy.

In men, they stimulate production of sperm and testosterone.

This happens on a specific and regular cycle in women. GnRH pulses have to be timed precisely or a woman's system may go haywire; eggs go unreleased and menstrual periods stop. Even three days of fasting can alter hormonal pulses. There is evidence that missing even a single meal can put the hormonal system on alert.

Why does eating less put women's bodies on alert? Scientists have long thought that a woman's body fat percentage regulates her reproductive system. They figured that, if fat stores dipped to around 11 percent, hormones could be disrupted and periods could stop.

For our ancestors, low food supply could be cause for concern and could disrupt family planning, so to speak. If you are losing body fat, the body might assume there is not much to eat, and prevent reproduction. But it's more than that; the female body seems to go on alert even before body fat drops. So bigger women may lose their periods and stop ovulating.

This is why experts think energy balance (calories you're eating and burning) may be more important here than body fat percentage. Consuming more calories than you burn is a negative energy balance, but it does not result only from eating or drinking less. It might also result from:

- too much stress

- too much exercise

- chronic inflammation

- illness

- infection

- poor nutrition

- too little rest and recovery

Any combination of these stressors could put any woman into excessive negative energy balance and stop ovulation. Psychological stress might also play a role in damaging hormonal health. The body cannot necessarily tell the difference between an actual real threat and a perceived threat brought on by feelings or thoughts and feelings. Threats of this sort can increase your levels of the stress hormone cortisol. Cortisol inhibits GnRH. Disrupting GnRH can create a cascade effect which may suppress the ovaries' production of progesterone and estrogen the hormones critical for reproduction.

If you're in a negative energy balance for long enough, particularly if you're overweight or under stress, reproduction can stop.

Low-energy diets can reduce fertility in women. And that only makes sense; the body may want emergency reserves. Human females are unique among mammalian world, one of the few which cannot terminate or pause pregnancy when conditions aren't right. It's called *embryonic diapause*, an unconscious process of a mammal's bodily responses to environmental factors such as food availability and temperature. In humans, once the placenta breaches the maternal blood vessels, the fetus is in control. The developing baby can block the action of insulin to hoard glucose. It can dilate the mother's blood vessels, adjusting blood pressure for more nutrients in a phenomenon called *maternal-fetal conflict*. Fertility during a famine could biologically be fatal. So women tend to carry a little extra weight as a biological necessity. Getting rid of it can be harder for women for this reason, and fasting may not be the answer, as we've seen. And there are more reasons for this than just a biological preparation for pregnancy.

1. Women might be more sensitive to nutrient changes and imbalances than men. This could be due to the protein-like molecule kisspeptin, which is essential to reproduction. Kisspeptin stimulates GnRH production in both sexes and is sensitive to insulin, leptin, and ghrelin. Those are the hormones which regulate and react to hunger and fullness. Women have more kisspeptin than men. More kisspeptin means women's bodies are more sensitive to energy balance changes. Fasting can cause women's kisspeptin to dip. When kisspeptin drops, it throws GnRH into imbalance, and that upsets the monthly hormonal cycle.

2. Restricting nutrients like protein can have different effects on women than on men. In general, females eat less protein than men. But protein has amino acids, which are crucial for reproduction.

If amino acids dip, that can negatively affect estrogen receptors and the hormone insulin-like growth factor (IGF-1). Both thicken the uterus' lining during the menstrual cycle. If the uterus lining fails to thicken, the egg cannot implant and pregnancy cannot occur.

Ergo, low-protein diets can reduce fertility.

Estrogen is good for more than just reproduction and the uterus.

The body has estrogen receptors in almost every part, including in the brain, the GI tract, and even the bones. Changing estrogen balance changes metabolic function in mood, cognition, recovery, digestion, bone formation, protein turnover, appetite and energy balance.

Estrogens modify the peptides which the body to feel full (cholecystokinin) or to feel hungry (ghrelin). Estrogens stimulate neurons which stop the production of appetite-regulating peptides.

Estriol, estradiol, and estrone are the estrogenic metabolites; three types of estrogen. Before menopause, estradiol is most prevalent. Estradiol drops after menopause, but estrone remains consistent. A drop in estradiol can trigger increased fat storage.

Lower estradiol may be linked to increase in fat storage, but it is probably not the only cause. Increases of fat around menopause may be due to lowered muscle mass, aging, and appetite changes. Low estradiol is linked to higher appetite.

So women in particular have a lot to think about when engaging in a fast. Given the basic information and the details particular to a female's specific biology, you should now be able to make the best choices of which fast is best for you, and how best to start it and how long to keep it going.

Remember, this is all about you.

But no matter which fast you choose, or how long you remain fasting, you're going to have to break that fast eventually. And when you do, you'll be facing some new challenges. Some of these face men and women both, others are particular to a woman's unique physiology. But we'll provide the information you need, that's why we're here. And you want to grow and be a healthier and happier person, that's why you're here. So let's proceed together to the next step on our journey.

Breaking a fast.

CHAPTER THREE: Breaking a Fast

When you're ready to break your fast, you have to be careful. Too much food too soon can lead to refeeding syndrome. If your body undertakes the shift from ketosis to carbohydrate-based foods, the body may release insulin for digestion. That process that requires calcium, phosphate, magnesium, potassium, and essential vitamins including B1. These deficiencies may lead to hypotension and heart failure and hypotension and often to sudden death.

When refeeding, your body also stimulates stem cell regeneration, as well as boosting hormones, immune system cells, and metabolic activity.

Guidelines on safely breaking a fast include:

- A period of light eating equal to half the duration of the diet

- Start with no more than 10 calories per kilogram of body weight per day

- Take vitamin and mineral supplements a half-hour before breaking the fast

- Drink pure fruit juice or bone broth to break your fast.

- Follow up with avocados, pureed soups, well-cooked vegetables. Avoid fruits and fructose

- Eat smaller portion

- Eat slowly, but more often

These are dietary guidelines. But fasting is as much about resetting the mind as it is about resetting the brain. Fasting is a good way to remind yourself that there are two kinds of hunger, physiological eating and psychological eating.

Physiological eating is, healthy, necessary, deliberate, and motivated by a physical need for food. Psychological eating, on the other hand, is unhealthy, unnecessary, habitual, and motivated by an emotional need for distraction or comfort.

So when breaking a fast, keep in mind that your relationship with food should fundamentally change from a psychological relationship to a physiological relationship.

In order to gain and secure over your eating habits and redefine your relationship with food, consider asking yourself these four questions:

1. Why? Why am I eating? If it's anything other than hunger, it's for the wrong reasons. Celebrating? Wrong reason? Stocking up for another fast? Wrong reason. Bored? Wrong reason.

2. What? What am I eating? Since new stem cells are created after a fast, break that fast with the right foods. Some prefer organic foods, some may adhere to a food regiment like the ketogenic diet.

3. How? How am I eating? Eat slowly, give your body time to digest. It will give you the feeling of being full and help prevent overeating. Avoid distractions when eating, focus on the food. Enjoy it, don't simply consume it. You're resetting your relationship with food.

Mindful Eating Exercises

1. The *raisin meditation* is generally done using a raisin, though it can be done with any type of food. The idea is to bring complete sensory consciousness of what you're eating. This consciousness extends from the first touch to the aftermath of the last swallow. This works best while breaking a fast, when your senses are at a peak and you'll be especially appreciative.

Touch the raisin, hold it, pick it up and consider its weight, texture, color. Think about the process it underwent to go from grape to raisin. Think about the crevices, and imagine the smoothness of its grape form. Smell it, reflect on the smell. Touch the raisin, consider its density its firmness.

Put the raisin slowly into your mouth. Feel the raison on your tongue. Bite into it and note the release of flavors, the change in texture. Chew it slowly, concentrate on the flavor, the deterioration of the grape between your teeth.

Swallow. Feel the contractions in your throat during the swallowing reflex. Follow the raison as it slides down your throat.

2. When eating, rest your fork between bites. Set it down and let go of it. This mindfulness exercise allows you to focus on what you're eating, to be fully present in the moment. And it will help you eat slower, encouraging more-thorough digestion and better health.

Best Foods for Breaking a Fast

Remember that when you're resetting your system, your new fuels will help shape your new cells. So it's vital to eat the right foods when you break your fast. It's even more important when breaking long-term fasts.

Here's a reliable recipe for breaking a fast:

- Start with a glass of apple cider vinegar and water

- Then enjoy a bowl of bone broth with two hard-boiled eggs, iron-rich greens such as spinach or kale. Keep the meal under 500 calories

Apple cider vinegar (ACV) in particular is beneficial to this process. It has a variety of benefits, including:

- Stimulation of the digestive process

- Levels alkaline PH levels

- Kills bad gut bacteria gut

- Stabilizes blood sugar

- Stimulates digestion

- Improves first-meal digestion

Here's a good recipe for an ACV drink which you may enjoy while fasting, but not for breaking a fast.

- Water (10 - 12oz)

- ACV (2 tablespoons)

- Pink Himalayan salt (1/2 teaspoon)

- Cream of tartar (1/2 teaspoon)

- Bottled lime juice (2 tablespoons)

- Stevia to taste

ACV capsules are also available.

Bone broth is popular for its hearty flavor and also offers these benefits:

- Rich in essential minerals

- Rich in electrolytes

- Rich in collagen

- Rich in glycine

- Rich in many anti-inflammatory amino acids

- Low in carbohydrates

Bone broth comes as a liquid or powder, both are mixed with a water base.

Kale and spinach are rich in essential nutrients and vitamins which fasting may deplete, including:

- Folate

- Iron

- Potassium

- Manganese

- Magnesium

- Copper

- Calcium

- Vitamin A

- Vitamin B2, B6

- Vitamin C

- Vitamin E

- Vitamin K

Kale and spinach are good either raw, cooked, or whipped into a vegetable or fruit smoothie. The benefits include:

- Better digestion

- Constipation prevention

- Blood sugar management

Eggs are easily digested, rich in protein and may curb the appetite (hard-boiled).

Nuts, chia seeds and others, pecan and almond and flax are popular these days for their essential proteins, fats, nutrients, minerals, and fiber including:

- Calcium

- Copper

- Selenium

- Iron

- Phosphorus

- Manganese

Fish and fish broth are terrific sources of unsaturated fat (the healthy kind) with various proteins, omega 3, and vitamin D.

Cauliflower, broccoli, and brussels sprouts are cruciferous vegetables, rich in nutrients, fiber, and vitamins, including:

- Vitamins A, C, K, B2, B5, B6, B9

- Manganese

- Magnesium

- Iron

Watermelon is easy to digest, rich in fiber, and only a semi-solid food (91% water), perfect for breaking a fast.

Bananas provide healthy carbs, potassium, fiber, vitamins B6 and C. They can also boost blood sugar.

Unsweetened yogurt, kimchi, and sauerkraut are fermented foods, boosting good gut bacteria and enzymes which are lost during a fast. Avoid any spicy kimchi meals.

Avocado, the fattiest fruit in the world is ideal for breaking a fast. It's low in calories, rich in omega-3 and -6 fat while being filled with vitamins, minerals, and antioxidants, including:

- Potassium

- Copper

- Folate

- Vitamin B6, C, E, K

- Antothenic acid

Keep your first post-fast first meal around 500 calories. If you're more active, consider eggs instead of broth for better muscle growth during the next week.

Breaking a Fast for Women

The rules for breaking a fast in a healthy way apply basically the same to women as to men. The biological imperatives are the same. But there are some specifics which will help women to break their fasts more effectively, in accordance to their particular biology, particularly regarding hormones and thyroid.

First of all, avoid things which don't break down easily, like garlic or unions. These ferment in the colon, which is good. But not so great the first thing after a fast. Avoid prebiotic fibers like artichokes for the same reason, they can create too much bad bacteria when what you want is good bacteria. Simple proteins are better.

Avoid dairy, even if a smoothie or shake seems like a good idea after a fast. Dairy's calcium and protein become acid and that could cause inflammation.

Avoid cruciferous veggies when breaking your fast. Just wait a few hours after you've broken your fast.

Avoid paring fats and carbs when breaking a fast. But this creates fat storage, even more so after a fast.

For women in particular, you should have a cortisol-breaking strategy before you break your fast, because women produce more cortisol during fasting. And it should be elevated during a fast, but not in conjunction with food, as this creates fat storage. So break your fast with low cortisol levels to prevent fast storage after a fast.

Consider drinking a little salt water before breaking a fast. Salt can indirectly drop your cortisol levels. Cinnamon tea will moderate cortisol levels and lower blood sugars. Yoga, meditation, deep breathing can bring cortisol levels down.

Only consume lean protein from a fish source or even a shellfish. Lean fish like halibut, or shellfish like shrimp. A lean protein shake (not from whey) is good. Lean white-meat chicken is ideal.

Hypothyroidism is common to women during a fast, and zinc affects thyroid receptors in the cells. This results in lower thyroid levels and prevents hypothyroidism. Shellfish has a lot of zinc.

Women need iodine after a fast. Seaweed is an excellent source of iodine. Sprinkle some seaweed chip on your shellfish or lean fish. Limit consumption between three and seven ounces, depending on your weight, at least when breaking a fast.

Avoid gluten. It can slow down your thyroid and your metabolism.

This fast-breaking period lasts about two hours.

That should get just about anyone back into a regular and healthy diet smoothly, allowing a continuous intermittent fasting lifestyle which can be especially good for women. But either man or woman, the reasons for losing weight are often the same for both genders. They seek healthier bodies and greater longevity, they want more vitality, more physical and mental strength and stamina.

And, even more often, they want to lose weight. We've already seen some of the frightening statistics about obesity, especially in women.

A study in the New England Journal of Medicine examined obesity in 176 countries. It found higher obesity rates among adult women all over the planet, regardless of economic or educational status. This suggest that women may be disproportionally affected by obesity and are more likely to suffer the consequences.

More than half of women in the Caribbean and urban Latin America are overweight (body mass index of greater than or equal to 25) or obese (body mass index equal to or greater than 30).

But to properly lose weight, one has to have a working knowledge, a functional understanding, of what they're dealing with. That's what this book (and the other books in our extensive library) is for. To make the most of renewed vitality, it's important to know what autophagy is and how it works. If you want to make the most of the yoga and exercises and other things to come in this book, you'll have to know how and why they work as they do, otherwise you're just a zombie doing what you're told. But that's not you, and that's not what this book is for. This book is meant to help you to reset your mind and your body. But remember that all of this is about you, nobody else. The book sets you on a journey which you must navigate, but with our help.

So, if you want to make the most out of your battle against fat (and its shadow partner, cholesterol) you have to know what you're dealing with.

CHAPTER FOUR: Fats and Cholesterol

You've heard these words, and you might even be obsessing about them. They've become catchwords for dietary evil. But they're both natural parts of the human body, and both are necessary for the normal functioning of several different bodily systems. It's important to know good fats from bad, good cholesterol from bad. You might have heard these terms bandied about as well. If you're going to start fasting and engaging in other fairly drastic dietary changes, you have to know what fats to embrace or avoid, which cholesterol can kill you and which can save your life.

Cholesterol

Cholesterol is a waxy substance which collects in the arteries. It is often mistaken for detrimental, but some cholesterol is crucial to good health.

There are two different types of cholesterol; low-density lipoprotein (LDL) and high-density lipoprotein (HDL). HDL carries cholesterol directly to the liver. There it's removed from the bloodstream so it cannot build up in the arteries. This is the so-called *good* cholesterol. LDL delivers cholesterol to the arteries where it may build up as plaque and cause a heart attack or stroke.

Triglycerides are the third major cholesterol component; unused calories your body stores as fat. Taking in more calories than you're burning allows triglycerides to collect and raise the risk of a heart attack.

Over 30% of Americans have high LDL (over 100). HDLs should be fewer than 40 (for men) or 50 (for women). Healthy triglyceride numbers are 150 or less. Your total cholesterol number should be at or less than 200.

Fats

Like cholesterol, fats come in both good and bad varieties. Good fats include monounsaturated and polyunsaturated fats. Bad fats include industrial-made trans fats. Saturated fats fall somewhere in the middle. The differences are chemical. Fats are structured as a chain of carbon atoms bonded to hydrogen atoms. The length and the shape of that chain, and the amount of hydrogen atoms, are what make a fat molecule. Good fats have fewer hydrogen atoms than saturated fats. They're liquid at room temperature, not solid.

The benefits of good (unsaturated) fats include:

- Major energy source

- Aids mineral and vitamin absorption

- Essential for muscle movement

- Necessary for building cell membranes

- Necessary for blood clotting

- Essential for necessary inflammation

Unsaturated fats

Unsaturated fats are liquid at room temperature. They're beneficial fats which:
Ease inflammation
Improve blood cholesterol levels
Stabilize the heart rhythms
Easily found in plant-based foods like vegetable oils, seeds and nuts.
The two "good" unsaturated fats are polyunsaturated and monounsaturated fats.
Monounsaturated fats have single carbon-to-carbon double bonds with fewer hydrogen atoms. They're found in such foods as:

- Canola oil

- Olive oil

- Peanut oil

- Nuts (hazelnuts, almonds, pecans)

- Seeds (pumpkin, sesame seeds)

- Avocados

- Sunflower oil

- Safflower oil

Polyunsaturated fats are essential fats found in cooking oils; necessary for bodily function but not made by the body. They're crucial to:

- Building cell membranes

- Nerve insulation

- Muscle movement

- Necessary internal inflammation

- Blood clotting

Omega-3 fatty acids and omega-6 fatty acids are types of polyunsaturated fat, which have two or even more double bonds. The numbers 3 and 6 refer to the distance between the beginning of the carbon chain and that chain's first double bond.
The benefits of omega-3 fatty acids include:

- Possible stroke and heart disease prevention

- Blood pressure reduction

- HDL increase

- Triglyceride reduction

- Heart rhythm control

- Reduction of some arthritis medications

- Reduction of dementia risk

Omega-6 fatty acids may be found in vegetable oils (safflower, sunflower, walnut, soybean, corn).
Polyunsaturated fats are found in rich supply in:

25

- Sunflower, soybean, corn, and flaxseed oils

- Fish

- Walnut

- Canola oil (for the polyunsaturated fat)

The American Heart Association recommends eight to ten percent of daily calories should come from polyunsaturated fats.

Saturated Fats

Saturated refers to the molecular makeup of the fat; the quantity of hydrogen atoms. This chain holds as many as possible, and so it is saturated with hydrogens.

Studies cannot verify a connection between saturated fats and heart disease. But there is a connection between polyunsaturated fat and heart disease.

Plenty of healthy foods (nuts and chicken) have some saturated fat. But less-healthy foods (beef, cheese, ice cream) have more saturated fat. It's found principally in animal food products and some plant-based foods have it as well (such as oils from coconut, palm and palm kernel).

Saturated fat can still be harmful in excess. The American Heart Association recommends no more than seven percent of caloric intake per day.

The biggest sources of saturated fat in the United States diet are:

- Whole- or reduced-fat butter, dairy desserts, milk

- Cheese and pizza

- Some meats (sausage, bacon, beef, burgers)

- Fast foods

- Cookies (grain-based sweets)

Replacing bad fasts with good fats may prevent resistance to insulin, which is a diabetes precursor.

Trans Fats

Trans fats (trans fatty acids) are created by the process hydrogenation (heating liquid vegetable oils near hydrogen gas). Partially hydrogenating vegetable oils makes them more stable and gives them a longer shelf life. Hydrogenating also hardens vegetable oils into solids (margarine and shortening). They can go from liquid to solid, so they're good for frying.

Trans fats offer no health benefits and there is no recommended safe consumption level. And they're officially banned from use in the United States and other countries.

Trans fats are common in small amounts in the fat found in dairy and beef. Risks of consuming trans fats include:

- Elevated bad LDL rates, lowered good HDL rates

- Damage to heart and blood vessels

- Increased inflammation, implicated in stroke, heart disease, diabetes, various chronic conditions

- Increased insulin resistance

Cholesterol and Women

Women are at greater risk for high cholesterol. Experts estimate that roughly 45% of women over 20 years old have total cholesterol numbers of 200 mg/dl or above, considered elevated. The American Heart Association found 76% of women don't know their cholesterol values.

Triglycerides are also riskier for women. Women's cholesterol levels fluctuate after menopause and they increase with age, creating greater risk of stroke and heart disease. Know your numbers and control them. High triglyceride levels predict a greater risk of heart disease in women.

A woman's HDL cholesterol level should be 50 mg/dl or under. Triglycerides should come to less than 150 mg/dl and total cholesterol below 200 mg/dl.

How Cholesterol Affects Women

Women generally have higher levels of HDL cholesterol due to the female sex hormone estrogen, which seems to boost good cholesterol. But menopause changes everything. Many women experience changes in cholesterol levels at this time in life. Total and LDL (bad) cholesterol rises and HDL cholesterol falls. Women who had good cholesterol numbers during their childbearing years may have elevated cholesterol in later years. Genetics and lifestyle can play roles as well.

This study of cholesterol in women brings us to a field of study which is often of particular importance to women, though its vital to the health of the male body as well. This is a vastly misunderstood but vital component of the human body. Like so much of what we study, it's rooted in our past and can dictate our future. And they have to be understood in order to be properly controlled and managed. And they may be of particular interest to women of any age.

Welcome to the wonderful world of your hormones.

SECTION 2: HORMONES AND HORMONAL IMBALANCE

CHAPTER FIVE: Hormones

Hormones. They get a bad break. They take the blame for every one of a woman's thoughts or actions, as if they were merely slaves to their hormonal function. If she's upset, happy, horny, it must be a female thing.

But of course that's a long-forgotten myth. Hardly. Some people still believe this, because they have no real understanding of what hormones are, how they function, what part they play in our lives, and what part we can play in their part on our lives. If you want to control them, you have to understand them.

Hormones travel through the bloodstream, helping organs and tissues function. Different hormones are generated to help different parts of the body perform different functions.

Endocrine glands secret hormones, necessary for the growth, development, reproduction, and several other bodily functions. These are your top ten essential hormones:

The hormones of thyroid, Thyroxine (T4) and Triiodothyronine (T3), are generated and released into the system by the thyroid gland. Their benefits include:

- Maintain metabolism

- Regulate weight

- Boost energy levels

- Regulate internal temperature

- Determine skin and hair health

Insulin is released by the pancreas and allows the body to use sugar from carbs for energy to use or store. Insulin prevents blood sugar levels from getting too low (hypoglycemia) or high (hyperglycemia).

Estrogen is the female sexual hormone released by the ovaries. It's responsible for menstruation, menopause, and reproduction. Excessive estrogen increases the risks of breast and uterine cancer, depression, moodiness, and a variety of other conditions. Too little estrogen can lead to:

- Acne

- Skin lesions

- Hair loss

- Weak fingernails

- Thinning skin

- other symptoms

Produced in the ovaries, progesterone is produced in the placenta (when a woman is pregnant), in the adrenal glands and ovaries. Progesterone stimulates and regulates various female bodily functions, including:

- Pregnancy preparation

- Pregnancy management

- Regulating menstrual cycle

- Stimulates sexual desire

Prolactin is released after childbirth. It enables the female to lactate and breastfeed.

Testosterone is a male sexual hormone. An anabolic (muscle-building) steroid, the benefits of testosterone include:

- Muscle building

- Developing reproductive tissues

- Increases muscle mass

- Increases body hair and other secondary sexual characteristics.

Testosterone deficiency can cause bone loss.

Serotonin is a rejuvenation hormone associated with:

- Learning and memory

- Sleep

- Mood regulation

- Muscular development

- Digestion.

Serotonin deficiency is closely associated with:

- Depression

- Migraines

- Insomnia

- Carbohydrate craving

- Weight gain

Too much serotonin may cause agitation, sedation, and confusion.

Cortisol, the hormone which maintains overall good health and energy, is produced by the adrenal gland. Cortisol controls physical and psychological stress. Under stress, cortisol increases heart rate, blood pressure, and respiration. Consistently high cortisol levels can cause high blood pressure, anxiety, ulcer, high cholesterol levels. Cortisol deficiency may cause chronic fatigue syndrome, alcoholism, and a variety of other conditions.

Adrenaline, known as an emergency hormone, released to counter stress. It is known to dilate blood vessels to the heart and the brain.

Somatotropin is known as the growth hormone which stimulates growth, cellular regeneration and reproduction, and it also boosts metabolism.

Here's a supplementary list of other hormones and what they do for your body:

The adrenocorticotropic hormone (ACTH) stimulates cortisol production.

Aldosterone is central to cardiovascular health.

Angiotensin is a common name for four hormones and each plays a vital role in blood pressure regulation.

Anti-Müllerian Hormone (AMH) aids in fertility and reproductive health in human females.

Calcitonin is among the body's most critical hormones. It controls calcium and potassium levels.

Cholecystokinin helps improve digestion.

Dehydroepiandrosterone (DHEA) is a precursor hormone. It has little biological effect on its own until it is converted into other hormones, when it is used for human reproduction.

Dihydrotestosterone stimulates male development and are contingent on testosterone levels.

Erythropoietin supports red blood cell production.

Estradiol is important to the female reproductive system. It's the strongest and most common estrogen for women of childbearing age.

Estriol is a minor estrogen hormone which promotes uterus growth. It also prepares a human female for giving birth.

Estrone is the third type of estrogen. It's the only estrogen made by the body after menstrual periods stop (menopause).

The hormone gastrin breaks down proteins and manages gastric acid release.

Ghrelin is the digestive hormone that controls appetite.

The peptide hormone glucagon regulates blood levels.

That's not to be confused with the glucagon-like peptide 1 (GLP-1). This hormone, produced in the small intestine, prevents glucagon production, resulting in lower blood sugar levels. GLP-1 also stimulates insulin production.

Gonadotrophin-releasing hormone (GnRH) secretes reproductive hormones including luteinizing hormone (LH) and follicle-stimulating hormone (FSH).

The human chorionic gonadotropin (HcG) hormone is vital to early pregnancy.

The hormone kisspeptin generates other hormones' release.

Leptin helps control appetite and weight.

Luteinizing hormone (LH) controls reproductive systems of males and females.

Melanocyte-stimulating hormone (MSH) protects skin from ultraviolet rays and promotes pigmentation development while controlling appetite.

Melatonin regulates the sleep cycle.

The hormone norepinephrine breaks down fat, increases blood pressure, and heart rate.

Oxytocin is vital for labor and childbirth, breastfeeding, bonding, social behaviors.

The parathyroid hormone affects calcium levels in the kidneys, intestines, and in the bones.

Peptide YY is produced in the small intestine when the body is full.

Prostaglandins help in fighting infection and healing damaged tissue.

Relaxin is produced in females in preparation for newborn delivery.

Somatostatin (SST) is a growth hormone which inhibits other hormones.

Thyroxine aids in muscle and heart functioning, brain development, digestion, and bone maintenance.

Vitamin D is actually a hormone to promote bone growth and calcium absorption.

That's a lot to digest, no pun intended. But remember that this book is like a workbook, a handbook for better living. It's not all meant to be memorized. You'll be coming back to parts of this book over and over again. It's a reference book, it's a manual meant for constant reference. So let all that data sink in and know that it's here for you. Until that time, there's more to know about hormones. Your very life may depend on it.

CHAPTER SIX: Hormonal Imbalance

This is where hormones go from the being the body's best friends to its worst enemies. Hormonal imbalance can change the whole chemical balance of the body and instigate all manner of dangerous conditions. Hormonal imbalances strike both men and women (women at a whopping 80%). But how do you know if you have a hormonal imbalance? And if you do, how do you know how to correct it?
Why, you read on!

Signs or Symptoms of a Hormonal Imbalance

Hormones are crucial to overall health. There's a variety of hormones to perform different functions. So it should come as no surprise that hormonal imbalance would have a variety of signs and symptoms of hormonal imbalance.
Some of the most common hormonal imbalances may cause any (but not necessarily all) of these signs or symptoms:

- Fatty hump between the shoulders

- Weight gain

- Weight loss

- Fatigue

- Muscle weakness

- Stiffness, swelling, or pain in the joint

- Muscle aches, tenderness, and stiffness

- Increased or decreased heart rate

- Sweating

- Greater sensitivity to heat or cold

- Frequent urination

- Constipation or more frequent bowel movements

- Increased thirst

- Increased hunger

- Depression

- Decreased sex drive

- Thinning or brittle hair

- Nervousness, anxiety, irritability

- Infertility

- Dry skin

- Blurred vision

- Stress

- Sleeplessness

- Puffy or rounded face

- Purple or pink stretch marks

Signs or Symptoms in Females

Adult females often have polycystic ovary syndrome (PCOS), which is a common hormonal imbalance. The typical female hormonal cycle also changes according to the stages of life:
- Puberty

- Pregnancy

- Breastfeeding

- Menopause

Symptoms of hormonal imbalance which are specific to females include:
- Heavy or irregular periods (including stopped or missed or frequent periods)

- Acne on the chest, upper back, or face, chest, or upper back

- Hirsutism (excessive hair on the face, chin, chest, or body)

- Skin tags

- Hair loss

- Vaginal atrophy

- Skin darkening (along neck creases, under the breasts, in the groin)

- Vaginal dryness

- Night sweats

- Headaches

- Pain during sex

- Menstruation won't begin

- Breast tissue won't develop

- Growth rate remains static

Symptoms and Signs in Males

Hormonal imbalance can be just as complicated and varied for men as for women. Insufficient testosterone and other imbalances can have a variety of symptoms and signs, including:
- Breast tenderness

- Loss of muscle mass

- Gynecomastia (development of breast tissue)

- Erectile dysfunction (ED)

- difficulty concentrating

- decrease in body and facial hair

- Hot flashes

- Loss of bone mass (osteoporosis)

Boys with hormonal imbalance may experience:
- High-pitched voice

- Impaired testicular, penile growth

- Lack of muscle mass

- Sparse bodily hair

- Gynecomastia

- Excessive growth of legs and arms, relative to the torso

Causes of Hormonal Imbalance

With the wide variety of hormones and functions, their causes are also widely varied, including:
- Prescription medications

- Cancer treatments (like chemotherapy)

- Hormone therapy

- Benign or cancerous tumors

- Pituitary tumors

- Eating disorders

- Stress

- Injury or trauma

The following conditions may originate with hormonal imbalances and may lead to other imbalances.
- Diabetes (type 1 and type 2)

- Diabetes insipidus

- Hypothyroidism (underactive thyroid)

- Hyperthyroidism (overactive thyroid)

- hyperfunctioning thyroid nodules

- Hypogonadism

- Addison's disease

- Thyroiditis

- Congenital adrenal hyperplasia (causing low levels of aldosterone and cortisol)
- Cushing syndrome (high cortisol)

Causes Unique to Women

Many causes of female hormonal imbalance relate to reproductive hormones. Common causes are:
- Premature menopause (primary ovarian insufficiency)
- Menopause
- Pregnancy
- Breastfeeding
- Birth control pills
- PCOS

Polycystic Ovary Syndrome (PCOS)

Polycystic ovary syndrome (PCOS), a hormonal disorder, is very common among women, especially of reproductive age. Women with PCOS have prolonged or infrequent menstrual periods or excess levels of the male hormone (androgen). Ovaries may develop small collections of fluid called *follicles*, and fail to release eggs regularly.

Early diagnosis and treatment (typically including weight loss) can reduce the risk of complications like heart disease and type 2 diabetes.

Symptoms of PCOS often appear around the first menstrual period, though it may develop later in life in response to bodily changes such as obesity or weight gain.

A PCOS diagnosis can be made with only two of these signs:

1. Irregular periods: Erratic menstrual cycles are by far the most common sign of PCOS.

2. Excess androgen: Symptoms of elevated male hormones include hirsutism, severe acne, male-pattern baldness.

3. Polycystic ovaries. Ovaries may be enlarged and fail to function regularly.

Obesity usually worsens symptoms and signs of PCOS. See your doctor if there are concerns about menstrual periods, infertility or signs of excess androgen (hirsutism, acne, male-pattern baldness).

The precise cause of PCOS is not known. Contributing factors may include:

1. Excess insulin, which could increase androgen production and cause difficulty with ovulation.

2. Low-grade inflammation. Women with PCOS have a type inflammation which is known to stimulate polycystic ovaries to produce androgens. This may lead to blood vessel and heart problems.

3. Heredity. New scientific studies show that genes may be linked to PCOS.

4. Excess androgen, which can result in acne and hirsutism (excess body or facial hair).

Complications of PCOS include:
- Infertility
- Gestational diabetes (high blood pressure induced by pregnancy)
- Miscarriage or premature birth
- Nonalcoholic steatohepatitis (severe liver inflammation caused by accumulated fat)

- Metabolic syndrome (the cluster of conditions which include high blood sugar, high blood pressure, and abnormal triglyceride and/or cholesterol levels)

Metabolic syndrome increases the risk of:
- Type 2 diabetes

- Prediabetes

- Cardiovascular disease

- Sleep apnea

- Depression, anxiety, eating disorders

- Endometrial cancer (uterine lining)

Obesity is associated with PCOS and can worsen complications of the disorder.

Tests for Hormonal Imbalance

There's no single hormonal imbalance test, since hormones are so many and varied. Visit your physician for something like that. Be prepared with a timeline and a list of symptoms, as well as any external factors like supplements, medications, stress, medications, which you may be taking. Your doctor may ask the following questions:
- How often are your symptoms?

- How do you relieve your symptoms?

- Have you recently lost or gained weight?

- Is there an increase of stress in your work or at home?

- Are you pregnant or hoping to get pregnant?

- Was your last period on time and of regular flow?

- Do you suffer from ED?

- Do you experience vaginal dryness or pain during sex?

Your doctor may want to do a blood test for thyroid health and testosterone, estrogen and/or cortisol levels.

Female patients may expect a pelvic exam and pap smear to check for tumors, cysts, or lumps. For men, the scrotum will likely be observed for lumps or abnormalities.

An ultrasound test may be done, using sonic waves to create images of the uterus, ovaries, testicles, thyroid, or pituitary gland.

You may also try a variety of at-home testing kits, available for a wide spectrum of conditions. These tests use blood or saliva to measure key thyroid hormones, sex hormones like testosterone and progesterone, and cortisol.

Some of these tests require the user to send a sample away in the mail. Results are often returned within a week or so. Most are FDA-approved.

Treatments for Hormonal Imbalance

Treatments for hormonal imbalance are as varied as their causes. Here are few common treatment options:

Estrogen therapy is popular for symptoms of menopause, such as hot flashes and other symptoms. This treatment employs small supplemental doses of estrogen. This kind of hormone replacement therapy (HRT) should only be done under medical supervision.

Vaginal estrogen comes in a tablet, as a cream, or as an insertable ring. The local treatments bypass the long trip through the bloodstream.

Hormonal birth control helps regulate the menstrual cycle. Types of hormonal birth control are:

- Birth control patch, shot, or pill

- Vaginal ring

- Intrauterine device (IUD)

It might also reduce extra body and facial hair and improve acne.

Anti-androgen medications are often effective. Androgens, male sex hormones, are present in women as well as men. Women with high levels might prefer medication to block the effects of androgen. Those may include:

- Facial hair growth

- Acne

- Hair loss

Testosterone theory suggests supplements for symptoms of low testosterone in males, and often for delayed puberty. This therapy is available as a gel, patch, or injection.

Thyroid hormone therapy incorporates supplements of the synthetic thyroid hormone levothyroxine (comprised of Unithroid, Synthroid, and Levoxyl) and may help achieve normal hormonal balance.

Metformin is a medication for type 2 diabetes and which has been helpful for some women presenting symptoms of PCOS. The FDA-unapproved treatment may lower androgen levels and encourage ovulation.

Vyleesi (bremelanotide) and Addyi (flibanserin) are FDA-approved medications for low sexual desire in women in their childbearing years. Vyleesi comes as a self-administered injectable, Addyi in a pill.

Side effects such as severe nausea and blood pressure changes.

Vaniqa (eflornithine) is often prescribed for excessive female facial hair. The cream does not remove existing hair, but it does slow new growth.

Natural Remedies and Supplements

There are no natural supplements which are proven to treat hormonal imbalance or menopause. But there are plenty of supplements for various symptoms. Melatonin can help sleep problems, glutathione and Coenzyme Q-10 (CoQ-10) and glutathione are terrific cellular supplements. Resveratrol and curcumin are powerful anti-oxidants and anti-inflammatories.

Many supplements have plant-based hormones resembling human hormones.

Many people use yoga or meditation when dealing with hormonal imbalances. We'll take a closer look at those soon.

Lifestyle Changes for Hormone Management

Lose weight. Experts agree that a ten-percent body weight reduction can make menstrual periods more regular. It can also increase the likelihood of getting pregnant. Weight loss may improve proper erectile function in men.

Eat well. A balanced diet is vital to anyone's overall good health.

To decrease vaginal discomfort, use lubricants and moisturizers free of parabens, petroleum, and/or glycerin.

Avoid hot flashes by identifying common triggers, which may include warm temperatures, spicy foods, and hot beverages.

Remove excess facial or body hair. Hair removal creams, electrolysis, or laser hair removal are popular.

Other Hormonal Imbalances

Acne is associated with hormonal imbalance, as it produces excess oil.

Hormonal imbalance is closely associated to weight gain, since hormones play a vital role in your metabolism. Cushing syndrome, along with other hormone disorders, may cause weight gain and obesity due to elevated cortisol levels in the blood. Increased appetite and subsequent fat storage are two natural results of too much cortisol. Severe hypothyroidism can lead to weight gain as well.

Diet and exercise remain the best way to manage weight, and intermittent fasting is a good strategy too, as we now know.

There are ways rebalance and control some hormones. Certain exercises and yoga practices which we'll soon look at do the same. Let's take a close look at hormones, as some of them are strongly grounded in heredity. Hormones are about more than age, environment, or diet. They're as much about the past as about the present or future. And if you're going to be in control of your hormones, you should know when you cannot control them at all; and how to control them if you can.

Hormonal Imbalances in Women During Fasting

Women who fasted intermittently can have a decrease of glucose tolerance. Women's metabolisms can suffer from intermittent fasting.

Rodent studies found that alternate-day fasting had significant hormonal changes on female rats. Studies on humans found that non-obese females had metabolic responses which may be not as robust of men of their age, indicating that fasting could be antagonistic or even dangerous to your health.

Intermittent fasting can cause hormonal imbalances in females if done incorrectly. Females may be very sensitive to signals of starvation. If the body senses it is being starved, it will increase production of the hunger hormones ghrelin and leptin.

When females experience insatiable hunger after food deprivation, they may be experiencing the increased production of those hormones. it is the female body's way of protecting a potential fetus, even when a woman is not pregnant.

Females may ignore these hunger cues, which causes the signals to get even louder. Or they ignore them, fail, then binge and follow it up with more deprivation and starvation again. The cycle can throw your hormones off and even stop ovulation.

In animal studies, female rats' menstrual cycles stopped and their ovaries shrank and they experienced more insomnia than male counterparts after two weeks of fasting. Male rats experienced lower testosterone production).

Intermittent fasting for longer periods can disrupt the female hormonal balance, causing fertility problems and worsening eating disorders like anorexia, bulimia, and binge eating.

Intermittent fasting may be hard on the female body if you jump in too quickly. If you are a woman or fasting for the very first time, you may prefer modified (or crescendo) intermittent fasting.

Crescendo fasting requires fasting only a few days. Females may get more benefit without throwing their hormones into a frenzy. This is a gentler approach which helps the body adapt to fasting. And if women do it right, it may be an amazing way to lose body fat, reduce internal inflammation, and boost energy.

Not every woman needs crescendo fasting, but it will promote success in most. Crescendo fasting entails:

- Fast for two to three nonconsecutive days a week (Tuesday, Thursday and Saturday)

- On fasting days, do light cardio or yoga

- Fast for 12 to 16 hours

- Eat normally on strength training/HIIT days

- Drink plenty of water (Tea and coffee with no sweetener or milk)

After two weeks, add one day of fasting.

Consider taking five to eight grams of BCAAs during a fast. A branched chain amino acid supplement gives fuel to the muscles and has few calories which can take some of the edge off of the fatigue and hunger.

Intermittent fasting may be of benefit many men, it can have a negative effect on women's metabolism and hormones. Females report serious problems, including metabolic disruption, binge eating, and lost menstrual periods. Early onset-menopause while intermittent fasting may occur in some women, even women in their early twenties.

Intermittent fasting can be disruptive of female hormones. Because hormones regulate key functions like metabolism, ovulation, and even mood, they are very sensitive to your energy intake. Changing how much and when you eat can negatively impact the reproductive hormones.

This can have a ripple effect, causing health issues.

One-way fasting affects the reproductive hormones of men and women. This is due to the hypothalamic-pituitary-gonadal (HPG) axis: The hypothalamus releases the gonadotropin releasing hormone (GnRH), telling the pituitary gland to secrete luteinizing hormone (LH) and also follicular stimulating hormone (FSH).

LH and FSH then turn and act upon the gonads. LH and FSH both stimulate production of progesterone and estrogen, necessary for ovulation and to support pregnancy.

In men, they stimulate production of sperm and testosterone.

This happens on a specific and regular cycle in women. GnRH pulses have to be timed precisely or a woman's system may go haywire; eggs go unreleased and menstrual periods stop. Even three days of fasting can alter hormonal pulses. There is evidence that missing even a single meal can put the hormonal system on alert.

Why does eating less put women's bodies on alert? Scientists have long thought that a woman's body fat percentage regulates her reproductive system. They figured that, if fat stores dipped to around 11 percent, hormones could be disrupted and periods could stop.

For our ancestors, low food supply could be cause for concern and could disrupt family planning, so to speak. If you are losing body fat, the body might assume there is not much to eat, and prevent reproduction. But it's more than that; the female body seems to go on alert even before body fat drops. So bigger women may lose their periods and stop ovulating.

This is why experts think energy balance (calories you're eating and burning) may be more important here than body fat percentage. Consuming more calories than you burn is a negative energy balance, but it does not result only from eating or drinking less. It might also result from:

- too much stress

- too much exercise

- chronic inflammation

- illness

- infection

- poor nutrition

- too little rest and recovery

Any combination of these stressors could put any woman into excessive negative energy balance and stop ovulation. Psychological stress might also play a role in damaging hormonal health. The body cannot necessarily tell the difference between an actual real threat and a perceived threat brought on by feelings or thoughts and feelings. Threats of this sort can increase your levels of the stress hormone cortisol. Cortisol inhibits GnRH. Disrupting GnRH can create a cascade effect which may suppress the ovaries' production of progesterone and estrogen the hormones critical for reproduction.

If you're in a negative energy balance for long enough, particularly if you're overweight or under stress, reproduction can stop.

Low-energy diets can reduce fertility in women. And that only makes sense; the body may want emergency reserves. Human females are unique among mammalian world, one of the few which cannot terminate or pause pregnancy when conditions aren't right. It's called *embryonic diapause*, an unconscious process of a mammal's bodily responses to environmental factors such as food availability and temperature. In humans, once the placenta breaches the maternal blood vessels, the fetus is in control. The developing baby can block the action of insulin to hoard glucose. It can dilate the mother's blood vessels, adjusting blood pressure for more nutrients in a phenomenon called *maternal-fetal conflict*. Fertility during a famine could biologically be fatal. So women tend to carry a little extra weight as a biological necessity. Getting rid of it can be harder for women for this reason, and fasting may not be the answer, as we've seen. And there are more reasons for this than just a biological preparation for pregnancy.

1. Women might be more sensitive to nutrient changes and imbalances than men. This could be due to the protein-like molecule kisspeptin, which is essential to reproduction. Kisspeptin stimulates GnRH production in both sexes and is sensitive to insulin, leptin, and ghrelin. Those are the hormones which regulate and react to hunger and fullness. Women have more kisspeptin than men. More kisspeptin means women's bodies are more sensitive to energy balance changes. Fasting can cause women's kisspeptin to dip. When kisspeptin drops, it throws GnRH into imbalance, and that upsets the monthly hormonal cycle.

2. Restricting nutrients like protein can have different effects on women than on men. In general, females eat less protein than men. But protein has amino acids, which are crucial for reproduction.

If amino acids dip, that can negatively affect estrogen receptors and the hormone insulin-like growth factor (IGF-1). Both thicken the uterus' lining during the menstrual cycle. If the uterus lining fails to thicken, the egg cannot implant and pregnancy cannot occur.

Ergo, low-protein diets can reduce fertility.

Estrogen is good for more than just reproduction and the uterus.

The body has estrogen receptors in almost every part, including in the brain, the GI tract, and even the bones. Changing estrogen balance changes metabolic function in mood, cognition, recovery, digestion, bone formation, protein turnover, appetite and energy balance.

Estrogens modify the peptides which the body to feel full (cholecystokinin) or to feel hungry (ghrelin). Estrogens stimulate neurons which stop the production of appetite-regulating peptides.

Estriol, estradiol, and estrone are the estrogenic metabolites; three types of estrogen. Before menopause, estradiol is most prevalent. Estradiol drops after menopause, but estrone remains consistent. A drop in estradiol can trigger increased fat storage.

Lower estradiol may be linked to increase in fat storage, but it is probably not the only cause. Increases of fat around menopause may be due to lowered muscle mass, aging, and appetite changes. Low estradiol is linked to higher appetite.

You might feel that you've learned as much as anybody without letters after their name would need to know about hormones. And one thing you must have learned is how central they are to our bodies and our lives on virtually every level. So there's no reason to stop short of knowing everything you need to know about them. You won't know everything there is to know about hormones, of course, but without understanding heredity's place in the story of the human hormone, you won't know what you can control and what can control you. This will make all the difference, as you'll soon see.

CHAPTER SEVEN: Hormones and Heredity

The word *hormone* derives from the Ancient Greek word for *impetus*. Hormones are the driving force of growth and mood changes, chemical behavior, eating, drinking, mating, fleeing and fighting.

There are numerous connections between lifestyle influences and hormonal imbalances, including medicinal and dietary. We've looked at some ways to treat these imbalances, many of them behavioral and chemical. But it's not all about lifestyle or intake. There are strong connections between hormones and heredity, and this must be considered when dealing with hormonal imbalances and how to deal with them.

Let's look at this fairly complex medical web of nature and nurture in a fairly straightforward way. Genes code for hormones and hormone receptors as well as hormone precursors. They contain necessary codes for hormonal synthesis, bodily transport and eventual elimination. Science has identified a lot of these specific genes, related to hormonal signaling.

The CRH gene codes for the corticotrophin-releasing hormone, for cortisol release as a stress response. Genetics plays a big part in depression and in cognitive ability. Hormones function genetically, even if we don't know precisely how to manipulate them to prevent resultant imbalances.

Genes code for hormones, and hormones, in return, regulate genes. Steroid hormones (estradiol, testosterone, cortisol, and progesterone) adhere to intracellular receptors that regulate the expression of the gene.

Can hormonal changes (puberty or menopause) activate or suppress genetic influences on a behavioral phenotype? Do changes in gene expression affect that influence? Which is in charge, behavior or genetics? Hormones and genetics interact, each playing their part. It's more interplay than cause/effect.

Genetic Syndromes / Endocrine Diseases

Genetic syndromes may or may not be connected to most hormonal disorders. These are medical conditions that are caused by gene mutations which are genetically inherited. They're only rarely related to the endocrine organs; once for every half-million to million cases.

The majority of parathyroid and thyroid diseases, for example, have no genetic component.

Closely associated genetic conditions may include:

- Neurofibromatosis type 1

- Multiple endocrine neoplasia (MEN) type 2

- Familial paraganglioma syndrome

- von Hippel-Lindau syndrome

Multiple Endocrine Neoplasia (MEN) Syndromes

Multiple Endocrine Neoplasia (MEN) syndromes are inherited syndromes which result from a mutated gene creating benign and malignant neuroendocrine tumors. The endocrine glands may overproduce hormone, which present as symptoms. Early diagnosis and quick treatment are recommended for treatment of the various MEN syndromes.

MEN-I: One or more glands develop excess normal tissue (hyperplasia) or adenoma (tumor). MEN-I often strikes the parathyroid, the pancreas, and the pituitary glands. It sometimes strikes the adrenal and thyroid glands, which produce and secrete hormones into the blood and blood.
Symptoms include:

- Peptic ulcer disease

- Low blood sugar

- Symptoms of pituitary difficulties, including headaches

- Symptoms of high serum calcium or kidney stones

- Hypercalcemia (pituitary dysfunction)

- Hypoglycemia

- Abdominal pain

- Aching or burning in the upper abdomen and lower chest, relieved by antacids, milk, or food.

- Headache

- Weakness

- Black stools

- Confusion or mental changes

- Vomiting and nausea

- Bloated feeling

- Anxiety

- Lack of coordination

- Vision problems

- Muscle pain

- Loss of appetite

- Loss of pubic and body hair

- Sensitivity to cold

- Coma from untreated hypoglycemia

- Low blood pressure

- Fatigue

- Unintentional weight loss

- Infertility, cessation of menses, failure to lactate (women)

- Loss of facial or body hair, loss of sexual interest (men)

Treatment depends on the glands. Surgical removal is a common treatment. A bromocriptine might be prescribed for pituitary adenoma. Hormone replacement therapy is often prescribed after glandular removal.

Pituitary and parathyroid tumors are usually benign, but malignancies may occur. It's often best to focus on treating the symptoms, like those of hypercalcemia, hypoglycemia, peptic ulcer, and pituitary dysfunction.

MEN-II: Multiple endocrine neoplasia II (MEN II) presents as thyroid cancer, usually accompanied by recurring cancer of the adrenal glands. MEN-II is caused by a mutation in the RET gene. It presents as multiple tumors appearing at different times. It affects men and women equally and it may strike someone of any age. There are two variants of MEN-II, designated A and B. MEN-IIA may cause medullary thyroid cancer, hyperparathyroidism, and pheochromocytoma. MEN-IIB is closely associated with neuromas (bumps on lips and/or tongue), and it also may cause pheochromocytoma and medullary thyroid cancer. Common symptoms of MEN-II include:

- Heart palpitations

- Severe headache

- Chest pain

- Sweating

- Abdominal pain

- Rapid heart rate

- Nervousness

- Weight loss

- Irritability

- Diarrhea

- Cough

- Cough with blood

- Personality changes

- Back pain

- Fatigue

- Increased thirst

- Nausea

- Loss of appetite

- Depression

- Increased urinary output

- Muscular weakness

Treatments include surgery, which is needed to remove the medullary carcinoma of the thyroid pheochromocytoma. Medullary carcinoma treatment includes removing the thyroid gland surrounding lymph nodes. Hormone replacement therapy is usually prescribed after surgery.

Family members should be screened for the related RET mutation.

Pheochromocytoma is usually benign. But the accompanying medullary carcinoma of the thyroid is a very aggressive malignant cancer. Early diagnosis and successful surgery often leads to successful treatment and cure.

MEN-IV: Multiple endocrine neoplasia type 4 (MEN4) is very rare, signaled by parathyroid and anterior pituitary tumors. MEN-IV are associated with tumors of the adrenal, renal, and reproductive organs.

Succinate Dehydrogenase (SDH) syndromes: The SDH gene suppresses tumor growth. A mutation in the gene creates a greater likelihood of paragangliomas and pheochromocytomas.

Von Hippel-Lindau syndrome is caused by a mutated VHL gene. It prevents tumor growth. Roughly 10-34% of patients with VHL syndrome develop pheochromocytomas or paragangliomas. They may also develop retinal angiomas (benign lesions with visual implications), hemoangioblastomas (benign tumors in blood vessel lining), neuroendocrine tumors of the pancreas, as well as renal cell cancers.

Neurofibromatosis type I originates with a mutated NF1 gene, which would inhibit tumor growth. Patients can develop benign skin and nerves tumors as well as abnormal patches of pigmentation in the skin. Cognitive abnormalities are common side effects, as are soft tissue sarcomas and some cancers. Over five percent of NF-1 sufferers also develop pheochromocytomas and paragangliomas.

And that brings us to the end of our considerable analysis of hormones. You now know what they are, how they function, what they do, and why. You know how to better manage them and what to expect from them. Like the rest of your body, hopefully you've learned to accept them and embrace them, working with them instead of against them. More and more, this perspective will be dominant. This book is about uniting mind and body, and each with itself. The body has many systems and all are being repositioned to properly work together.

So now we can move forward to the next part of our analysis, the next crucial step toward overall wellness and general good health.

So let's bring on the detoxes and the cleanses. But be ready, as things may get wild … wet and wild!

SECTION 3: DETOXING

CHAPTER EIGHT: Cleanses and Other Detox Programs

We've looked at some of the most drastic forms of cleansing and detoxing the bodies, including fasting. But while those are long-term practices (even intermittent fasting is basically a long-term protocol which includes short-term fasting) there are short-term remedies for detoxifying the body, and they include DIY and clinical approaches of various complexity.

Cleanses are perhaps the most popular non-fasting method of detoxing, and there different types of detoxes. There are alternatives to cleanses too, some of them of considerable interest.

Flushing

Flushing is a popular cleansing method. Instead of the slow purge of a fast, a flush is fast and thorough. Enemas are an inexpensive, common, DIY way to clean out your gut and bowel. Kits are available at almost any drug store, pharmacy, or grocery store.

Different enemas use different solutions, often depending on the malady. Solutions are either:

- Water (for general blockage)

- Saltwater (for constipation)

- Garlic (for candida and parasites)

- Coffee (general, use organic / mold-free)

- Chamomile (for healing and cleansing)

- Probiotics (for gut inflammation)

- Apple cider vinegar (for healing)

- Lemon juice (for pH balance)

- Soap (for constipation)

- Mineral oil (for constipation)

Despite benefits, at-home enemas have possible drawbacks.

Lemon juice and coffee are highly acidic and may damage the intestinal lining. Improperly cleaned enema tools can cause bowel infections. Enemas eliminate the gut's good bacteria as well as the bad, which can lead to greater digestive disruptions. Excessive solution may cause bowel stretching and even tearing. Nausea and even vomiting are common during and/or after a cleanse. Too many enemas can weaken the bowel muscles and may disrupt normal bowel movements, and that can create a dependence.

The Coffee Enema

As long as we're so deep into the subject (pun intended), let's take a look at the coffee enema, one of the leading at-home enemas.

Even drinking coffee remains a controversial practice (never mind consuming it otherwise). Over the decades, coffee has taken the blame for liver damage and then praised for its benefits to the same. It's a powerful antioxidant, which is only coming to light. It's been suggested as an alternative to alcohol.

A coffee enema has been called a great method to clean out the lower intestines. Coffee's antioxidant properties make it a great cleansing solution, as its impressive levels of theobromine, theophylline, palmitate, kahweol, cafestol, and of course caffeine. These elements also have positive effects on internal inflammation, which is often a digestive problem that requires an enema.

Coffee enemas have been shown to have these benefits:

- Flushing out bacteria, heavy metals, fungus, and yeast from the digestive system
- Cleansing the liver and colon
- Restoring bowel function
- Lowering inflammation
- Relaxing bowel muscles
- Opening blood vessels
- Opening bile ducts
- Curing bowel disorders
- Increasing bile production
- Increasing bowel function
- Healing bowels
- Increasing immunity
- Stimulating glutathione S-transferase in the liver
- Repairing digestive tissue
- Cleansing the liver
- Improving blood circulation
- Cleaning out diverticulitis
- Improving energy levels
- Helping cellular regeneration
- Relieving digestive issues (constipation, bloating, cramping, and nausea)
- Improving gut health

And so, they're often used to help manage such conditions as:

- Parasites
- Cancer
- Overdoses
- Candida virus
- IBS (irritable bowel syndrome)
- Liver dysfunction
- Constipation

- Various other digestive disorders

It always suggested to perform any enema immediately after a bowel movement. Some suggest an activated carbon charcoal binder be consumed both before an enema and after to bind any toxins before the release for a much more efficient elimination.

Enemas are sometimes recommended once a week. Healing patients from digestive disorders sometimes do one a day. Very ill patients (cancer patients, for example) may have several enemas per day.

All enemas carry some risk, as we've discussed: colon tearing, dehydration, electrolyte imbalance, dizziness, and weakness. Note: Enemas are not recommended for pregnant women, children or those with allergies to caffeine or coffee. You might think that last one goes without saying, but you'd be surprised what some people will do.

Clinical Colons

There are also clinical approaches, which include colon therapy clinics. Some are small and intended for brief visits. Others are more like spas, they include massages, baths, and appropriate nourishment. More elaborate spas provide a two-day cleanse, often with a private room.

Cleanses

Let's put away the tubes and plastic bags and take a look at cleanses, the most popular method of at-home detoxing. They're widespread and varied, with new cleansing recipes and techniques.

These cleanses are so new and inventive, in fact, that most haven't been clinically tested and they don't get or seek the approval of the Food & Drug Administration (FDA).

The reputed benefits of detoxification include:

- Weight loss

- Improved energy

- Headache relief

- Muscle aches

- Constipation

- Fatigue

On the other hand, the human body has ways of detoxifying itself, including urinating, defecating, sweating. The digestive tract, kidneys and liver, break down toxins and prepare them for elimination.

It's also true that the body's natural processes can't keep up with our modern, toxic environment. We're not built to endure such an unnaturally toxic world: Fossil fuels have corrupted our skies and waters, plastic fills our oceans (along with oil spill, radioactive overspill and leakage). Steroids and pesticides from industrial farming and ranching techniques have poisoned the foods we eat. The foods that aren't poison are poison themselves; sugar substitutes, processed and genetically modified foods. Tobacco is still modified with deadly chemicals.

To combat all these toxins, cleanses may last from a single day to an entire month.

Cleanses for Women

- NutriFlair D Mannose 1200mg: with dandelion and cranberry extract

- Body Organic Apple Cider Vinegar Pills: For bloating relief, weight loss

- ACV Apple Cider Vinegar Gummies: Natural energy supplement, ACV
- Pristine Food's Max Detox Colon Cleanse Weight Loss Pills for Women: Colon Cleansing
- Snap Keto Detox Pills Advanced Weight Loss Bundle: For colon cleansing and fat burning

- Apple Cider Vinegar Gummies with Mother: For weight, detox, organic ACV
- Potent Apple Cider Vinegar with BHB Salts: Boosts ketosis, ACV, detox
- LEANFIT 14 Day teatox Made for Woman Detox Cleansing Tea: Reduces bloating
- Research Labs Resistance Bands Set w/ 15 Day Colon Cleanse & Detox

Caveats of Cleansing

Weight loss from cleanses (as it is from long-term fasting) is often temporary. And cleanses won't heal much in the body either. Athletes should not cleanse, as they use their body's stored carbohydrates. Athletic bodies don't use fat as fuel, as their bodies often don't carry enough stored fat. Athletes should not cleanse during recovery from sports injuries. The body needs those nutrients. This is why people who are fasting should limit strenuous exercise.

Pros and Cons of Detoxing

Cleansing requires commitment; of money, of time, of personal health. Weigh the pros and cons and, as always consult with your doctor before changing your exercise protocol or diet. Pros include increased vitamin and mineral intake, as well as new insight into food sensitivities via elimination and then reintroduction.
The cons include lack of energy, disruption of glucose levels in the blood, and metabolic rate disruption. Gastrointestinal distress and frequent bowel movements are also common. These diets are also protein deficient. And, as we've discussed, cleansing makes too much exercise unwise. This may lead to sloth, atrophy, weight gain, and other conditions.

Tips for Detoxing

1. Limit your alcoholic intake. Your liver processes roughly ninety percent of alcohol in your body. When the liver metabolizes alcohol it becomes acetaldehyde, a cancer-causing chemical. The liver coverts that to harmless acetate, which is then eliminated from the body. Excessive alcoholic intake damages the liver, rendering it unable to process acetaldehyde to acetate. This leads to various cancers which include liver cancer. Fatty buildup, inflammation, and scarring are other ways that alcohol may damage the liver.
Health authorities recommend a maximum of two drinks a day (men) and one drink a day (women). This is not a recommendation to start drinking if you don't already drink now.
2. Get more sleep. The body is busy when at rest, involved in assorted detoxification processes. It's beneficial for the brain as well as for the psyche. Getting enough sleep during a fast is especially important. The brain recharges and reorganizes during sleep. It also removes toxins, including the protein beta-amyloid, which is a major contributing factor in the development of Alzheimer's disease.
Sleep deprivation may contribute to:
- Type 2 diabetes

- Anxiety

- Stress

- Heart disease

- Obesity

- High blood pressure

Experts recommend between seven and nine hours of sleep every night.
A number of things may prevent or interrupt sleep, including:

- Artificial light from electronic devices

- Erratic scheduling

- Caffeine

- Anxiety

- Stress

3. Drink more water. Water has health benefits crucial during a cleanse, including:

- Waste product removal

- Thirst quenching

- Joint lubrication

- Body temperature regulation

- Nutrient absorption

- Digestive aid

- Natural detoxification

Experts suggest 125 ounces (3.7 liters) for men and 91 ounces (2.7 liters) for women.
4. Limit sugar intake. Excessive sugar can cause or contribute to cancer, obesity, diabetes, and heart disease. These diseases prevent natural detoxification when they damage the organs such as the liver and the kidneys.
5. Increase antioxidant consumption. Oxidation is when molecules lose an electron and matter breaks down, as in the case of rusting metal. Molecules which lose electrons become free radicals. Some free radicals can be beneficial (in the digestive process) an excess of free radicals may tear the walls of veins and arteries. Alcohol pollutants, chemicals found in cigarette smoke, and unhealthy dietary habits may create an excess of free radicals. Free radicals are associated with deadly diseases and conditions including dementia, asthma, heart and liver disease, as well as various cancers. Antioxidants introduce new electrons, correcting free radicals and making them functional molecules again.
Popular antioxidants include:

- Lutein

- Vitamins A, C, E

- Selenium

- Lycopene

- Zeaxanthin

    These are commonly found in:

- Spices

- Cocoa

- Fruits

- Berries

- Vegetables

- Green tea

- Coffee

- Nuts

7. Listen to Your Gut. It's crucial to overall health, central to digestion and critical to detoxification. Good gut health requires good bacteria called *prebiotics*. They generate short-chain fatty acids, nutrients beneficial to your overall health.

Antibiotics, poor diet and dental hygiene may create an imbalance of bad and good bacteria. This can weaken the immune and detoxification systems. It may also increase the risk of inflammation and related diseases.

Foods rich in prebiotics include:

- Artichokes

- Onions

- Garlic

- Oats

- Asparagus

- Tomatoes

- Bananas

8. Limit salt intake: Excessive salt forces the body to retain fluids. This is complicated by liver or kidneys conditions. With too much salt and too little water, the body generates an antidiuretic hormone that works to prevent urination. This causes bloating and discomfort. Increased water intake flushes water weight caused by too much salt, washing out the salt too.

Too much sodium can be balanced out with potassium-rich foods including:

- Bananas

- Kidney beans

- Spinach

- Squash

- Potatoes

9. Reduce inflammation. Inflammation has its place in the body, but excessive internal inflammation may contribute to:

- Cancers

- Heart disease

- High blood pressure

- Type 2 diabetes

- Stroke

Exercise may be tricky during a cleans, but it can certainly help control inflammation. Experts recommend from 150 to 300 minutes of moderate exercise (like brisk walking) per week. Or between 75 and150 minutes of vigorous physical activity (like running) per week. These are for normal, non-cleansing weeks.

10. Use more spices: Cooking with and eating sulfur-rich foods such as eggs, broccoli, garlic, and garlic. These promote glutathione production and assist the body to excrete heavy metals like cadmium. Glutathione is known as a master antioxidant. Chlorella is an algae that helps to eliminate insecticides, phthalates, heavy metals and other toxins.

11. Use natural cleansers: Vinegar and baking soda are as effective as industrial cleansers and they lack many harmful chemicals.

These chemicals and the risks they may pose include:

1. Phthalates, found in air fresheners, dish soap, and toilet paper, among other products. Endocrine disruptors. Higher phthalate levels correspond to reduce sperm count.

2. Perchloroethylene (or *perc)* is found in carpet and upholstery cleaners, spot removers and dry-cleaning solutions. One of the Environmental Protection Agency's (EPA) possible carcinogens. Side effects include dizziness, loss of coordination, among others.

3. Triclosan is often found in liquid dishwashing detergents and so-called *antibacterial* hand soaps. Triclosan is also a possible carcinogen. Its runoff is even dangerous to algae.

4. Quarternary Ammonium Compounds, or *quats*, are in antibacterial household cleaners, fabric softener liquids, and dryer sheets. They are known skin irritants and may be associated with asthma and various other respiratory conditions and disorders.

5. 2-Butoxyethanol is common in multipurpose cleaners, and in window and kitchen cleaners. It has been associated with pulmonary edema (resultant from excess water in the lungs), sore throats, narcosis, severe liver and kidney damage.

6. Ammonia is abundant in porcelain and metal polishers, and in glass cleaners. It may have immediate effects on sufferers from asthma, lung issues, or bronchitis, or other breathing problems. It may also interact dangerously with other chemicals.

7. Chlorine, a thyroid disrupter, is found in laundry whiteners, toilet bowl cleaners, mildew removers, and household tap water.

8. Sodium Hydroxide is common in oven cleaners and drain openers. It can be extremely corrosive to nose, throat, skin and eyes.

But here are some healthier cleaning alternatives for the home!

- Choose all-natural, fragrance-free, organic products

- Forgo air fresheners

- Take dry-clean clothing, bedsheets, and drapes to a wet cleaner

- Buy cleansers which use liquid carbon dioxide (CO_2)

- Avoid any antibacterial cleaners

- Use alcohol-based hand sanitizers which do not include triclosan

- Use vinegar as a fabric softener

- Use antifungal, antibacterial tea-tree oil (mixed with vinegar and added lavender for a pleasant scent) as an all-purpose cleaner

- Use diluted vinegar and newspaper to clean windows and mirrors

- Use vodka for polishing mirror and metals

- Use toothpaste to polish silver

- Use vinegar and baking soda to clear clogged drains

Unfortunately, commercial cosmetics, shampoos, deodorants, and moisturizers often contain questionable chemicals such as:

1. Parabens: Chemicals that preserve shelf-life. Parabens are found in body wash, makeup, face wash, night cream, and shampoo. They create hormonal imbalances by mimicking estrogen and are linked to breast cancer and fertility/reproductive issues.

2. Phthalates increase flexibility and are found in cosmetics, deodorants, hair spray, and lotions, and hair spray. They are known endocrine disrupters and can even cause some birth defects.

3. Fragrance is an umbrella term for a collection of chemicals often found in moisturizers, hand creams, and hair products. It may cause reproductive issues, allergies, hormone disruption, and infertility.

4. Sodium Lauryl Sulfate (SLS) and/or Sodium Laureth Sulfate (SLES) are common in shampoo, body wash, and bubble bath. They may cause skin irritation and trigger allergies.

5. BHT are synthetic antioxidants meant to extend shelf life. They're often found in diaper creams, lipstick, and moisturizers. They are likely carcinogens, hormone disrupters, and may cause severe liver damage.

6. Retinyl palmitate and Retinol are found in anti-aging skincare creams, as well as moisturizers. They can speed tumor growth on the skin and even damage DNA.

7. Lead is a heavy metal and neurotoxin common in lipstick and lip gloss, and even in Vaseline. Lead is associated with behavioral and learning difficulties.

8. Formaldehyde is common in many cosmetics. Formaldehyde is a known carcinogen and it's closely linked to asthma, neurotoxicity, and developmental toxicity.

Bakuchiol, a new natural alternative, may have incredible anti-aging benefits. It gives you similar results to retinol without the irritation.

Here are some healthy alternatives to the dangerous cosmetics and soaps. The publishers of this book do not promote nor endorse these products and we suggest you do your own personal and private research.

- Pure Deodorant

- Adaptive Moisture Lotion

- Citrus Mimosa Hand Cream

- Citrus Mimosa Body Butter

- Volume & Shape Mist

- Hydrating Body Lotion

- Sea Salt Spray

- Daily Shampoo

- Citrus Mimosa Body Wash

- Sheer Lipstick

- Kid's Body Wash

- Baby All-Over Wash

- Citrus Rosemary Body Oil

- Nourishing Day Cream

- Antioxidant Soft Cream (Day Cream)

- Calming Diaper Rash Cream

- Dew Skin Tinted Moisturizer

- Overnight Resurfacing Peel

- Tetrapeptide Supreme Cream

- Tripeptide Radiance Serum

- Ultra Renewal Eye Cream

- Sheer Lipstick

- Sheer Lip Gloss

- Color Intense Lipstick

Don't be afraid to come back to that and other lists as often as you need to. Think of this book as a workbook of sorts, a reference guide, a recipe book for overall good health to be read and reread, referred to as necessary.

And, to limit the need of going through the previous list, lets move on to some prefabricated cleanses which might be easy, convenient, affordable, and ideal for your needs.

CHAPTER NINE: Popular Cleanses

Cleanses take on a good many from, as we've seen. And it should come as no surprise that companies would be ready with premeasured and packaged cleanses to get the job done quickly, conveniently, and properly. Yes, water makes a great cleanse, but there is also a variety of cleansing for different purposes and from different producers. Let's review some of the better ones, those prepacked to deliver maximum nutritional impact and value. Remember that we are not associated with these producers. We are here for you, not them. We're here to let you know what's available, and one or more of these may be perfect for your specific needs. And always consult with your doctor before altering your diet or exercise protocols!

Juice Cleanses

Holistic nutritionists suggest juices cleanses can help the body take a break from heavy and potentially allergenic foods in favor of more easily digested and assimilated nutrients found in pure fruits and vegetables. The juices hydrate and detoxify and hydrate simultaneously.

Raw Generation offers plenty of juice cleanses, as well as a signature Protein Cleanse. Available in three-, five-, and seven-day options, the cleanse proports that it will clean the body and still not sacrifice proper consumption of protein, and without sacrificing the subsequent energy. The options sell for somewhere between roughly $100 and $250. They contain 40 grams of plant protein and six juices.

Pressed Juicery offers over 20 juice blends in three bundles of cleanse packages, each sells for about $30 dollars.

Suja offers a signature 3-Day Juice Cleanse for about $100, which features a seven-juice cleanse and healthy breakfast recipes.

Juice Generation offer thee Cooler Cleanses, available in one-, three-, and five-day packages ranging in cost from roughly $60 to roughly $300. The cleanses focus on juices. With their Blend It Yourself offering, the ingredients are delivered to mix at home.

Juiced offers a convenient and affordable juice cleanse intended to energize and jumpstart healthier lifestyle habits. Offering blended, raw fruits and veggies for daily consumption for up to a full week, the company's Jumpstart Cleanse costs roughly $30 a day. The cleanse seeks to improve stress response, break sugar cravings, boost mental clarity and focus, and more. The regiment suggests seven juice drinks and unlimited raw fruits and vegetables per day.

Project Juice's organic juice cleanses include three five-day options. The user may also create a customized regiment. Their beginners-level and experienced-level cleanses cost about $75 per day and each includes six juice drinks a day. The company's premium package, the Immunity Reboot Cleanse, includes two potent wellness shots every day at about $85 per day.

Lemonkind offers a 3-Day Reset Core Juice Cleanse featuring two-dozen juices (eight per day for three days). The cleanse is designed to detoxify the body, break bad habits, and jumpstart a healthier diet. The regiment offers a juice drink every two hours, making it easy to follow and more satisfying.

Squeezed offers various options to transition into a cleanse. Programs range from one day to seven days at a cost of about $30 per day. Raw fruits and vegetables are offered during the week.

Three Cleanses to Avoid

Warm lemon water and a few bottles of juice may provide less than 1000 calories, which will leave a lot of people weak, hungry, and irritable. It may cause headaches anti-sociability. Juices the fruits robs them of their nutrients and fiber.

The tea cleanse is known to create stomach cramps and sleep deprivation. And tea is a laxative, so while it may evacuate residual waste, it can't change fat into muscle or change the ratio of one to another.

The Master Cleanse makes some pretty outrageous claims. It offers only six to 12 glasses of a drink consisting of water, lemon juice, maple syrup, and cayenne pepper. Users stick to this regiment for up to ten days. The cleanse claims to shed 20 pounds in that ten-day period. The Master Cleanse also claims to help dieters overcome their psychological need to eat. Still, ten days is longer than most any expert will suggest you go without eating.

Dedicated Cleansing Kits

A product called zuPOO claims to flush the bowel of between five and 20 pounds of excess fecal matter. A powerful blend of vitamins, herbs, minerals, and barks include:

- Cascara Sagrada: Effective against constipation, an immune system booster, promotes good bacteria

- Bentonite clay: Draws waste out of the body and carries it to expulsion, using the essential and beneficial minerals calcium, magnesium, iron, sodium, silica, copper, and potassium

- Aloe ferox: a well-known colon cleanser

- Milk thistle: Supports liver function and tissue health

- Cayenne pepper: Encourages saliva for good digestion and to fight bad breath; stimulates enzyme production, critical for digestive system functionality

- Slippery Elm Extract: For bloating, abdominal pain, and straining, and improvements in the consistency of stool. It can improve digestion and aid in weight loss.

The formula is taken in capsules, one or two before bed. Gas may build up as flushing begins, after roughly 12 hours.

Tips for Cleansing

Fiber is important. Eat enough brown rice and organic fresh fruits and vegetables and fruits:
- Beets

- Radishes

- Broccoli

- Spirulina

- Artichokes

- Chlorella

- Seaweed

- Cabbage

Protect and cleanse your liver with these herbs:
- Burlock

- Milk thistle

- Dandelion root

- Glutathione

- Green tea

- Vitamin C

Experts recommend:

- Drink two quarts or more of water daily

- Deep breathing to oxygenate the system

- Emphasizing positive emotions for stress relief

- Hydrotherapy (hot five-minute shower followed by 30 seconds of cold, three times, then nap for at 30 minutes or more)

- Saunas for sweating to eliminate waste

- Dry-brush your skin or use foot spas to remove toxins through the skin.

Once your body is cleansed, it's time to move on to picking the right diet. There are a number of good ones, any of them ideal for women as well as men. We'll look deeper into certain dietary needs and concerns which women have soon enough. Until then, every woman can benefit from understanding and even adopting some of the diets we'll now look at in greater detail.

Keep in mind as you read that the ketogenic diet and the Mediterranean diet recur again and again, indicating their efficacy. Women in particular should consider one of these two, but there's lots of other good information here too. So let's get to it, shall we?

SECTION 4: DIETING

CHAPTER TEN: Ketogenic Diet

You already know the importance of a good diet by now. You also know that a good diet is effective for weight loss but also for weight management. Some diets are particularly good for intermittent fasting.

Fasting itself is a crash diet. But a diet is a regiment, and one of today's most popular regiments, and one best suited to intermittent fasting, is the ketogenic diet.

Ketosis, or the ketogenic diet, is often associated with autophagy. I restricts intake of carbohydrates and stimulates the use of reserves for energy. In the ketogenic diet, about 75% of your body's calories come from fat. Five to ten percent come from carbohydrates. The shift causes the body to change certain metabolic pathways and begins using fat for fuel rather than the glucose which is derived from carbohydrates. This shift in metabolism is called *ketosis*.

Your body generally uses carbohydrates as the preferred fuel source, this allows fat to collect. Denying the body carbohydrates forces the body to use fats for fuel. The body reprograms itself to use fat as the preferred source of fuel, creating brain-feeding ketones. Fat stores are utilized and can no longer build up so readily.

The ketogenic diet has a low carb content, moderate protein content, and high fat content. Ketosis takes about two weeks to occur.

Staple ketogenic foods include:

- Meat

- Fish

- Butter

- Eggs

- Heavy cream

- Low-carb vegetables

- Cheese

- Seeds

- Avocados

- Nuts

- Oils

A lot of those foods probably seem familiar from the chapters on cleansing and fasting. That's verification that the ketogenic such a good diet for before or after fasting. The ketogenic diet eliminates nearly every source of carbohydrates:

- Rice

- Grains

- Beans

- Fruits

- Milk

- Potatoes

- Cereals

- Sugars

- High-carb veggies

The ketogenic diet is known to increase fat burning, lower insulin levels, and producing ketones. It can instigate muscle gain, fat loss, and improved disease markers. A ketogenic diet can be more effective for weight loss than a low-fat diet. One study had volunteers on the ketogenic diet who lost over two times more weight than those on a low-calorie, low-fat diet. Calories in both groups were reduced equally.
A 2007 study had a low-fat diet group which lost 4.6 pounds (2.1 kg) and a low-carb diet group which lost 15.2 pounds (6.9 kg). Over three months, the low-carb diet group lost three times more weight than the low-fat diet group.
The ketogenic diet works through a series of processes to promote weight loss:

- Higher protein intake

- Gluconeogenesis (conversion of protein and fat into carbohydrates for fuel)

- Appetite suppressant

- Improved insulin sensitivity

- Improved metabolism and fuel utilization

- Increased fat burning

- Decreased fat storage

The ketogenic diet is shown to have positive, even restorative effects on conditions such as:

- Metabolic syndrome (type 2 diabetes, obesity, heart disease)

- High blood pressure

- High blood sugar levels

- High waist-to-hip ratio (excess belly fat)

- Low insulin levels

- Low levels of HDL (good) cholesterol

- High levels of LDL (bad) cholesterol

Many of these risk factors may be improved or eliminated with some lifestyle and nutritional changes. Note: Studies have found that the ketogenic diet may have negative effects in children. Research also indicates that saturated fat intake (as in the ketogenic diet) may increase levels of LDL cholesterol, which is a risk factor for heart disease. Other studies show connections between some fats and various forms of cancer.

Ketogenic Diet and Metabolic Disease

The ketogenic diet can affect some metabolic disease markers, which include:
- Fewer carbohydrates: This means lower blood sugar and insulin

- Decreased resistance to insulin: This can cause high triglyceride levels, fat storage, and inflammation
- Ketone bodies: They serve to protect the body against epilepsy, cancer, Alzheimer's, and other diseases
- Reduced inflammation: Reducing metabolic syndrome
- Fat loss: Especially abdominal fat, a staple of metabolic disease
- Restoration of insulin function: Insulin fights inflammation

Ketogenic Diet's Risks and Drawbacks

Note: The ketogenic diet is not suitable for sufferers of:
- Pancreatitis
- Carnitine deficiency
- Liver failure
- Fat metabolism disorders
- Porphyrias
- Pyruvate kinase deficiency

Dieters may also get the *keto flu*, a collection of flu-like symptoms including:
- Low energy
- Nausea
- Digestive discomfort
- Increased hunger
- Poor exercise performance
- Sleep issues
- Poor mental function
- Dehydration

And there might be risks to the kidneys and liver after extended periods of ketogenic dieting, though the research is lacking.

A ketogenic diet isn't always easy to stick to. A low-carbohydrate diet or carb-cycling may be preferable. Athletes may not like the reliance upon fat, as we said, because they rely more on carbs. Vegetarians and vegans may resist the reliance on dairy and meats.

Too many ketones may cause ketoacidosis (DKA). DKA is prevalent in type 1 diabetes and possible in type 2 diabetes, when ketone levels escalate. DKA is considered a medical emergency and may result in a coma.

DKA warning signs include:

- Nausea
- Dry mouth
- Consistently high blood sugar
- Fruit-like odor of the breath
- Frequent urination
- Breathing difficulties

A ketogenic diet centers around the following foods:
- Eggs: Organic, pasteurized, whole
- Poultry: Chicken or turkey
- Shellfish: Shrimp and scallops, oysters
- Fatty fish: Wild salmon, herring, mackerel
- Meat: Venison, bison, pork, organ meats, grass-fed beef
- Full-fat dairy: Cream, butter, and yogurt
- Full-fat cheese: Brie, mozzarella, cheddar, goat cheese, cream cheese
- Nuts and seeds: Walnuts, almonds, peanuts, macadamia nuts, peanuts pumpkin seeds and flaxseeds
- Nut butter: Natural almond, cashew, and peanut butters
- Healthy fats: Olive, coconut, avocado & sesame oil; coconut butter
- Avocado:
- Non-starchy vegetables: Broccoli, mushrooms, tomatoes, greens. peppers
- Condiments: Pepper, salt, herbs, lemon juice, vinegar, spices

Keto-friendly beverage choices include:
- Water: For hydration
- Sparkling water: For flavor
- Unsweetened coffee: With heavy cream, not sugar
- Unsweetened green tea

The following foods should be restricted:
- Baked goods: Cookies, breads, rolls, crackers, and doughnuts
- Sweet, sugary foods: Maple syrup, ice cream, sugar, candy, coconut
- Sweetened drinks: Soda, juices, flavored teas, sports drinks
- Pasta: All noodles
- Grain products: Wheat, rice, oats, cereals, tortillas
- Starchy vegetables: corn, potatoes, butternut squash, pumpkin, sweet potatoes, peas

- Beans and legumes: Black beans, chickpeas, lentils, kidney beams
- Fruit: Grapes, bananas, citrus, pineapple
- Sauces: Barbecue sauce, sweet salad dressing, dipping sauces
- Some alcoholic beverages: Beer, sugary mixed drinks
- Unhealthy fats: Margarine, shortening, vegetable oils (corn, canola)
- Processed foods: Processed meats, packaged foods, fast foods
- Diet foods: Artificial colors, preservatives, sweeteners such as sugar alcohols and aspartame

A One-Week Sample Keto Menu

Note: The following recipes are based on reasonable portions. Proportions of one ingredient to another depend on taste. We're basing these meals on some standard dietary measurements. Salad recipes are to include two cups of greens, salad dressings include two tablespoons. Nut butters or cream cheese should be limited to one tablespoon. Recommended cheese portions should be two slices or one ounce. Fruit and vegetable portions should be between one and five pieces, depending on the size. Meats are generally six to eight ounces per portion. All the diets recommend six to eight 12-ounce glasses of water daily.

This menu, put together by dietary experts, offers less than 50 grams of carbohydrates per day.

A 7-Day Sample Menu for the Keto Diet

Monday
- Breakfast: Two eggs scrambled, served on a lettuce and topped with sliced avocado
- Lunch Grilled salmon a small salad
- Dinner Pork chop with mashed cauliflower and cabbage slaw
- Snacks: Sunflower seeds or celery and green pepper slices with guacamole

Tuesday
- Breakfast: Hard-boiled eggs, coffee
- Lunch: Tomatoes stuffed with tuna salad
- Dinner: Meatballs with zucchini noodles, cream sauce
- Snack: Macadamia nuts, sliced cheese and roast beef roll-ups

Wednesday
- Breakfast: Cheese and vegetarian omelet, with salsa
- Lunch: Sashimi and miso soup
- Dinner Roasted chicken with sautéed mushrooms and asparagus
- Snacks: Smoothie (almond milk, almond butter, greens, and protein powder), Greek yogurt (full-fat) with crushed walnuts, almonds, or pecans

Thursday
- Breakfast Smoothie made with almond milk, greens, almond butter, and protein powder
- Lunch: Chicken tenders (almond flour) served on a greens, cucumbers and goat cheese

- Dinner: Grilled shrimp with lemon butter sauce, asparagus

- Snacks: Hard-boiled eggs, sliced green pepper a goat cheese

Friday
- Breakfast: Two fried eggs, bacon, side of greens

- Lunch: Hamburger (grass-fed) with a lettuce wrap, avocado, side salad

- Dinner: Baked tofu and cauliflower rice, peppers and broccoli with peanut sauce

- Snacks: A palmful of walnuts with a small portion of berries, celery sticks with almond butter

Saturday
- Breakfast: Avocado halves filled with eggs, baked

- Lunch: Poached salmon / avocado rolls in seaweed (no rice)

- Dinner: Beef kebabs (grilled) with peppers, served and sautéed broccolini

- Snacks: Kale chips, pork or turkey bar

Sunday
- Breakfast: Scrambled with vegetables, salsa

- Lunch: Sardine or tuna salad made served in an avocado half

- Dinner: Broiled trout, sautéed bok choy

- Snacks: Seaweed strips with cheese, turkey jerky

That's a week of satisfying and keto-friendly meals. But everybody likes to snack every now and then. Hard-boiled eggs

The Ketogenic diet has gotten a lot of attention, which is only fitting. Elements of the diet recur in other diets. And there are lots of other popular diets. So let's take a look at some of them now.

CHAPTER ELEVEN: Other Popular Diets

The Paleo Diet

The paleo diet (or the *stone age* diet) is based on foods similar to those which were available during the paleolithic era (between 2.5 million and 10,000 years ago). These foods include lean meats, fish, fruits, vegetables, seeds, and nuts. Since farming became popular about 10,000 years ago, grains, dairy products, and legumes are included.

The paleo diet holds that the human body is basically the same as it was during the paleolithic era, but our environment has drastically changed (known as the *discordance hypothesis)*.

The paleo and the ketogenic diets have similar goals, including a full body detox. You may want to gain muscle mass, lose fat, or maintain your optimal body weight. Or you may simply be seeking meal-planning assistance.

The paleo diet features some variation, making it flexible. The new paleo dieter can look forward to enjoying these foods:

- Fruits

- Vegetables

- Lean meats (grass-fed or wild game)

- Nuts and seeds

- Fish (salmon, albacore tuna, mackerel, any that are rich in omega-3 fatty acids)

- Olive oil or walnut oil

The paleo diet avoids these foods:
- Grains: Barley, wheat, and oats

- Salt

- Legumes: Peas, beans, peanuts, lentils

- Refined sugar

- Potatoes

- Dairy products

- Processed foods

A Typical Paleo Diet Daily Menu

Just a reminder: These recipes also follow reasonable-portion measurements. Salad recipes are based on two cups of greens. Limit salad dressings to two tablespoons. Cream cheese or nut butters should be limited to one tablespoon. Cheese portions should be limited to two slices or one ounce. Vegetable and fruit portions between one and five pieces, depending on the size. Meat portions are generally six to eight ounces. All diets recommend six to eight 12-ounce glasses of water each day.

With that in mind, here's a look at the first of several different sample menus, this one delineating what you might eat during a typical day following a paleo diet:

- Breakfast: Broiled salmon, cantaloupe

- Lunch: Broiled pork loin, salad (romaine, cucumber, walnut, carrot, tomato, lemon juice dressing)

- Dinner: Beef sirloin tri-tip, steamed broccoli or spinach, salad (greens, avocado, unions, tomatoes, almonds, with lemon juice dressing) and strawberries.

- Snacks: One orange, celery stalks and carrot sticks

A One Week's Sample Paleo Menu

Monday
- Breakfast: Smoothie (almond milk, kale, Apple, banana, avocado)

- Lunch: Tossed salad with fried seabass, pumpkin seeds, olive oil dressing

- Dinner: Roasted chicken with stuffing (onions, carrots, rosemary)

Tuesday
- Breakfast: Scrambled eggs with tomatoes, pumpkin seeds, and spinach

- Lunch: Salad with roasted chicken, olive oil dressing

- Dinner: Salmon (baked) with asparagus and broccoli

Wednesday
- Breakfast: Banana with blueberries and almonds

- Lunch: Green salad and salmon, olive oil dressing

- Dinner: Stir-fry beef with peppers and onions

Thursday
- Breakfast: Broccoli (fried in cocoanut oil) and a poached egg with toasted almonds

- Lunch: Tossed salad with tuna, boiled eggs, sesame seeds, olive oil

- Dinner: Baked chicken wings or legs, with steamed broccoli

Friday
- Breakfast: Smoothie (cocoanut milk, mixed berries, spinach)

- Lunch: Omelet with tomato, broccoli, butternut squash, with mixed salad

- Dinner: Salmon stir-fry with peppers, broccoli, baby corn

Saturday
- Breakfast: Bacon and eggs with tomatoes, pan-fried in olive oil

- Lunch: Chicken / vegetable soup, with turmeric

- Dinner: Lamb chops (not fried) with spinach and red cabbage

Sunday

- Breakfast: Omelet with tomato, mushroom, onion

- Lunch: Mixed salad with chicken, avocado, seeds, olive oil

- Dinner: Beef stew and vegetables.

Between meals, drink water and get plenty of exercise. The diet recommends drinking water with some physical activity every day. The paleo diet may offer special benefits over others, including:

- Better appetite management

- Greater weight loss

- Improved blood pressure

- Lowered triglycerides

- Greater glucose tolerance

The Mediterranean Diet

The popular Mediterranean diet is known for managing longevity and better health and for the prevention of various diseases. The diet is based the foods from the countries around the Mediterranean Sea, including Italy, France, and Greece, and France. These foods include:

- Olive oil

- Fish

- Healthful fats

- Whole grains

- Legumes

- Nuts

- Vegetables

- Fruits

- Red wine

- Purple grapes

- Dark chocolate

The diet de-emphasizes foods such as:

- Dairy

- Eggs

- Meat

- Processed meats

- Packaged or processed foods

- Sugary foods

- Refined oils

- Refined grains

The Mediterranean diet has a high percentage of calories from monounsaturated fats (like olive oil) so this diet may not be right for people who are watching their fat intake.

A One Week's Sample Mediterranean Menu

Note: With every day, a breakfast option of Greek yogurt with walnuts and blueberries is allowed.
Monday
- Breakfast: Mediterranean omelet (add chopped herbs like oregano, basil, or tarragon)

- Lunch: Mediterranean chicken pasta

- Dinner: Cod & asparagus bake

Tuesday
- Breakfast: Yogurt and honey fruit cups with crushed walnuts

- Lunch: Quinoa and tabbouleh salad

- Dinner: Mediterranean chicken with olives, tomatoes, and capers

Wednesday
- Breakfast: Mediterranean broccoli and cheese omelet (with Italian bread)

- Lunch: Mediterranean Pork with orzo

- Dinner: Shrimp and veggies with feta skillet

Thursday
- Breakfast: Mediterranean stuffed tomatoes

- Lunch: Mediterranean Cobb Salad

- Dinner: Chicken and veggies with goat cheese skillet

Friday
- Breakfast: Vegetable omelet (with goat cheese)

- Lunch: Mediterranean Chickpeas with feta cheese

- Dinner: Parmesan chicken served with artichoke hearts

Saturday
- Breakfast: Mediterranean veggie puff (spinach, red pepper, cheddar)

- Lunch: Mediterranean lemon chicken orzo soup (with feta or Parmesan, side of toast)

- Dinner: Mediterranean pizza

Sunday
- Breakfast: Feta and asparagus frittata, tossed salad

- Lunch: Mediterranean Chicken with Rice

- Dinner: Pistachio Baked Salmon (pistachios, dill, brown sugar)

Snacks for the Mediterranean diet include reasonable portions of olives, fruits, nuts, or Greek yogurt.

The Atkins Diet

The Atkins diet offers low-carbohydrate fare designed to help you lose weight. It may also prevent or combat other health problems, including heart disease and high blood pressure.

Fifty years after the diet's creation, we have two Atkins diets. The original is now called Atkins 20 (with a net carb intake of 20 grams. The new Atkins 40 allows 40 grams of net carbs.

Both versions of the diet include proteins, vegetables, and healthy fats. Some people do consider the Atkins as a forebearer of the ketogenic diet.

The Atkins diet something called the *Food Guide Pyramid*. It prioritizes food from bottom (consumed more) to top (consumed less). It features whole grains like oats, rice, and barley.

The pyramid excludes *white foods*:

- Pasta made with white flour

- White rice

- White bread

- White potatoes

- White sugar

The Atkins diet comes in phases, with net carbs varying in each phase.

Phase 1: Induction. The strictest phase, wherein dieters entirely forgo:

- Alcohol

- Bread

- Fruit

- Starchy vegetables

- Grains

- Dairy products (besides butter and cheese)

Phase 1 includes 20 grams net carbs daily (the FDA recommendation is 300). The concept is to increase fat-burning ability. It is motivational and often effective.

Phase 2 introduces some whole-food carbohydrates to pursue ongoing weight loss, including:

- Legumes

- Nuts

- Berries

- Yogurt

- Tomato juice

Phase 2 includes between 25 and 50 net carbohydrates daily until the dieter is within ten pounds of target weight.

Phase 3 adds a variety of carbohydrates, including starchy vegetables, whole grains, and fruits. Phase 3 includes between 50 and 80 net carbohydrates daily for roughly a month after the target weight is reached.

Phase 4 is for lifelong maintenance, offering a low-carb diet of 80 to 100 net carbs daily.

The Atkins diet uses the now-familiar process of ketosis.

Women on the Atkins diet lost ten pounds on average, lowered their blood pressure, and improved triglyceride levels in study done by the Journal of the American Medical Association.

The Atkins diet, however, has some of the same drawbacks the ketogenic diet has. High fat intake is dangerous to the heart, liver, kidneys, as well as other organs and systems.

A One Week's Sample Atkins Menu

The Atkins diet offers between 60 and 70% fat, between 20 and 30% protein, and up to ten percent carbs. Net carb intake is only 20 to 40 grams daily, which come mostly from mineral- and vitamin-rich vegetables. The following sample diet averages roughly 20g daily net carbs.

Monday
- Breakfast: Scrambled eggs with sautéed onions and cheddar cheese
- Lunch: Deli ham with mixed greens and avocado, five large black olives, sliced cucumbers, blue cheese dressing
- Dinner: Baked Catfish, broccoli and butter
- Snacks: Atkins Peanut Butter Fudge Crisp Bar, 3/4 sliced zucchini and provolone cheese

Tuesday
- Breakfast: Sausage scramble
- Lunch: Tuna salad with greens, cherry tomatoes
- Dinner: Lean pork chop, cauliflower and cheddar cheese
- Snacks: Sliced red bell peppers and ranch dressing, celery and cream cheese

Wednesday
- Breakfast: Omelet with Swiss cheese and spinach
- Lunch: Grilled chicken and baby spinach, tomato, avocado salad
- Dinner: Sauteed beef and vegetables over romaine leaves
- Snacks: Strawberry shake, sliced ham with cream cheese and a spear of dill pickle

Thursday
- Breakfast: Omelet with cheese and spinach with avocado, salsa
- Lunch: Atkins frozen chicken pot pie
- Dinner: Hamburger with pepper jack cheese, tomato, avocado, romaine lettuce
- Snacks: Atkins vanilla shake, zucchini with Monterey jack cheese

Friday
- Breakfast: Scrambled eggs with shredded cheddar cheese and salsa
- Lunch: Atkins frozen chili con carne, mixed greens tossed with Italian dressing
- Dinner: Half a cobb salad, ranch dressing
- Snacks: Atkins cafe caramel shake, sliced bell pepper and ranch dressing

Saturday

- Breakfast: Stuffed bell pepper (eggs scrambled with onion and spinach)

- Lunch: Tuna salad (dill pickle, celery, mayo)

- Dinner: Italian sausage, grilled bell pepper and union, with baby spinach, mushroom slices, blue cheese dressing

- Snacks: Atkins strawberry shake, portobello mushroom cap stuffed with salsa and pepper jack cheese

Sunday

- Breakfast: Pumpkin pancakes

- Lunch: grilled chicken breast over romaine hearts and radishes, creamy Italian dressing

- Dinner: baked salmon and broccoli

- Snacks: Snap peas with cheddar cheese, celery with cream cheese

The Diabetes Diet

Theis diet is designed for healthy eating and managing blood sugar. The diabetes diet includes eating healthy foods in moderate amounts at regular mealtimes. It's low in calories and fat while being rich in nutrients. The diet includes fruits, whole grains, and vegetables. It's a terrific diet for people on diabetes. It's also recommended for fasting, longevity, weight management and weight loss. The diet can reduce the risk of cardiovascular diseases and some cancers. Low-fat dairy can reduce the risk of osteoporosis.

Other benefits of the diabetes diet include:

- Control of blood sugar levels

- Control of stroke and heart disease risk

- Control of high blood pressure

- Control pf high blood fats

- Prevention of hyperglycemia, a risk factor for kidney, heart, and nerve damage

The diabetes diet includes three meals per day at regular mealtimes. This helps insulin use. These meals focus on good fats, fish, fiber, and healthy carbs.

You may not realize that there are healthy carbs. Sugars are simple carbs, starches are complex carbs (which break down into glucose). This diet focuses on healthy carbs, including:

- Vegetables

- Fruits

- Low-fat dairy (milk and cheese)

- Whole grains

- Legumes (beans and peas)

Fiber-rich foods include plant foods and others that the body can't digest or absorb and which help to moderate blood sugar levels. These high-fiber foods include:

- Fruits

- Vegetables

- Nuts

- Whole grains

- Legumes (peas, beans)

Fish is recommended twice per week (tuna, mackerel, salmon, sardines). The omega-3 fatty acids may prevent different types of heart disease. Grill, steam, roast, or poach the fish.

Just as there are healthy carbs, there are also good fats. These are the polyunsaturated and monounsaturated fats which may lower cholesterol levels. Foods rich in good fats include:

- Olive, canola, and peanut oils

- Nuts

- Avocados

Things to Avoid on the Diabetes Diet

This diet excludes trans fats, or saturated fats. These fats are common in animal protein and high-fat dairy products like bacon, sausage, hot dogs, beef, butter, and palm kernel and cocoanut oils. Trans fats are found in baked goods, processed snacks, stick margarines, and shortening.

Diabetic dieters should avoid known sources of cholesterol, including egg yokes, high-fat dairy products, organ meats, high-fat animal protein. The diet includes 200 milligrams (or less) of cholesterol daily.

This diet calls for than 2,300 mg of sodium per day, less for sufferers of high blood pressure. That's a lot of sodium.

Diabetes Diet Meal Plans

The American Diabetes Association has the *plate plan*. It works by splitting the plate into quarters; half the plate for vegetables (of the non-starchy type, such as carrots, spinach, tomatoes), a quarter for protein (tuna, chicken, lean pork) and a quarter for whole grains (like rice) or a vegetable (starchy, like potatoes or green peas). Avocados and nuts may be added in small portions. Fruit or dairy can also be added, and a glass of unsweetened coffee or tea and a glass of water.

A Sample Diabetes Diet Menu

This sample menu offers 1,200 to 1,600 calories per day.

- Breakfast: Whole-wheat bread with jelly, shredded wheat cereal with one-percent percent low-fat milk, one piece of fruit, one cup of coffee

- Lunch: Roast beef sandwich (wheat bread, lettuce, tomato, low-fat American cheese, and mayonnaise) one apple, water

- Dinner: Salmon, small baked potato, carrots, green beans, one dinner roll, unsweetened iced tea (add milk to taste)

- Snack: Popcorn with margarine

The Hormone Diet

Hormonal imbalance and weight loss are each affected by diet. Hormonal fluctuations can have a big effect on stress, sluggishness, weight gain, lagging libido, and various other health problems. Some favor a version of the Mediterranean diet, good for weight loss and energy levels.

It's the *glyci-med* diet. It begins with the Mediterranean diet and adds foods low on the glycemic index (these are foods that raise blood sugar slowly, whereas foods that are high on the index raise blood sugar quickly).

The hormone diet is great for sufferers of heart disease, hypertension, and diabetes. The hormone diet includes:

- Lean protein (eggs, fish, chicken breasts)

- Most fruits and vegetables (flaxseeds, chia seeds, most nuts)

- Olive oil (as well as unsaturated oils like canola)

- Whole grains (brown rice, buckwheat, quinoa)

The hormone diet eliminates or minimizes:

- Fried foods

- Caffeine

- Full-fat dairy

- Processed meats

- Artificial sweeteners

- Alcohol

- Peanuts

- Saturated fat

- Hi-GI carbohydrates

This diet doesn't include fasting. Dieters eat every four hours or so. Healthy meals represent 80% of the diet, leaving two meals out of ten as *cheat meals*. Some prefer six days on the diet and then take a *cheat day*.

Dieters advance to a medium-level regiment after a few weeks. Greater effort makes for better results. It's best to do it progressively. Don't jump ahead to an advanced level without tackling the easier levels. This is true for all the diets and regiments in this book.

For this level, dieters forgo sugar, caffeine, alcohol, diary, gluten, and all oils for two weeks. They're replaced with supplements such as vitamin D3, calcium, magnesium, and omega-3 fatty acids.

The hormone diet recommends organic, whole foods, not processed and freshly cooked.

The diet isn't a fast, so regular exercise shouldn't be problematic. The diet suggests a half-hour, once a day, six days per week. Interval training, full-body strength training, and yoga are recommended.

The diet is convenient for vegetarians and vegans and those who eat gluten-free. These organic and gluten-free ingredients are often more expensive. Expensive hormone tests might be recommended, and they might not be covered by insurance.

This diet favors:

- Cruciferous vegetables, which help your liver metabolize estrogen as well as prevent estrogen-dominant cancers. They include cabbage, Brussels sprouts, kale, cauliflower, bok choy.

- Salmon and Albacore tuna, which help make male sex hormones such as testosterone, and omega-3 fatty acids. Salmon may stabilize hunger hormones and appetite

- Avocados, which are rich in beta-sitosterol, balancing cholesterol and cortisol levels. Plant sterols are very influential on progesterone and estrogen, the hormones which are responsible for regulating the menstrual cycle and ovulation.

Organic vegetables and fruits don't include the hormone-disrupting pesticides and chemicals such as glyphosate, which are known endocrine-disrupters that reduce fertility and also may have other harmful side-effects.

High-fiber carbohydrates (veggies, fruits, whole grains) remove extra hormones and they facilitate chemical bonding and removal of active, unbound estrogens. Carrots, squashes, sweet potatoes, and other root vegetables are often very popular choices.

Probiotics are good gut bacteria. Prebiotics, on the other hand, are fibrous foods those bacteria eat and thrive on. Your gut is your biggest endocrine organ. It creates and secretes roughly 20 hormones, each of which plays a role in metabolism, appetite, and fullness. Prebiotic foods include:

- Raw oats

- Dandelion

- Garlic

- Asparagus

- Apples

- Bananas

- Almonds

- Chicory

- Kimchi

- Yogurt

- Jerusalem artichokes

Some foods may complicate these hormonal imbalances. They include processed and fried foods, as well as sugar and sugar substitutes. These impact the balance of the hormones ghrelin and leptin. Alcohol is a hormonal disrupter, from estrogen metabolism to blood sugar level.

Vegetarian and Vegan Diets

A vegetarian diet can be effective and health and meet all your nutritional needs. They're known for various health benefits, and they include lessening the risk of some cancers, diabetes, and heart disease. A vegetarian and/or vegan diets echo a lot of things in this book, fasting included. There are varying types vegetarian diets too, catering to differing tastes and needs. Lacto-vegetarian diets eschew eggs, poultry, meats, fish, but not dairy products such as milk, butter, cheese, and yogurt.

The ovo-vegetarian diet cuts out seafood, poultry, pork, beef, and dairy products, but it does allow eggs. The lacto-ovo diet does not include poultry, meat, and fish, but it does allow eggs and dairy products. The pescatarian diet includes fish, but it excludes meat and poultry, eggs and dairy.

Vegan diets eschew poultry, eggs, meat, fish, dairy products, and foods which contain any of these products.

The flexitarian diet is plant-based but it includes reduced portions of eggs, dairy, meat, fish, and poultry, but only on occasion.

The vegetarian diet focuses on healthy, plant-based, including fruits and veggies, nuts and legumes, and whole grains. Sugar-sweetened juices and refined grains are to be avoided.

The following vegetarian diet includes portions based on a 2,000-calorie-pe-day diet. As with all the recipes in this book, observe the proper measurements: Fruits and vegetables at about one and a half to two cups (though it's a bit higher, two to three here, as there's no meat), dressings are recommended at two tablespoons, pieces or slices of fruits or veggies at between one and five, salads are two cups of greens. The diet offers grain and dairy portions that diets like the ketogenic diet don't offer. A maximum of six and a half ounces of whole grains are recommended. Dairy is limited to three cups per day, protein foods allowed up to three to four ounces daily. The vegetarian diet includes oils (from nuts or olives) at about 25 to 30 grams daily.

The vegetarian (and vegan) diet requires more supplementation, as they eliminate or reduce the natural sources of:

- Calcium and vitamin D: For strong teeth and bones, found in dark green vegetables and soy

- Vitamin B-12: For red blood cell production, anemia prevention

- Protein: For healthy skin, bones, muscles and organs

- Omega-3 fatty acids: For hearth health

- Iron and zinc: For red blood cells

- Iodine: For thyroid hormones

Monday
- Breakfast: Overnight baked eggs bruschetta (in a casserole dish)

- Lunch: Arborio rice with white bean soup

- Snacks: Fruit and cheese kabobs with yogurt

- Dinner: Vegetarian pizza

Tuesday
- Breakfast: Poached eggs with tomato, onion, and cumin

- Lunch: Roasted sweet potato salad, vinaigrette dressing

- Snack: Portobello bruschetta with rosemary aioli

- Dinner: Vegetarian enchiladas (eggplant, summer squash, corn)

Wednesday
- Breakfast: Parfaits (yogurt, nuts, fruit)

- Lunch: Mediterranean bulgur bowl (cheeses, veggies, bulgur wheat)

- Snack: Deviled eggs

- Dinner: Lentil tacos

Thursday
- Breakfast: Apple Pancakes

- Lunch: Pitas stuffed with roasted sweet potatoes and chickpea pitas

- Snack: Mini peppers stuffed with cheese and chives

- Dinner: Ricotta primavera (garlic, herbs, green and red pepper, and ricotta cheese)

Friday
- Breakfast: Oatmeal waffle

- Lunch: Mushrooms stuffed with Monterey jack cheese with garlic toast

- Snack: Roasted beetroot and garlic hummus

- Dinner: Vegetarian pad Thai

Saturday
- Breakfast: Portobello mushrooms Florentine

- Lunch: Quinoa-stuffed squash (pumpkin seeds, garbanzo beans, quinoa)

- Snack: Chewy Honey Granola Bars

- Dinner: Black bean tortilla pie

Sunday
- Breakfast: White cheddar and black bean frittata with salsa

- Lunch: Spinach quesadilla

- Snack: Homemade guacamole

- Dinner: Grilled veggie burgers (cumin, garlic, chili powder)

Now here's a seven-day vegan menu. Limit snacks to whole fruits or vegetables. Recipes should follow similar recipes available online.

Monday
- Breakfast: Fruit smoothie

- Lunch: Hummus wrap

- Dinner: Spaghetti with charred tomatoes, shishito peppers

Tuesday
- Breakfast: Peanut butter and banana oatmeal

- Lunch: Portobello mushroom soup

- Dinner: Pizza burrito

Wednesday
- Breakfast: Avocado toast

- Lunch: Mashed chickpea sandwich (with veggies)

- Dinner: Black bean enchiladas

Thursday
- Breakfast: Fruit smoothie

- Lunch: Black bean burritos

- Dinner: Taco bowl

Friday
- Breakfast: Berry cobbler overnight oats

- Lunch: Balsamic spinach wrap (salt, balsamic, smoked paprika, maple syrup) over spinach and avocado

- Dinner: Veggie pizza

Saturday
- Breakfast: Avocado toast

- Lunch: Mediterranean wrap

- Dinner: Enchilada burrito

Sunday
- Breakfast: Banana overnight oats

- Lunch: Flatbread and white bean puree with steamed asparagus

- Dinner: Veggie burger

This brings us to diets for women, particularly those over 50. There are particular needs and circumstances which make their lives more challenging, and we're here to help them meet those challenges. Younger women may want to pay particularly close attention, as they may be able to avoid maladies common to women later in life (heart disease, bone loss). Women of any age can benefit as much from these dietary considerations as they could from the previous analysis of hormones, autophagy, and fasting. But let's get particular in this next chapter and take a closer look at the diets of women, especially those 50 or over.

CHAPTER TWELVE : Diets for Women Over 50

When women reach 50 years of age, certain physiological and psychological changes occur, often leading to:

- Weight gain

- Insomnia

- Loss of bones

- Indigestion

Women begin losing one percent of lean body mass every year after the age of 40 unless they keep physically active. To maintain body muscle, physical activities like walking, jogging, and yoga, are suggested.

With waning hormones, changes in physical activity, and weight gain, women's bone health often fails as they age. Women of that age should:

- Get plenty of vitamin D, calcium, protein

- Should quit smoking

- Stay active

- Stick a diet heavy in vegetables, fruits, fish, whole grains and fat-free dairy

- Limit sugary, fried, or processed foods

- Avoid crash dieting

- Avoid fasting

Here are some meals and snacks which are idea for women over 50:

Any good diet for women over 40 should have enough zinc. Anybody will get plenty of that by enjoying a hardboiled egg with a glass of milk. It's good for improved eyesight and stronger bones and muscles. But it's a bit high in cholesterol, so don't eat this for every meal every day!

A good diet for women has a proper supply of calories. They can do this by adding Choco chips berries to their diet:

- One cup of grain cereal

- 57 grams of dried cranberries

- 57 grams of choco chips

- 30 grams of seed of sunflower

Nut butter snacks include peanut butter, almost butter, any nut butter. A tablespoon with a cut apple is ideal for fiber and protein.

Foods which are cooked in fish oil work well for women after 40. The omega 3 fatty acid help prevent dementia, heart attack, stroke, and can enhance memory.

Pistachios are high in good cholesterol, important for women over 40. They may combat calcium deficiency.

Apple and potato peels are great for women past 40 for their nutritional value.

A dark chocolate shake is just a milk shake (or fruit smoothie) with two squares of dark chocolate. The resveratrol will augment concentration and focus.

These diets are good for what women over 50 are most concerned about; bone strength, memory loss, weight management, and muscle growth. They are all:

- Easy to follow (besides a few guideline and some simple shopping lists, the diets don't require supplements)

- Adaptable (according to personal preferences and nutritional needs)

- Not too restrictive

- Nutritionally balanced

- Evidence-based

The Mediterranean diet is considered by experts as one of the healthiest diets for almost anyone, especially women over 50. It's popular for its positive effects on various chronic and age-related illnesses such as diabetes, heart disease, mental decline, and cancer. One study proved that the diet is associated with a 30% reduced risk of obesity in peri- and postmenopausal women. The flexitarian diet is also recommended for women over 50 because it's easy to follow.

But we've already dedicated a pretty good amount of page space to those, so feel free to go back and reread, or simply read on!

The DASH in the DASH diet stands for *dietary approaches to stop hypertension.* It's a single diet designed to treat or even prevent high blood pressure (hypertension). This makes it a great diet for women over 50. The diet is notable for low sodium content and high potassium, calcium, and magnesium content, known to reduce blood pressure.

Some people on the diet limit sodium to 2,300 mg a day, others as little as 1,500 mg, in accordance with the American Heart Association's recommendations.

The DASH diet is mainly comprised of fruits, vegetables, and low fat dairy, with moderate amounts of legumes, whole grains, nuts, seeds, poultry and fish. Red meat and sugary foods are only occasionally allowed. Cured or processed meats are excluded.

The MIND diet is considered best for brain health. Risk factors for dementia are greater for women than men. Roughly two-thirds Alzheimer's disease patients are women. So the MIND diet was designed to reduce Alzheimer's risk, as well as reducing the risk of other age-related mental problems.

MIND stands for Mediterranean Intervention for Neurodegenerative Delay. It combines elements of the DASH and Mediterranean diets, shown to support brain health. It emphasizes leafy greens, whole grains, beans, berries, olive oil, and fatty fish. Fried food, red meat, cheese, butter, and sweets are strongly discouraged.

Multiple studies support the efficacy of the diet. Even people who follow the diet only moderately tend to show a slowed rate of mental decline.

Chronic restrictive dieting can lead to bone loss, weight gain, and eating disorders. Intuitive eating is a program to reform diet mentality and rebuild a more positive relationship with the body and with the foods that body wants and gets. The diet was created by dietitians claiming that chronic dieting causes not only physical and but also psychological harm.

Intuitive eating features ten foundational principles, including things like making peace with food, honoring health, and coping with emotions without using food. There are no banned foods, no rules regulate portion sizes or meal timing. The goal is to relearn how to listen to the body's hunger and fullness cues. This means the dieter no longer depends on a particular diet for mental or physical nourishment.

A recent study showed a close association between intuitive eating and improved psychological health with a reduced risk of eating disorders. Other research indicates that those who follow this plan could be more likely to maintain healthy weight, even though weight loss may not be the goal.

These diets have significant overlap (as a lot of things in this book do). They offer minimally processed, nutrient-rich foods high in minerals, vitamins, lean protein, fiber, healthy fats, and antioxidants.

Women over 50 ought to pay special attention to specific nutrients, like protein, calcium, vitamin D, and the B vitamins.

Collagen and Diet for Women

Collagen is the body's most abundant protein. It's in our skin, bones, muscles, digestive system, tendons, and blood vessels. It's like a glue which holds the body together. And collagen production ebbs as we age. So our dietary needs change as well, especially in the 40s.

Foods high in protein provide the body with the amino acids it needs to make more protein. Women over 50 should be sure to get plenty of:

- Vitamin C: Found in kiwi, citrus fruits, and pineapple

- Copper: Found in cocoa powder, organ meats, and portabella mushrooms

- Glycine: Found in gelatin, chicken and pork skin

- Zinc: Found in beef, oysters, and crab

Four Collagen-rich Meals

Salmon rice bowl: These healthy, antioxidant-rich meals support your body's production of collagen. They take about 40 minutes to prepare and great for premeal prep. Double the serving sizes to have enough for the whole week.

Salmon is a terrific source of omega-3 fatty acids, great for joint and bone health and for brain function. Lemon, kale, sweet potato, and avocado are all collagen boosters.

Sweet potato tacos with spicy avocado dressing: Chicken provides the protein, sweet potatoes, avocado, onion, and lime finish the tacos.

Kale Caesar salad with chicken features kale or spinach, rich in nutrients. Add nuts or seeds for some crunch.

Sweet potato nice cream is like the filling from a sweet potato pie without the crust, and frozen. A great collagen-boosting dessert.

Here's what you'll need to make these delicious meals:

- Sweet potatoes

- Spinach

- Kale

- Shallots

- Garlic

- Avocado

- Red onion

- Garlic

- Scallions

- Banana

- Lime
- Chicken breasts
- Salmon
- Almond milk
- Flax milk
- Parmesan
- Plain goat milk yogurt
- Quinoa
- Red wine vinaigrette
- Black beans
- Almond butter
- Cocoa powder
- Vanilla extract
- Anchovy paste
- Dijon mustard
- Worcestershire sauce
- Whole-grain bread
- Tortillas
- Collagen peptides
- Salt
- Pepper
- Cumin
- Smoked paprika
- Chili powder
- Cinnamon
- Olive oil

Symptoms of collagen deficiency include:
- Achy joints
- Fine lines and wrinkles
- Leaky gut
- Irritable bowel syndrome symptoms
- Skin dryness

- Blood pressure issues

- Cellulite

- Hair thinning

Other foods rich in collagen include:
- berries

- tomatoes

- butternut squash

- asparagus

- avocado

- Brussels sprouts

- legumes

- eggplant

Some spices to add include:
- Turmeric

- Green tea

- Ginger

- Maca, acai, and spirulina

How Your Nutritional Needs Change as You Age

Eating healthy is especially important as you age. Aging is closely associated to changes in the human body, including thinner skin, muscle loss, and less stomach acid. These changes may make someone prone to nutrient deficiencies, others may affect your senses and overall quality of life.

Roughly 20% of the elderly have atrophic gastritis, chronic inflammation damaging the cells which produce stomach acid. Low stomach acid may affect nutrient absorption, including calcium, vitamin B12, magnesium, and iron. The elderly also have a reduced need for calories. They need as much nutrients if not more, while eating fewer calories. Another issue is the reduction in the body's ability to recognize hunger and thirst. This could make someone prone to dehydration and unintended weight loss.

Older adults need fewer calories since they tend to move and exercise less, so they carry less muscle. Eating the same amount of calories can generate weight gain, especially true in postmenopausal women, as the decline in estrogen levels can promote belly fat storage.

So it's important for any senior to eat whole foods like fruits, veggies, fish, and meats. Nutrients which become important as you age include vitamin D, protein, calcium and vitamin B12.

Constipation is a problem common to people over 65, and it is two to three times more common in women. This is because women of that age move less had may take medications of which constipation is a side effect. Eating fiber may help, as it passes through the gut undigested, helps to form stool and promote regular bowel movements.

In five studies, scientists found that dietary fiber stimulated bowel movements. A high-fiber diet can prevent diverticular disease, a condition especially common to the elderly. Diverticular disease is often viewed as a disease of the Western diet. It's incredibly common, affects half of people over 50 years old in several western countries but it's practically absent in populations with higher fiber intakes. Diverticular disease affects less than 0.2% of people in Africa and Japan.

11 Foods for Looking Younger

1. Extra Virgin Olive Oil

- Lowers blood pressure

- Reduces risk of heart disease

- Helps to prevent metabolic syndrome

- Fights cancer

- Younger skin

- Anti-inflammatory

- Sun damage protection

2. Green Tea's benefits include:
- High in antioxidants

- Fight diabetes

- Insulin resistance

- Fights inflammation

- Fights heart disease

3. Fatty Fish
It's the long-chain omega-3 fats in fatty fish like salmon which are so beneficial against inflammation, heart disease, ulcerative colitis, among others. It may protect against sun damage to skin as well. Salmon has the carotenoid antioxidant astaxanthin, responsible for salmon's pink color.

4. Dark Chocolate/Cocoa
Dark chocolate has lots of antioxidants, even more than blueberries, cranberries, or acai berries. It may increase insulin sensitivity. reduce blood pressure, and improve arterial elasticity. Chocolate contains flavanols, protecting the skin from sun damage. Flavanol-rich dark chocolate doubles the amount of time a person could stay in the sun before burning. It did not occur in those who ate chocolate with fewer flavanols.
Choose dark chocolate with at least 70% cocoa solids.

5. Vegetables
Veggies are nutrient-dense and low in calories. They contain antioxidants to reduce the risk of cancer, heart disease, and cataracts.
Many veggies are high in beta carotene and other carotenoids which protect against solar radiation and free radicals, which lead to aging skin. Pumpkin, carrots, and sweet potatoes are the best sources of beta carotene. Some are rich in vitamin C, important for collagen production and a powerful antioxidant. In one study, people given 180 mg of vitamin C every day for four weeks, skin's antioxidant activity was increased by 37%. Veggies with the most vitamin C include bell peppers, leafy greens, broccoli, and tomatoes. A study of 700 Japanese women found that the women who ate more yellow and green vegetables had fewer facial wrinkles.
Vegetables provide sun protection and may prevent free radical damage to skin. This is largely due to their strong antioxidant effects.

6. Flaxseeds

Flaxseeds contain lignans, which may lower cholesterol and insulin and reduce blood sugar levels, and may decrease the risk of prostate and breast cancer. They are also a terrofoc source of the omega-3 fatty acid ALA, which protects the skin from solar radiation and can reduce skin damage from the sun. In various controlled studies, women who ate flaxseeds or flax oil for three months showed smoother skin and improved hydration.

7. Pomegranates

Pomegranates are among the healthiest fruits. They have more antioxidant power than green tea. They decrease inflammation and may help prevent the damage from high blood sugar. They may also improve results for sufferers of colon cancer. They can also protect the skin from sun damage and increase collagen production.

8. Avocados

Avocados are packed with fiber, heart-healthy fat, and various vitamins and minerals essential for health. They contain polyhydroxylated fatty alcohols. These fight inflammation, protect skin from the sun and repair damaged DNA.

The monounsaturated fat and antioxidants zeaxanthin and lutein provide DNA and skin protection.

9. Tomatoes provide impressive health benefits, thanks to high lycopene content. Lycopene is a carotenoid which reduces the risk of stroke, heart disease, and prostate cancer. It may also protect the skin from solar rays. One study showed that women who consumed foods rich in lycopene and other antioxidants showed a measurable decrease in wrinkle depth after four months. Cooking tomatoes with olive oil or other healthy fats boosts the body's absorption of lycopene.

10. Spices

Spices contain plant compounds which have beneficial effects on health. Some might help skin look younger. Cinnamon increases collagen production, which can lead to increased skin elasticity and firmness. It can also reduce skin damage resultant of advanced glycation end-products (AGEs), that form when blood sugar gets too high. Research suggests capsaicin, found in chili peppers, can reduce age-related changes occurring in skin cells. Ginger is rich in gingerol, an anti-inflammatory compound which may help prevent age spots which develop from sun exposure.

11. Bone Broth

Bone broth has become popular among the health conscious. It's made by boiling the bones of meat, fish, or poultry for long periods to release minerals and protein. One component is collagen, credited with beneficial effects on bone and muscle health. Collagen breaks down into gelatin when it's cooked, rich in amino acids proline, glycine, and hydroxyproline. Controlled studies show that collagen can improve skin moisture, firmness, and elasticity, and may reduce wrinkles. In another study, wrinkle depth in postmenopausal women was significantly reduced when they took a collagen supplement plus skin-supporting nutrients such as vitamins E and C and E for three months.

Diet Packages for Women

Here's a survey of the top diets marketed to women in the United States and other Western countries. Nutrisystem is widely known and respected, offering:

- Free home delivery

- A+ BBB rating

- Nutritionally balanced meals

- Pizza, pasta, muffins and more

- 160+ menu items

- No calories or carbs counting

- Plans for diabetics and vegetarians

- 100% money back guarantee

BistroMD is highly rated by users and offers:
- Seen on The Biggest Loser and Dr. Phil

- Programs for men and women

- Free diet analysis

- Science- and research-based

- Healthy, delicious meals

The South Beach diet is among the most famous, offering:
- Over 60 Keto-friendly selections

- Free diet analysis

- Flexible and easy to follow

- Free shakes and shipping

For some, Jenny Craig is the first (and last) name in dieting. But it does have some drawbacks and some benefits, including:
- Expensive

- Hard to get started, a little confusing

- Dedicated personal consultant

- One- and two-week plans

Weight Watchers is also world-famous, though it also has good points and bad, including:
- No diet meal delivery

- Point counting

- Community support

- Personal coaching

Whew! Again, don't be overwhelmed by all this information. Make notes, bookmark things to come back to. You don't have to know or understand these things all at once. Some of this information is meant to be referred to, again and again. So take what you've learned and know that you can always find whatever information you need.

Right here.

And here's a bit more, as our analysis takes us from diet to it's own shadowy partner, the dietary supplement. And this only makes sense. Diets are intended to provide sustainable levels of nutrition, but they often fall short in one way or another. Whatever diet you choose, supplements may be necessary or at least advised. And once again, you have to know what you're looking for and where to find it. So let's take a look at some of the crucial elements and minerals and vitamins you might be missing out on during a fast or even a specialized diet. You can't afford to miss out on this next chapter or the information in it any more than your body can afford to miss out on the nutrients we're about to discuss.

CHAPTER THIRTEEN: Natural Supplements

Now we move into the realm of vital vitamins, nutrients, and minerals, and where you can find them. Organic, holistic, or natural healthcare is more widespread than you may think. The World Health Organization (WHO) reports that between 65% and 80% of the global populace have used or currently use holistic, naturopathic medicine as primary healthcare. Thirty-eight percent of adults and even 12% of children in the US have received some type of alternative medicine.

Volumes have been written about these proteins, vitamins, minerals, and herbs. Each has several purposes, benefits, as well as side effects. We strongly recommend (as always) that you work with you physician before bringing anything new to your diet. We'll include any significant risks. But we'll focus on the benefits, as they relate to; autophagy, fat burning, fasting, cellular regeneration, and hormonal balances.

Proteins, Enzymes, Vitamins, Minerals, Nutrients

Amino Acids: Called *the building blocks of all proteins*, they're metabolism intermediates and should be ingested daily.

Beta-carotine: One of the carotenes or carotenoids, it combats high blood pressure and boosts immunity. It is most applicable functions to our purposes here. It also enhances immunity, reproductive health, proper cell communication, and it is powerful antioxidant.

Vitamin B Complex: Compromised of eight compounds: biotin, folate, thiamine, niacin, riboflavin, vitamin B6 and B12, biotin, and pantothenic acid.

Thiamine: (Vitamin B1) aids in metabolism of amino acids and carbohydrates.

Riboflavin: (Vitamin B2) converts fats, proteins, and carbs into energy.

Niacin: (Vitamin B3) helps to synthesize cholesterol and fat and aids in metabolism of fats, carbohydrates and proteins.

Biotin and pantothenic acid: (Vitamin B7 and vitamin B5) convert fats, proteins, and carbohydrates into energy.

Vitamin B-12: Required for using amino and fatty acids and fatty acids to make DNA.

Vitamin B-6: To make proteins and metabolize certain enzymes. Vitamin B-5 helps preserve gastrointestinal and immune function. Patients recovering from heart attacks are advised not to take vitamin B complex.

Conjugated Linoleic Acid: (CLA) helps burn body fat, fight high blood pressure and cardiovascular disease, lower high cholesterol and triglycerides, reduce inflammation and boost insulin resistance.

Coenzyme Q10 (CoQ10): Found in all mitochondrial cells. Roughly 95% of your energy is produced by those cells. CoQ10 is most abundant in internal organs, where they're most needed. CoQ10 is used to treat obesity, high blood pressure, heart disease, high cholesterol, and immunity disfunction. CoQ10 is an energizer and an energizer and antioxidant, preventing and scavenging free radicals.

Curcumin: Anti-inflammatory agent which is also has antioxidant, anti-carcinogenic, anti-inflammatory, and antimicrobial properties. It's used to treat cardiovascular and liver diseases, and gastrointestinal disorders. Curcumin reduces and scavenges free radicals. Curcumin shows promise for treating diabetes, cholesterol, and supporting good heart health.

Vitamin C: Promotes wound-healing and develops and maintains connective tissues. It has anti-diabetic and anti-cholesterol properties and is a powerful antioxidant and booster to overall detoxification and metabolism.

Vitamin D: Used treat conditions of the blood vessels and heart, including high blood pressure and cholesterol. It can be beneficial for weight and is used for a host of other diseases and conditions too long to detail here.

Vitamin E: Popular for treating and preventing blood vessel and heart diseases including heart attack, hardening of the arteries, diabetes, high blook pressure, and other maladies. Vitamin E is used to improve physical endurance, increase energy, and reduce muscle damage after exercise. It's also a powerful antioxidant.

Glutathione: Glutathione is recycled in the body until toxic overload is too great. Glutathione cycles other antioxidants as well collecting and cooling free radicals. Toxins cling to glutathione, and it carries them to the bile and stool to be eliminated. High glutathione levels reduce muscle damage and recovery time, and they increase endurance and strength, shifting metabolism toward muscular development and away from fat production.

Magnesium: Essential to good health, it's the fourth most-abundant mineral in your human body. About half of total body magnesium is in the bone. The other half is found mostly inside cells of body tissues and organs. It maintains normal muscle function, heartbeat, regulates sugar levels and promotes normal blood pressure. It may be connected to protein metabolism and energy.

Melatonin: A powerful sleep aid, it may help with weight loss. It's used to treat diabetes and high blood pressure. Melatonin is not safe for use by children or during pregnancy.

Quercetin: A powerful antioxidant that protects against high blood pressure, heart disease, and various respiratory infections.

Resveratrol: An antioxidant, anti-inflammatory substance found in dark chocolate and red wine, green teas, and some nuts. Resveratrol protects against LDL oxidation and lowers cholesterol. Resveratrol may reverse obesity and diabetes and reduce inflammation. Resveratrol turns on the cell's survival pathways. This prevents damage to individual cells. It also aids in weight loss, nutrient intake, and could remove accumulated toxins.

Zinc: An essential trace metal, it's useful in treating type 2 diabetes.

Herbs

Alfalfa: An excellent laxative and diuretic, it fights urinary tract infections and detoxifies the urinary tract. It neutralizes intestinal acids and eases such digestive problems as indigestion and gastritis. Alfalfa has enzymes which are ideal for digestion. It can stabilize blood sugar levels and lower bad cholesterol. Alfalfa is a powerful source of essential vitamins including the B complex as well as A, D, E, and K, crucial for blood clotting.

Artichoke Leaf: Artichoke leaf treats chronic gastrointestinal conditions, as well as some liver and gallbladder conditions involving high blood fat. It's an excellent choleretic and antioxidant.

Cascara Sagrada: A powerful laxative and improves the colon walls' muscle tone.

Corn Silk: Used to treat congestive heart failure, diabetes, and high blood pressure.

Ginger: Relieves indigestion, gas pains, diarrhea, and stomach cramping. It stimulates blood circulation, removing toxins to cleanse the bowels and the kidneys.

Pollen Extracts: Known for anti-inflammatory powers and smooth muscle relaxation.

Reishi: Enhances the immune system and improves blood circulation. Reishi is also used to treat anxiety and high blood pressure among other things.

Supplements for Women

Calcium and vitamin D are the most important nutrients for bone health. Calcium builds and maintains healthy bones. Vitamin D helps you absorb calcium. But older adults absorb less calcium. The gut absorbs less calcium with age.

Vitamin D can be made from the skin when exposed to sunlight, but aging may cause thinner skin, reducing vitamin D intake.

Vitamin B12 is a water-soluble vitamin known also as *cobalamin*. It is essential for the production of red blood cells and maintenance of healthy brain function. Studies show that 10 to 30% of people over 50 have reduced ability to absorb vitamin B12, often causing a deficiency.

Older people may also have conditions which reduce stomach acid production, leading to less vitamin B12 absorption. Atrophic gastritis is a condition which may cause this. Older people on a vegan or vegetarian diet are less likely to get vitamin B12, because it's more abundant in animal foods like fish, eggs, dairy, and meat. These contain crystalline vitamin B12, not bound to food proteins. Other nutrients which may benefit anyone as they age, including:

Potassium: Associated with lower risk of kidney stones, high blood pressure, heart disease, and osteoporosis, all common to the elderly.

Omega-3 fatty acids can lower triglycerides and high blood pressure, both risk factors for heart disease, the number one cause of death among the elderly.

The elderly are at risk of magnesium deficiency because of insufficient intake, medication, and age-related changes to the functioning of the gut.

Iron deficiency is very common in elderly people. This can cause anemia, when blood doesn't supply sufficient oxygen to the body.

Most of these nutrients are found in vegetables, fruits fish and lean meats. Vegetarians or vegans will benefit from an iron or omega-3 supplement. Iron is found in a wide variety of vegetables, but plant sources are not absorbed as well as meat. Omega-3 fats are found mostly in fish.

Studies have found the elderly have lower hunger hormones levels and higher fullness levels, so they may get hungry less often and feel full more quickly. A study with 11 elderly people and 11 young adults found that the elderly had lower levels of hunger hormone ghrelin before meals. Several studies found that the elderly have higher levels of fullness hormones leptin and cholecystokinin and leptin.

How many calories are burned at rest, your resting metabolic rate (RMR), decreases by one to two percent every decade after the age of 20.

A review of 10 studies found that increasing vegetables was linked to a waist reduction in women of 0.14-inch (0.36-cm). Another study, of 26,340 men and women between 35 and 65 years of age-linked eating vegetables and fruits with reduced waist circumference, lower body weight, and less body fat.

A two-year study of 245 women revealed that those who slept seven hours a night or more were 33% likelier to lose weight than women who slept less than seven hours per night. Better sleep quality was also closely linked to weight loss success.

So that's a virtual dictionary for necessary vitamins, nutrients, proteins; what they do and where to find them. Keep the chapter bookmarked for easy reference, as you'll go back to it repeatedly. When ready, move on to the next step on your journey toward wellness. After fasting, autophagy, defining our goals as to fat and cholesterol, choosing a diet and the right supplements, it's now time for the next big step on your journey to total wellness. And this next section can be even more vital to women than for men, for a variety of reasons we'll take a closer look at.

Roll up your sleeves, it's time to exercise.

SECTION 5: EXERCISE

CHAPTER FOURTEEN: Exercising During Fasts

Some of this analysis has touched on exercise, when it was well-advised and when it was not. We never recommend lethargy, but over-exertion when resources are depleted may have dangerous or perhaps deadly effects (on the heart and other vital organs and body functions). There are risks, benefits, specific regiments that are better for some kinds of fasting than for others.

Exercising for Intermittent Fasting

Exercising is important during intermittent fasting, when taking in calories. Exercise invigorates autophagy and resets the body for a more energetic, vigorous lifestyle. It redirects your body's energies toward muscle growth. Muscle loss is a risk of any kind of fasting.

It's more than just the advantages of exercising, but the detriment to the body if you don't exercise during intermittent fasting.

Lethargy during fasting resets the body to a lethargic pace. The body reads it as a signal of weakness, that the body is too weak to do a healthy fast.

In the paleolithic past, fasts were always followed by a hunt, so the body expects some activity. Change the body's expectations it will deliver on those expectations. Lethargy signals the body to forego developing body mass. That will affect hormonal production, slow metabolism, increase weight gain and lethargy.

This may convince the dieter that fasting is unhealthy and should be abandoned. That furthers more destructive habits of overeating and lethargy, further unbalancing blood sugar levels, things that inspired the fast to begin with.

Weight lifting is a good exercise for fasting, because of its focus on muscle development. It's terrific for intermittent fasting, since there are always biological resources to divert to muscle growth.

During intermittent fasting, general daily exercise is probably best. Your body is already enduring extreme changes with the fast. Anything up to twenty-four hours in considered intermittent. Walking is a good moderate form of exercise. Jogging is a bit more high impact, and anybody ought to check with their doctor before beginning to job. It can be hard on the hearts and joints. Since fasting may deplete essential minerals like calcium, take care before running for extended periods.

Moderate calisthenics such as push-ups, sit-ups, and pull-ups are also perfect for exercise during intermittent fasting.

Some intermittent fasting requires abstinence (from caloric intake) for more than 24 hours, so it requires deliberate application for minimal risk and maximum effectiveness. The longer the fast is, the more care needs be taken.

1. Walking: For long fasts, walking is even more important. It works muscle groups and burns calories, it instigates autophagy and increases metabolism. It's good for digestion. It's good for the respiratory and circulatory systems. It clears toxins out of the body through perspiration, urination, and bowel movements. Walking is also a great distraction for the hungry faster. Walking is reflective, meditative, and calming.

The fasted morning walk is a bodybuilder's trick for eliminating body fat. Consume zero calories to let the body use only reserves when walking. After fasting, the body is ready to use its resources. A fasted jog or cycle session uses body fat. Insulin is generally low in the morning, aiding in burning fat.

2. Weights: As we've said, lifting weights preserves muscle during long fasts. Strategies for weight lifting are different depending on if the dieter is fasting long-term or intermittently.

The longer the fast, the more care must be taken with exercising. If you're fasting for 16 hours, go on lifting as you normally do. You may even up your reps, if you feel comfortable.

Here are a few tips if you're fasting for long periods and you have concerns about muscle loss:

- Lift at higher intensities to lower the reps in a cycle

- Do not lift to failure

- Do not max-out repetitions during a long fast

- Do not max-out on effort

- Emphasize full-body exercises instead of isolated reps

Autophagy affects every cell and muscle of the body. So spread that energy over every part of your body. Fasting resets the body, and you want the body to reset to a total body focus.

Cardio: *Easy cardio* is ideal while fasting. Cardio means endurance training, ideal for fasting (which requires its own kind of endurance). Keep cardio intensity in the so-called *aerobic zone*, the heart rate at which your body burns calories from body fat. Here's an equation to finding your ideal aerobic heart rate: Your age subtracted from 180. If you're 40 years old, your ideal aerobic rate of 140 beats per minute. At 20 years old, your ideal BPM (beats per minute) is 160. Don't exceed your BPMs during a fast.

You won't feel taxed, and that's good. It means your body is using fat as fuel.

With longer fasts, avoid intense endurance training, sprinting, and jogging.

And it's not just what you eat, it's when you eat it. All these diets suggest regular mealtimes. When exercising, that should be timed to your eating windows. Time workouts deliberately as well. A study in women illustrated that resistance training led to muscle gains contingent on intake of protein and calories. Don't break a fast just after a workout.

Exercise During Long-term Fasting

The longer the fast, the less you should exert yourself. It's also worth repeating that, for muscle-building, fasting may not be the best approach. Fasting will help you to slim down, and working out will certainly help you to bulk up. But those are two goals, each with its own strategy.

For maintaining muscle mass during a fast, let your reps and cycles and weights be proportionate to the length of the fast. Longer fasts mean a bit less exercise. Consider a two-day full body regiment at the most during an intermittent fast.

Workout in the middle of your eating window to allow you to have a good meal and replenish lost nutrients at home.

Experts suggest 30 minutes of cardio, two or three times a week. For weight loss and management, an hour per day of light exercise is often suggested.

An Important Note

We're about to introduce exercises so you can use what you've learned and put it to physical use. It's likely that you've been reading this book alone (as most books are written). But while you can read these yoga, exercise, meditation, and hypnotism instructions and memorize them, that would conflict with the goals of clearing the mind. And nobody I know can read and meditate simultaneously.

There are two recommendations.

One is to record your voice. It's easy to download a smartphone voice-recording app. Read the directions here into the app, then play them back to yourself. This allows you to clear your mind and to perform the complex maneuvers these practices may require. The benefits of this approach include convenience (nobody needs to be inconvenienced) privacy (prized fasters and dieters) and self-control (recording at a pace which suits you).

The drawbacks include the absence of guidance or input. These things often require some expertise to maximize benefits and avoid injury. It can also be a bit isolating.

The other approach is include another person in these meditations, workouts and exercises (especially hypnosis).

A second person can provide encouragement, and maybe even expertise. But a second person can improvise and can also contribute a perspective that no prerecorded voice can offer. A human being is more flexible than a prerecorded voice, and flexibility, you may have noticed, is key to a lot of what we're talking about.

And having a partner means you can be a partner to them, which will only help you master the exercises from a different perspective.

But you may not have a partner. If not, don't let that discourage you and certainly don't let yourself quit. If you have to do it alone, do it alone. You can move on to classes and coaches later, if you like.

Exercise Apps

Don't forget the apps! These can help extend your exercise routines beyond even what we have here. They may be a good substitute for a class or a partner too. These are the best ones we found, with a bit about what features to offer. Remember that, as with all our lists of apps or other products, we have no connection to them. We don't endorse any product or brand. We are simply providing the best information possible so you can make the best decisions possible.

Keep in mind that, unlike previous apps, these apps are not all free. Some of them are quite pricey, actually.

Apple Fitness Plus is popular, and their subscription fitness service works with their watch and the iPhone and other devices. Their subscription is $9.99 per month.

PEAR Personal Fitness Coach is free and available for Android or iOS. The subscription is $5.99 per month. Its specialties are:

- Hands-free and eyes-free audio coaching

- Guided workouts at a wide variety of levels

- Wide choice of packages

- Performance tracking

- Sharing data with other apps

Fitbit Coach is available for iOS and Android for a subscription of $39.99 per year or $7.99 per month. It allows the user to:

- Recommend exercise activities

- Log daily activities

- Enjoy dynamic workouts which become more difficult depending on data input

Workout Trainer is free for iOS and Android and offers different subscription rates starting at $6.99 per month. It includes:

- Exercises and training routines for newcomers and veterans.

- An easy-to-answer questionnaire

- Personalized exercises and workout plans

- Notifications and reminders

- Tracking streaks

- Tracking stats

- One-on-one specialized trainers

Peloton is available for iOS and Android for $12.99/£12.99 monthly. This app helps you take advantage of everything Peloton offers without the treadmill. The app is:

- Free

- Available for a free 30-day trial

- Popular for guided workouts in everything from yoga to cardio to stretching.

- Ideal for group workouts

- Perfect for tag joining

  Fit Radio, for IOs and Android, offers these unique features:

- It generates new, inspirational playlists

- It offers a wide different of workouts

- Seven-day free trial

Shred is available for iOS and Android for a monthly rate of $12.99 a month. It offers intense workouts and is a good supplement app to a gym workout. Some benefits of the app are:

- Different workout types

- Supportive community

- Activity logging

- Interactive visuals

- 7-day free trial

Seven is free for iOS and Android and offers:

- Training in seven-minute-a-day programs

- Connections to friends for progress tracking

- 3D guides

- Subscription club ($9.99 monthly or $79.99 annually)

JEFIT is free for iOS and Android. It specializes in strength training and bodybuilding. Special features include:

- Thousands of routines

- Exercise log

- Detailed instructions

- Workout planner

- Progress tracker

  Oh, one more thing before we start exercising …

You're probably losing strength and muscle as you age. The average adult loses three to eight percent of muscle mass every decade after the age of 30. The loss of strength and muscle mass is called *sarcopenia.* Eating more protein is recommended to maintain muscle and fight sarcopenia.

A study followed over 2,000 elderly people over three years. Those who ate more protein daily lost 40% less muscle mass. A review of 20 different studies found that eating more protein may slow muscle loss while increasing muscle mass and helping to build more muscle. A protein-rich diet combined with resistance exercise may be the most effective method of fighting sarcopenia.

Here are some workout tips for first-time female gym bunnies!

Women going into a gym for the first time are often intimidated. This is due to the gym stigma of physical perfection, most women's the lack of knowledge and lack of confidence. But there's no reason to feel that way. These tips are specifically designed for women hitting the gym for the first time.

First of all, remember that your trip to the gym is for you, nobody's benefit but your own. You're not competing with anybody or trying to impress anyone. Blot the others out of your mind and do what you need to do for you, your body and your mind. In fact, even as you imagine everybody is looking at you and judging your imperfections, virtually all of them are thinking the same thing about themselves being judged by others. But you're not judging them, so why should they be judging you? Remember that everyone at the gym started somewhere.

Bring your headphones and create a playlist that will keep you motivated and feeling good. It'll help you zone out distractions and focus on your own workout.

Schedule your workout, keep your bag packed with your most comfortable workout clothes, and make sure you actually go. The reason most people don't workout is that they don't go to the gym.

If you're a complete novice, start slow. You might not realize how much you're straining your muscles until much later, when the cramping and pain set in. Also, don't forget to stretch before and after your workout. This is particularly important for a beginner and for a woman.

A treadmill is a good warmup exercise after you've done a few stretches. Ten or 15 minutes is a good way to get the heart pumping and the blood flowing. If you've never been on a treadmill before, and this is likely if you've never been to the gym, don't be afraid to ask for guidance. In fact, you'll want some guidance on every new machine you use to make sure you use it properly and avoid injury.

Cardio might be too intense for beginners. If so, be flexible and go back to stretches and the treadmill until you're ready to move forward. Never push your body beyond its endurance, especially not at the earliest stages of working out.

Thirty minutes twice a week is good for a beginner's workout. Elliptical machines, treadmills, stair climbers, stationary bikes, and rowers are good low-intensity, beginner's machines.

Move on to 15 minutes of cardio when ready, then gradually start increasing that time.

For women older than 40, bone density may decrease, due to various dietary and hormonal changes. Cardio exercise is terrific for bone growth.

A good full-body workout might include back rows, shoulder presses, crunches, leg curls, leg presses, and chest presses. Consult with a personal trainer if you're not sure how to do these beginner-level exercises. Female beginners might try two-to-three sets with eight to then repetitions. Start with light weights to build up to heavier weights.

Women possess lower levels of the muscle-building hormones. This makes weight training so handy for increasing muscle, metabolic rate, and bone density.

Now let's get to work!

Belly Fat Exercises

1. Burpees: These are great for the core, lats, chest, quads, shoulders, triceps. It includes explosive plyometric movement to get the heart pumping!
Note: When doing these exercises, open with each foot lined up to be under its corresponding shoulder. With the burpee, you stand (feet being shoulder-distance apart) and ease your hips back. Lower down into a slow squat. Put both hands flat on the mat just outside of where your feet were. Push both feet back and straighten, letting your chest touch the floor. Push to lift into a plank. Now reverse the procedure and pull both feet back. Stand up, as quickly as you performed the first half. The speed is part of its effectiveness. This exercise includes elements of the power-squat and the push-up.
Some accentuate it by using a medicine ball. Set the ball on the floor between both hands as you plank, then pick up the medicine ball when you stand.
2. Mountain Climbers: Similar to burpees, this exercise works different muscle groups while focusing on the core.
Assume the high-plank position you took in berpees, wrists directly under the shoulders. Keeping your core tight, draw your belly button back and in, toward the spine. Drive the right knee forward and in toward the chest, then return the foot and straighten the leg, back to a plank position. Drive the left knee in toward the chest, then return the leg to the plank position. Alternate the two sides until satisfied.
3. Overhead medicine ball slams are terrific for the endurance, for the core, for the heart rate. The heavier the ball, the better.
Stand with your at feet hip-width (instead of shoulder-width), holding the medicine ball in both hands. Stretch your arms over your head, stretching the body. Slam the ball forward and down, making sure to bend your knees a bit as you hinge forward. Squat to pick up the medicine ball and stand again. Raise the ball to start the cycle again.
4. Russian twists are terrific for the core and they also improve strength and definition.
Start on the floor in a sit-up position, a medicine ball in both hands held against your chest. Raise both feet, then lean back at a 45-degree angle. Twist your torso left and right, still holding the medicine ball.
5. Running on an incline remains a terrific way to burn fat. Running is good cardio, and an incline can increase the burn up to 50%. Start with a walk or a jog for five or ten minutes, then begin jogging or perhaps running. Slow to a walk for five minutes more to then jog from five to ten, then alternate again. Extend the running portions to twenty or thirty minutes or more, keeping the walking stretches to ten or cutting them down to five.
6. Rowing machines are terrific for working up the heart rate, burning calories, and melting fat while you build muscles in the shoulders, back, arms, core, and legs.
An effective four-minute cycle start with 20 seconds of rowing and ten seconds or rest. Remain in the rowing position during your rest, noting the meters or miles traveled. Go through the cycle eight times, improving your distance each time. After the eighth rest, go for a fast 500 meters and time it. The next time, beat that number.
7. HIIT puts forth the notion that intense cardio in short bursts, not sustained periods of low-intensity cardio, are ideal for burning fat.
Do a 10-minute warm-up, then 30 seconds of as many repetitions of any one thing as you can: Squats, push-ups, single-arm rows, or kettlebell swings. Rest for 30 seconds, then pick a different exercise for the next 30-second round. Do ten rounds with ten different exercises. Be sure to choose exercises that work varying muscle groups.
8. Strength Training is great for losing weight. Weight lifting isn't really designed to burn fat, it's just a perk. Moderately heavy weights are generally used for weight management or cardio. Very heavy lifting is good for adding muscle mass. But there is a place between them that's great for burning fat.

If you're not lifting weights, get some and start. Just a few hand weighs will be fine at first. You can do your rounds at home. If you are lifting, increase the weight and the duration of the workouts. This can create the afterburn effect, when fat is being even after the end of the workout.

9. Walking is great for the mind and the body. It's excellent for metabolism and for autophagy, for all the body's systems.

Experts recommend 45 to 60 minutes of walking daily for improved metabolism. It can also prevent overtraining. Overtraining can lead to excessive cortisol production, the stress hormone contributing to belly fat. One hour of rapid walking a day can burn one pound of fat a week.

From diet to exercise, our journey can only take us to one logical place, and that's Yoga. Yoga and fasting interconnect in a number of intriguing and educational ways.

Yoga is also a preferred way for women to exercise and stretch and also to meditate. 75% of yoga practitioners are women.

So let's unroll the mats and get ready to take our next step down the road to total wellness. From autophagy to fasting and breaking fasts, through dieting and cleansing and dieting, to exercise and now to yoga. It's the necessary step to even more lofty practices for which yoga (and only yoga) can best prepare you.

SECTION 6: YOGA FOR FASTING

CHAPTER FIFTEEN: Yoga for Fasting

Yoga is over 5,000 years old, and it's becoming more popular all the time. Consider these statistics:

There are more than 300 million yoga practitioners in the world.

Yoga is the most common complementary health approach in the US, with over 6,000 yoga studios and over 18,000 registered US yoga schools.

UK national interest in yoga rises by 73% ever year, and roughly 460,000 Brits go to yoga classes weekly. The UK pilates and yoga market was worth in excess of £875 million in 2018. The UK's national yoga industry employs over 16,000 people and teaches between 20,000 and 30,000 yoga classes weekly. The number of yoga practitioners is continuously rising, with no signs of slowing down. There were over 55 million US yoga practitioners in 2020.

- Weight reduction

- Stress

- Mental clarity

- Calmness

- Increased body awareness

- Mental relaxation

- Better concentration

Yoga remains popular in India, where it started, but is rising in popularity in Indonesia, Spain, Portugal, with the US fifth on the list. Italy, Costa Rica, the UK, and Morocco are in the top 10.

Fasting Meets Yoga

Yoga and fasting have a lot in common. Each entails discipline and stamina. Both are great for psychological wellness and physical fitness. Yoga requires the meditative mindset critical to a successful fast.

And both focus on detachment, rising above to achieve a higher mental and physical state.

Yoga and fasting require resistance to temptation, to forego instant gratification. If yoga is your focus, your main challenge could be to overcome lethargy. If fasting is your main objective, you may try to overcome hunger. Yoga is terrific for either, and there are some yoga regiments with a fasting-friendly approach.

Fasting allows the digestive systems to rest and reinvigorate. Most people run their systems all day every day and don't think twice, much less give their bodies a deliberate rest. And this book is about being deliberate, mindful.

Fasting rids the body of extra mass, water weight and fecal matter, or fat from around the belly. Fasting rids the body of such obstructions. It does takes more than either fasting or yoga to keep extra weight from returning. Losing weight increases the body's elastic, more capable of the flexibility yoga requires. Yoga stretches the muscles to keep them growing, which is considerable during a fast.

Fasting has meditative qualities. It calls users to recalibrate their relationship with food, and with their need and desire to eat. It allows a faster more walking and thinking time. A lot of fasting is religious, some political; fasting's main purpose is to focus the mind by focusing on the body. The benefits of fasting are broader, including a deeper state of awareness. In Tantra Yoga, one of the niyamas is closely related to food. A ten-day detox is part of Inspya Yoga's teacher training.

Even when outside of a religious and spiritual context, fasting often brings mental clarity. This is so due to the autophagy in the brain which improves performance. Clearing the mind is the hand, yoga is the key, spiritual realization is freed when the first two meet.

As with fasting, diet and exercise, everything work together to improve a well-balanced system. Yoga offers strength along with improved flexibility. Strength and focus improve in all areas of life.

Yoga and fasting both give any person a feeling of accomplishment, and immediate rewards. The body feels better during and after yoga, as in fasting.

Yoga is perfect for intermittent fasting. Yoga suggests a break between meals; eight hours. This allows the excretory system to function. That's the same as having breakfast, dinner, but no lunch. That's already a favored intermittent fast, which we read earlier.

Yoga embraces water and juice fasts, and dry fasts for as long as several days. A healthy person may wet fast for as long as five days. Over seven days isn't recommended.

Here are a few tips on keeping your yoga regiment smooth and effective while fasting.

Motion is key to yoga, and physical activity of some kind is important while fasting. There will be times when you are too unmotivated or weak for energetic movement that yoga sometimes requires. There is always *seva* (selfless service), *pranayama* (breathing exercises), concentration and meditation. You might spend some time reading about yoga. It's part of the practice. If you consistently lack enough energy for a mild yoga session, you may be lacking in healthy carbs or fats, or proteins.

Be sure the timing's right. Be wary of the wrong time or the wrong day. Timing and regularity are crucial to working out while fasting. If you're lacking energy routinely in the evenings, get up early and do yoga before your work day. If you are skipping lunch during an eight-hour fast between meals, you might spend the lunch period doing yoga. If work days are too busy, you can double-up on the yoga sessions over the weekends. If you're too tired and your diet is adequate, maybe you're working too hard. Meditation can be a good yoga alternative.

If you're committing to a yoga regiment, start slow. If you're new, find some guidance. There are classes for people at various levels, so it will be easy to find the right one for your needs. But don't get trapped in a slow class. The idea of fasting and the other practices we discuss here is to keep up and move ahead, to progress. The more you can take, the more you should take.

Beginners might start with a few rounds of sun salutation, as well as five other positions of choice. Then investigate static, gentler practices such as Yin Yoga (holding each pose for three to ten minutes). It's is ideal for releasing connective tissues and bands around the muscles. This gives the body a chance to relax, promotes circulation and clears blockages.

These practices help reduce *rajas* (passion, confusion) and *tamas* (darkness, chaos) while promoting *sattva* (purity). Fasting includes keeping bodies and surroundings clean, abstaining from gossip or lying, controlling emotions like anger.

Some *Pranayama* (breathing exercises) can be performed while fasting. Diaphragmatic Breathing (yogic breathing) calms the mind and helps focus. *Bhramari Pranayama* (bee breath) deepens concentration and prepares for meditation.

Here are other good poses for yogic fasting:

- *Paschimottanasana* (Seated forward fold)

- *Balasana* (Child's pose)

- *Setu Bandhasana* (Bridge pose)

- *Ardha matsyendrasana* (Seated spinal twist)

- *Bhujangasana* (Cobra pose)

- *Shavasana* (Corpse pose for relaxation)

We hope you've achieved a greater understanding of yoga; what it is, why you may do it, and how to make the most of it during a fast. You may also know how yoga will help optimize the effects of your fast.

Before we unroll our yoga mats, let's take a quick survey of some popular yoga apps.

Yoga Apps

Yoga Studio is top-ranked with several impressive benefits, including:
- High-quality content
- Excellent value
- Ease of use
- Numerous custom classes
- Ideal for back pain
- Focus on flexibility, balance, relaxation, and strength
- Customized flow
- Schedule classes
- Over 280 poses
- Customizable music tracks
- Weekly subscriptions

Down Dog is popular for these features:
- Useful as the user progresses
- Routines for all levels
- Varying practice durations (from ten to 110 minutes)

Daily Yoga specializes in community support and motivation. The app's popular features include:
- Weekly motivational activities
- Multi-week programs
- 200 yoga classes, 500 asanas, 50 workout plans
- New videos and programs regularly added

Glo is popular with yogis and those too busy for regular classes. The app offers:
- Classes of just five, ten, or 20 minutes
- User-friendly app
- Challenging or beginner-friendly classes

Simply Yoga is great for kids and adults at the beginner level. It offers:
- Sequences of 20, 40, or 60 minutes
- Easy-to follow directions

- 21-day and 30-day challenges

That should get you started on finding the best yoga app. Now let's put all your new knowledge about into practice with a program specially designed for yoga during fasting.

30+ Yoga Benefits for Women

1. It protects the spine: The spine is crucial to the human body, but it can be an especially tricky area for women. Pregnancy puts an enormous strain on the spine, as do the constant extra weight of female breast tissue. Yoga is a great way to maintain spinal health, these positions in particular:
- Flexion (rounds the spine forward)

- Extension (rotates the spine backward)

- Rotation (twists the spine)

- Side bending (elongates the spine on one direction)

- Axial extension (elongates the spine in the other direction)

2. It may increase happiness: Yoga may help anyone find inner peace. Women need that more and more as their lives become more hectic and demanding. These practices are great for peace and calm.
- Padmasana

- Dansana

- Gomukhasana

- Sucirandhrasana

3. Supports pregnancy: Yoga's fertility benefits include hormonal balance, stress release, increased sexual stamina and intimacy. Regular yoga practice is known to increase hormonal imbalance and ovulation. Studies show women who practice yoga may have double the chance of a successful pregnancy due to increased circulation to reproductive organs and relieved stress.
4. Increases flexibility: These yoga postures are perfect for flexibility:
- Tadasana (mountain pose)

- Veerbhadrasana (warrior pose)

- Trikonasana (triangle pose)

Further, you may try the aasanas to lower your blood sugar.
5. Improved sex life: Studies found that women's sexual desires increased during 12-week yoga protocol. The most significant results were found among women under 45 years old, and the quality of their orgasms was said to have improved.
6. Organ Functioning: Yoga massages your internal organs and boosts the body's ability to prevent disease. A yoga expert will come to know their body better, and will know when something is wrong, the better to prevent disease.
7. Glowing, healthy skin: Yoga is a good combatant of depression and stress, and those can create or agitate skin problems, including warts, acne, and wrinkles.
8. Improves posture: Yoga has certain benefits especially for women, pregnant women in particular. Yoga is great for posture, which can be a special problem for women especially as they age. It's also great for post-partem weight loss. Yoga during pregnancy may reduce complications.
9. Increased metabolism: Yoga is great for metabolism, which maintains healthy weight and controls hunger. This is important for women, who naturally hold emergency fat reserves.

10. Joint protection: Yoga is wonderful for strengthening the connective tissue as it stretches muscles. This is important to women, who may be prone to arthritis. An estimated 22.7% (54.4 million) of US adults have diagnosed arthritis, with a higher age-adjusted prevalence in women (23.5%) than men (18.1%).

11. Body sculpting: Yoga can focus development on certain isolated parts of the body, good for women who might be conscious of one part or another and wish to channel their efforts there.

12. Weight loss: Yoga can burn a lot of calories without overstressing the body, great for women and men alike.

13. Boosts emotional health: Yoga is meditative and good for depression and stress relief.

14. Blood pressure management: Yoga enables oxygenation and circulation, leading to safer blood pressure levels.

15. Blood sugar management: Women can be prone to diabetes. The following positions may be ideal for controlling blood sugar levels:

- Danurasana (means of bow pose)

- Paschimottanasana (means of forward bend)

- Sarvangasana (means of shoulder stand)

- Halasana (means of plough pose)

- Bhujangasana (means of cobra pose)

16. Menstruation issues: Women experience hormonal changes during menstruation which can make them anxious. Yoga helps relieve the discomfort and pain which often comes during this period, including:

- Irritability

- Insomnia

- Depression

- Discomfort

- Headaches

17. Fertility: Pregnancy yoga is a set of specially designed poses to helps women through pregnancy with less discomfort. It can also help with the birth and even postpartum stages. Yoga during pregnancy can help with back pain, common to pregnant women. Postnatal yoga should start around six weeks after birth, and it strengthens the pelvic floor muscles and abdominal muscles. Yoga helps regain a pre-pregnancy physique faster and easier.

18. Muscle toning: Yoga is great for building muscle without bulking up, the long, lean muscle women often seek.

19. Improved breathing: Yoga positions for better breathing include:

- Padangusthasana

- Marjaryasana

- Bitilasana

- Utttana Shishosana

- Parigasana

20. Fights gestational diabetes: Studies show that 30 minutes of yoga per day for a month can reduce blood glucose in pregnant women who suffer from diabetes. Yoga reduces stress, which plays a role in maturity-onset diabetes.

21. Pain management: Yoga is ideal for a lot of things which plague women, including:

- Arthritis

- Back pain

- Carpal passage disorder

- Stress

- Weakness

- Stiffness

22. Sharpening memory: Yoga is great for memory improvement.

23. Balance problems: Yoga is perfect for developing better balance. Muscle strengthening also helps with imbalance.

24. Quickens injury recovery: A stronger body and mind are more resilient to injury.

25. Quality time with friends: Yoga groups and classes are a good way to socialize, something women need in their increasingly demanding professional and home lives.

26. Weight Management: Yoga increases metabolism, stretches and tones muscles, and these help with weight management.

27. For all ages: Yoga is as effective for the young as for the old. Women have unique challenges in aging, such as bone loss, for which the forgiving nature of yoga is a perfect exercise.

28. May beat migraines: It's anecdotally proven, if not scientifically. But women may be prone to migraine headaches (two to three times more so, due largely to hormones).

29. Increased energy: Yoga boosts energy which lasts longer, and without energy drinks. Women's increasingly frantic and demanding lifestyles often require the extra energy yoga provides.

30. Relationship benefits: It's a good shared practice, quality time with your intimate. And the connection of yoga and arousal are clearly established.

31. Improved sleep: Various yoga positions are designed and proven to promote a good night's sleep.

32. Healthy immune system: Yoga can improve the immune system, something women need especially as they age.

33. Tension relief: Yoga relieves tension on every level; physical, psychological, even emotional. Again, the demanding nature of women's lives require this kind of relief.

34. Improved discipline: The mind and the body are more responsive, more agile during a yoga regiment. Your stamina will increase, and that contributes to more strident discipline.

35. Solves digestion problems: Yoga is great for stretching and clearing the gut.

36. Beautiful skin: Yoga increases circulation and encourages collagen production for better skin. Some of the best positions for this are:

- Padmasana

- Dhanurasana

- Adho Mukha Svanasana

- Shavasana

- Sarvangasana

- Halasana

37. Enhances concentration: Yoga helps focus concentration in men and women both. It's meditative, reflective, and designed to increase concentrative skills.

Begin with the child's pose, sitting on your calves on the mat (or a block) with knees together or wide, then lean forward, arms extended and forward, head down. Close your eyes an let your body get heavy. Inhale into your lower back, hold for a count of three before exhaling slowly. One more breath in, feel the back broaden, then exhale slowly through the mouth and nose. Do it a third time.

Walk your hands to the right and stack your left hand on top of your right for a side body stretch on the right side. Anchor your left sitting bone down, breathe the ribcage wider as it fill s with air. Walk your hands to the left and stack the right over the left. A deep breath opens the other side of the ribcage. Hold the position and breathe slowly.

Bring hands to center and come to an all-fours position, breathing as you arch the spine and roll your head on your shoulders, loosening up any tension. Slowly roll the spine up as you drop your head to stretch your spine. Dip the tailbone. Again, arch the spine with the head up, then roll the spine and dip the head and tailbone. Create space in the upper back and shoulders as you go through these movements.

Do this a few more times, breathing slowly as you do.

With your head down and spine rolled, arch the spine but keep the head down, Raise your tailbone as high as you can, hand on fingertips and feet on tiptoes. Head down, stretch the spine, arching as you push the tailbone upward. Stretch the legs and arms in rotation, lowering one heel to the mat and then the other, lowering one palm and then the other. Prioritize lengthening the spine. Spread you fingers and toes wide apart.

Slowly drop down to rest on your knees. Pull your right leg forward under your chest, foot on the mat hear your right hand. Breathe as you lung, leaning forward on the right leg as you reach up and arch your back. Breathe in, and as you breathe out extend your elbows backward and goal post your arms, extending your chest as you lean back. Swoop forward and repeat the motion, slowly arching back as your arms extend and your chest protrudes.

Do this several times, breathing slowly.

Then, put your feet together and stand, body still folded forward, hands on the mat. Bend the knees a bit and clasp your arms, holding opposite elbows. Sway from one side to the other, stretching the spine, arms and shoulders. Point the crown of the head downward.

Sweep the arms down around and up, stretching your arms back and extending your chest as you breathe in and out. Inhale, reach up, then exhale and fold forward. Extend your left foot back, right foot forward with knee up beneath your torso. Left hand flat on the mat with arm extended, right arm reaching up to the ceiling. Hold that twist position as you breathe slowly.

Exhale as you return to all fours position. Now do the same to the other side, extending your right foot back, left foot forward with knee up under the torso. Support with the right hand as the body twists to the left, arm reaching up. Hold and breathe slowly.

Again, arch your spin and push your head back (up cat) before pushing your head and tailbone down and rolling the spine upward (down cat), inhaling on the up and exhaling on the down.

Retain the position and swing the arms up in front and up to the ceiling, inhaling, before exhaling and bringing them back down around the sides. Once at the mat, inhale and draw the arms up again. Repeat the cycle as desired. Hold the position midway, with arms up, leaning back to open your heart space while you awaken the muscles in back of your body.

Stand up, feet a bit apart, knees slightly bent as you fold forward again. Clasp your hands behind your head, fingers interlocking. Gently sway to one side and then the other, lengthening the neck as you breathe.

Let your hands drop to the mat, then stand up and bring them up, arms extended up. Exhale and cactus your arms back and to your sides, leaning back. Feel the shoulder blades come together. Lower your arms and fold forward as you exhale.

Return to all fours, extend your right leg back and left leg forward, foot flat and knee raised under the torso. Support with your right hand on the mat and twist, reaching up with the left hand. Hold the twist and breathe slowly. Feel the muscles loosen, the spine stretching. Sense your organs being squeezed clean. Go a bit deeper into the twist with every breath.

Exhale and return to all fours. Extend your left leg back and right leg forward in another lunge position, support with your left hand, and twist up with the right arm extended to the ceiling. Hold the twist position, leaning back a bit with every breath before lowering your arm and returning to all fours.

Do an up cat and a down cat, lifting your knees into the downward-facing dog, legs and arms straight, fingertip and tiptoes, tailbone extended upward. Modify it by walking the hands back, nearer to the feet, elevating the tailbone. Bend one knee, lowering the other heel to the mat, then reverse it. Sway your hips gently from side to side.

Move into a plank position, back and legs straight, arms straight with shoulders over wrists, fingertips and tiptoes extended. Breathe slowly as you hold that pose.

Drop your knees to the mat, then your belly and your chest, palms on the mat at your side, elbows extended upward behind the back in a baby cobra pose. Let your tailbone move toward your heels as you slowly push up, arching your back while keeping your arms bent at the elbow. Raise your hands off the mat, bring them around to your sides and then behind your back. Interlock your fingers tightly and gently move your hands to the left and then to the right, gently stretching each side. Pull back toward your tailbone, opening the shoulders as you stretch the spine. Hold the position and breathe slowly.

Pull back onto your knees, sit on the heels of your feet as you fold forward, face down and arms extended. Your folded hands form a diamond shape, palms down on the mat. Breathe in slowly and out again. Return to a seated position, hands to heart's center. Breathe in and out slowly.

Remember to unwind from your yoga session. Spend some time with quiet meditative time or affirmation. Prepare for the rest of our day and transition into it with calm and confidence.

Now let's move on to a yoga regiment ideal for fasting, good for men and women both!

CHAPTER SIXTEEN: A Program for Yoga During Fasting

Yoga amplifies the resets of autophagy that happens during fasting. This program cleanses the mind and body in powerful ways.

As always, consult a doctor and follow prescribed guidelines and don't strain to the point of injuring yourself.

The program is flexible. If you're gearing up for a one-day fast, practice only the first day's exercises. Stay flexible through the first week, stopping if you need to. Yoga and fasting both require smooth, gradual assimilation. When you're doing both at once, they're even more important. Re-evaluate around the third day to see if you should break your fast and repeat the three days the next week, to take it further if you can. Good change is gradual.

This is a three-, four-, or five-day program; you will remove one food from your diet to replace it with a yoga practice. The duration can be flexible upon.

The program offers two yoga classes to choose from, one rigorous and one gentle. The intensity of the rigorous classes slowly decreases as your energy reserves do the same. Repeating the program, you may switch classes, creating a nearly endless combination of classes. Do only one class per day, don't double up.

The program includes a meditative option for every day, since meditation is an important part of both fasting and yoga. And in the same way that being active properly resets the body, meditation resets the mind. Such meditative practices dominate the next chapter, but they also belong here as part of a week-long program.

This program is perfect for anyone interested in the physical and mental benefits of fasting, yoga practitioners of any level, and anyone wanting to supplement their current health regiment.

This program entails doing one yoga position after the next, but you may not know all those positions by name. We'll favor describing the action, naming the positions when it doesn't disrupt the flow.

Day 1

Gentle Option: Toxic Twist

This is the first exercise for a reason; it's perfect for resetting the body. It's challenging and will get your juices flowing, kickstarting your new detoxification regiment.

Twisting the body cleanses the kidneys and the liver. This class offers twists in different variations. Drink lots of water during and after the toxic twist or its rigorous option.

Start with a downward-facing dog position, feet and hands on the floor, legs straight and head down. Exhale. Lower your body flat on the matt, touching down before curling your back and lifting your head up, hands on the mat outside your chest, (the tall cobra position). Arch your back, raising the head, inhaling, then lowering back down as you raise your chest off the matt. Keep knees and hands on the matt, arms are straight, head is down, breathing is deep. Return to downward-facing dog.

Raise your left leg up behind you, stretching it as far as possible, keeping your leg straight and your toes extended. Then bring the left leg back and in to touch your knee to your chest. Place your left foot on the mat and lift your body, raising the hands above the head. Lower your clasped hands to the heart and look down.

Place your right hand on the mat and twist, reaching up with the left hand and exhaling. Hold the position and stretch. Return your left hand to the floor, exhaling. Return your right hand to the mat and straighten your right leg behind you, returning to downward-facing dog.

Exhale as you straight your body and lower your belly and then your chest to the floor, exhaling. Curl your back in tall cobra position, hands on the mat as you pull/push yourself up with your back arching and your head back, inhaling. Hold the position.

Exhaling, keep the hands and knees on the floor and then push yourself back, head facing down. place your weight on your calves, your knees wide apart. Turn your palms up to twist your arms, shift your hips a little to the left, then the right.

Do the same to the other side.

Raise your right leg up behind you as far as you can, keeping your leg straight and toes extended. Bring your right leg back and in, touching the right knee to the chest, hands still on the ground. With your right foot on the floor, lift your body and raise the hands above the head. Lower your clasped hands to the heart, head down.

Set the left hand on the mat and twist to reach upward with your right hand, exhaling. Hold the position and stretch. Return the right hand to the mat, exhaling. Return the left hand to the mat and straighten the right leg behind you. Return to downward-facing dog.

Exhale and plank, then lower the belly and then the chest to the floor. Curl the back up in tall cobra, hands on the mat as you pull/push yourself up with back arching and your head back, inhaling. Hold the position. Exhaling, keep hands and knees on the mat and push yourself back, your back parallel to the floor and your head facing downward. Your weight should be on your calves in this position, with you knees wide apart. Turn the palms up to twist the arms and shift your hips a little to the right, then the left.

Repeat as desired.

Rigorous Option: Soft Heart with A Twist; Chaturanga Free Practice

Trusting your legs and your core to be strong, yoga lets the heart to be soft. The movement eases the heart space is the back bend. Twists and side bends expand the space in the ribcage and heart. This practice is wrist-friendly.

Start with your arms up, knees bent slightly. Lower your body to rest on your knees. Bring your right knee forward and up, foot flat on the mat as you raise your left arm up straight. Lean to the right, stretch your left arm as you breathe deeply. Hold the position.

Twist and lower your right arm to touch your right elbow to your left leg, just the outside the left knee. Your left hand points up toward the ceiling, palm flat. Now raise the right arm and place the right hand flat against the left, palm-to-palm. Let the right hip to move toward the left knee. Press the left elbow into the right knee. Turn the face rightward toward the ceiling and look up. Expand the capacity of the lungs, the capacity of the heart. Exhale. Straighten the back and reach up, arms straight. Lower the hands, palms to the mat as the left knee rises. Inhale as you half-lift the body, your right leg is straight, fingertips and toes on the mat.

Bring the feet together, legs slightly bent at the knees. Exhale as you lean fully forward and drop the head, hands touching the mat near both feet. Reach up and stand, legs slightly bent as before. Legs still bent, lower the arms and then reach back behind you (the airplane position).

Bring the arms forward and then up in front of you until they're reaching straight up to the ceiling and, in the same motion, raise the right leg. Find your balance at the outside of the left foot. Let your right hip to descend, twist to the right with the left arm in front and the right arm stretched out behind you. Reach down with the left hand and press it against the outside of the upraised right knee, right arm still outstretched behind you. Pull the right knee in with the left hand. You may choose to let the left arm float, that will work the core even more.

Release and return to a standing position, facing forward. Return to the original position, arms upraised and knees slightly bent.

Now do the same for the other side.

Start with arms up, knees slightly bent. Lower the body to rest on the knees. Bring the left knee forward and up, foot on the mat and raise the right arm up straight. Then lean to the left, stretching the right arm as you breathe deeply. Hold the position.

Then twist and lower the left arm to touch the left elbow to the outside of the right knee. The right hand is pointing up toward the ceiling, palm flat. Now raise the left arm and place the left hand flat against the right, palm-to-palm. Let the left hip to move toward the right knee. Press the right elbow into the left knee. Turn the face leftward toward the ceiling and look up. Expand the capacity of the lungs, the capacity of the heart. Exhale. Straighten your back and reach up, arms straight. Lower both hands, palms to the mat as your right knee rises. Inhale as you half-lift your torso, left leg straight, toes and fingertips on the mat. Bring feet together, legs slightly bent at the knees. Exhale as you lean fully forward and drop the head, hands touching the mat by the feet. Reach up and stand, legs slightly bent as before. Legs still bent, lower the arms and then reach back behind you (the airplane position).

Bring the arms forward and then up in front of you until they're reaching straight up to the ceiling and, in the same motion, raise the left leg. Find your balance at the outside of the right foot. Lower your left hip, twist to the left with the right arm in front and the left arm stretched out behind you. Reach down with the right hand and press it against the outside of the upraised left knee, the left arm still outstretched behind you. Pull the left knee in with the right hand. As with the other side, you may choose to let the right arm float, that will work the core even more.

Release and return to a standing position, facing forward. Return to the original position, arms upraised and knees slightly bent.

Repeat as desired.

Meditative Option: Meditate & Cultivate Calm

This 15-minute-long meditation is perfect for beginners and advanced meditators and anyone in between. The practice focuses on enjoying the meditative process without getting hung up on meditating correctly. Remaining connected to the breath will make you will feel calmer, lighter, and clearer.

Sit comfortably with legs crossed, knees out and ankles in. A good tip to have the knees in line with the hips, or even lower. That's central to the lotus position, to keep the knees low. Use a pillow or yoga block for greater comfort if you like. Place the hands on the knees with palms up, take a deep breath, Feel the tailbone lower, as if connected to the earth. Feel your heart rise up, through your head and up as if connected to the heavens.

Take a deep breath brough the nose and right into your heart center. Relax the shoulders and exhale.

Repeat as desired.

Day 2

Gentle Option: Reset Refuge; Bliss Out and Be Blessed

Experience the bliss of this smooth and soft and practice. This class combine hip openers and gentle flow, self-massage, twists, *mudra* and *pranayama* and enhance the body, soul, and mind.

Stand on the knees, facing forward. Pull the right knee back to a 45-degree angle behind you, pelvis lowered, right leg in front and bent at the knee, foot on the mat. Lean back and inhale while extending the arms to the sides, then bending the elbows to raise the hands upright at the sides of the head. Keep the elbows at a point behind the shoulders.

Set the left hand on the left knee and twist, bringing the right arm across to the left side of the body. Bend the right arm and press the right elbow against the outside of the left knee. Make a fist with the right hand and cover it with the left hand, left elbow up. With the right elbow against the left knee, twist to the left with greater force. Turn the torso up and toward the left. Take a deep breath right in to the belly and then slowly and gracefully release. Don't rush that.

Walk (or inch) the left foot toward the right, then lower yourself down by straightening the right leg and pressing the left knee to the mat. The left calf is also against the mat, horizontally in front of you. Beware of any pain in the left knee.

With both hands on the mat, lean forward over the left calf, head down and forward. Hold and breathe deeply. Place the elbows and lower arms flat on the mat in front of the left calf and foot.

Let this be a soft pose. Release unnecessary tension in the body and dive into the breath. Direct the breath to the place of sensation, the left hip or inner thigh, which is what you're stretching most. Hold that pose. Often and surrender, release and receive.

Slowly lean back, pulling the left leg back and replacing the left knee to the mat, Push up until you're standing on your knees, your spine upright.

Now let's do the same to the other side.

This time, pull the left knee back to a 45-degree angle behind you, pelvis lowered, left leg in front and bent at the knee, foot on the mat. Lean back and inhale while you extend your arms to your sides before bending the elbows to raise both hands upright at the sides of the head. Keep your elbows behind your shoulders.

Set the right hand on the right knee and twist, bringing the left arm across to the right side of the body. Bend the left arm and press the left elbow against the outside of the right knee. Make a fist with the left hand and cover it with the right hand, right elbow up. With the left elbow against the right knee, twist to the right with greater force. Turn the torso up and toward the right. Take a deep breath right in to the belly and then slowly and gracefully release. Don't rush that.

Walk (or inch) the right foot to the left, then lower yourself down by straightening the left leg and pressing the right knee to the mat. Now the right calf is also against the mat, horizontally in front of you. Again, watch out for any pain in the right knee.

With both hands on the mat, lean forward over the right calf, head down and forward. Hold and breathe deeply. Place the elbows and lower arms flat on the mat in front of the right calf and foot.

Once again, let this be a soft pose. Release unnecessary tension. Direct the breath to the place of sensation, this time the right hip or inner thigh, which is what you're stretching most. Hold that pose. Often and surrender, release and receive.

Now slowly lean back, pulling the left leg back and replacing the left knee to the mat, Push up until you're standing on the knees, spine upright.

Repeat as desired.z

Rigorous Option: Yoga Alchemy; The Axis

In this practice we'll look at locating the true center of the being, the essence nature, the divine self. We'll begin with potent core work, vigorous, decidedly physically, to draw attention from the external to the internal; away from turbulent emotion to implacable, incorruptible self.

Start in a downward-facing dog position, with feet and hands on the mat, legs and back straight, pelvis upraised. Raise the right leg up and back and bend at the knee, extending the toes toward the left side of the body. Stretch and hold, breathing deeply. Keep the shoulders square. Keep the left foot strong, the left leg straight and firm. Hold the position and breathe deeply.

Return the right leg to an extended position behind you, straight and strong, before pulling it back in all the way to the chest. Extend the right leg again, back and up and straight. Hold it before bringing it back in to the chest. Repeat this five times, slowly and pausing between positions.

When you bring the right knee in the last time, place the right foot on the mat, keep the left leg extended behind you. Lean back and raise both arms up and back, keeping them straight. Reach upward, stretching the muscles. Hold the position and breathe deeply. Avoid tension in the upper body.

With the hands up, hook your thumbs together and wave the hands and fingers to stretch under-utilized arm muscles. Gently draw the arms back a bit more as you open your heart center. Release them and let the arms stretch out to the sides to open the chest. Hold and breathe deeply.

Raise your arms, then bring them together over your heart. Place both hands on the mat and pull both knees in.

Now let's do the same thing to the other side.

Assume downward-facing dog, feet and hands on the mat, legs and back straight, pelvis upraised. This time raise the left leg up and back and bend at the knee, extending the toes toward the right side of the body. Stretch and hold, breathing deeply. Keep the shoulders square. Keep the right foot strong, the right leg straight and firm. Hold the position and breathe deeply.

Return the left leg to an extended position behind you, straight and strong, before pulling it back in all the way to the chest. Extend the left leg again, back and up and straight. Hold it before bringing it back in to the chest. Repeat five times, pausing between positions.

When you bring the left knee in the last time, place the left foot on the mat, keep the right leg extended behind you. Lean back and raise both arms up and back, keeping them straight. Reach upward, stretching the muscles. Hold the position and breathe deeply. Avoid tension in the upper body.

With hands up, hook the thumbs together and wave the hands and fingers to stretch under-utilized arm muscles. Gently draw the arms back a bit more as you open your heart center. Release them and let the arms stretch out to the sides to open the chest. Hold and breathe deeply.

Raise your arms, then bring them together over your heart. place both hands on the mat and pull both knees in.

Repeat as desired.

Meditative Option: Meditate with Gratitude

Here one sits to reflect on what one is grateful for; the things which bring joy and calm in a frantic world. You can do this as an option to the other yoga practices, or do it before or afterward or even both.

This is a very simple exercise. Sitting in the lotus position, comfortable with back straight and hands on the knees with palms upturned, simply focus on your breath as you would in any transcendental meditation session. Feel the breath come in, hold it in the lungs, feel it being expelled in an exhalation. Feel the sensation of the oxygen entering the lungs, the bloodstream, passing through the body.

But with this exercise, once you're relaxed and in tune with the body, focus on slowing down the breath. Do it gradually, and not to extremes. The idea is to slow the process, to be more mindful, to have more control of the mind over the body, and this is what meditation is all about, especially for our purposes here. You can take as much time as you want, go as slow as you want. But remember to come out of it slowly. Any jarring shift into hyperactivity could be dangerous. Good change is gradual, and a transitional period into and out of this exercise is highly recommended.

Day 3

Gentle Option: Gentle Renewal Flow

This class renews energy, stretches the body, and gently tones muscles. There's a flow from one posture into the next. It includes postures like Warrior 2 and Triangle Pose, then single-leg balancing, along with long holds of hip-opening postures like the Half Pigeon and the Frog/Garland Pose (*Malasana*).

Start with downward facing dog, with feet and hands on the mat, legs straight, hips up and head down. Exhale. Be a step behind the breath, surrender to it. Step both feet toward your hands. Rise halfway, gently. Fold deeply, head down and hands on the mat. Inhale as you rise, stretching the arms out at the sides and then up over the head as you stand up straight. Hands together, exhale as you fold forward, bringing the arms in as you lower to the mat, head and hands down (while keeping legs straight). Raise your left leg into the air, inhaling, lean back and into a lunge position with the left leg back and straight and the right knee in front of you, right foot on the mat. Lower the right knee to the mat and arch the spine, raising the arms up and back into a crescent moon position.

Twist right and extend the arms to your sides, exhaling. Inhale as you raise the arms upright again and turn to face forward, Hold the left wrist with the right hand and lean to the right while you exhale. Inhale and return to crescent moon position, leaning back with the arms still outstretched above and behind you. Lean forward and return to downward-facing dog.

Now go through it again, this time for the other side.

This time raise the right leg in the hair, inhaling, lean back and into a lunge position, with the right leg back and straight and the left knee in front of you, left foot on the mat. Lower the left knee to the mat and arch your back, raising the arms up and back into a crescent moon position.

Twist right and extend the arms to the sides, exhaling.

Repeat as desired.

Rigorous Option: Deep, Slow, Mindful Flow

This thorough, full-body class moves at a reasonable pace, but it's still fairly challenging and rigorous. The class seeks to cultivate a balance between ease and effort. It involves twisting and heart-opening balance. Breath is a priority, and the class is suitable for all levels.

Start in a plank position. With fingers and toes on the mat, legs and body straight, hands outside the shoulders. Pull the left leg in so that the outer thigh is against the stomach. Inch the left foot inward so it's to the right of the left hand, but keep the left knee further left of the arm. Your calf should not be in a straight up and down position, but angled so that the knee is projecting to the left. If you think of the leg as two hands on a clock, from the perspective that would read 11:25, not 12:35.

Lean forward just a bit to stretch the muscles and unlock the joints. Now move the left foot to center so that the calf is straight up and down.

Back into a plank position, lower yourself halfway down, inhale and push the head up and back, arching the spine. Take a few deep breaths in this position. Push the toes down and the head back, stretching the core.

Lift the hips and tuck in the head, back into a downward-facing dog position. Lift the heels and stay on tiptoes as you lean the heels to the right and return them to the mat. The feet are now horizontal to the body. Feel the beath from the left hand to the left hip joint. Hold the position and breathe deeply. Then shift the heels from the right to the left, keeping the toes firmly fixed on the mat. This time feel the pressure from the right hand to the right hip. Hold and breath before returning to downward-facing dog.

Walk step the feet back to the hands and slowly rise to a standing position.

Repeat as desired.

Meditative Option: Living the Dream; A Vision Meditation

This option has the practitioner looking into the future to envision an ideal condition or situation for their lives. This prepares the mediator for the life they want.

Sitting comfortably (or laying down) and obtaining a calming, regular breathing rhythm, close your eyes to imagine yourself stepping into an elevator. The doors close and you rise; you rise above the worries and complications of your current circumstance. You let go of the pressures and constraints of your present reality. Look up above the doors and see the lights advance, right to left as it takes you higher and further from your anxieties and stresses.

Now the elevator stops and the doors slide open. You are now looking at your idealized life. For you, this is heaven on Earth. What do you see? Is it tropical or mountainous or metropolitan? Where do you live? How is it decorated?

Who's there with you to share it? Where are you? How are you all dressed? There are no constraints, no limits, it's the very maximum of whatever your heart desires. How do you feel?

When you've spent time there, know you'll have to return to your present reality. And transition here is as important as anywhere. Wave goodbye to your family and friends for the time being, knowing you'll see them again soon. Take that elevator back to the ground floor, where you're once again grounded in reality. Both feet may be on the ground, but your head and your heart may remain in the clouds. And isn't that a wonderful thing?

Day 4

Gentle Option: Yin Yoga for Stress Relief

This class offers stress relief through a series of nourishing yin postures which are sequenced so as to unwind your whole being, returning it to a balanced state. The practice will ground you in breath awareness and will take you through a sequence of yin poses to quiets the mind. These postures are carefully chosen to help the joints, relieve lower back pain, and stimulate the parasympathetic nervous system to decrease stress and release anxiety.

This is just one of several stress relief posses which can be held for prolonged periods of time and are great for easing tension. It's the sphynx pose, or the seal pose (they're actually a bit different). Lay flat on the mat, facing downward, with toes extended, elbow and lower arms on the mat in front of you.

For the least amount of back-bend, stack your forearms in front of you with each hand over the opposite elbow. Lower your forehead to rest on your forearms.

For more bending of the spine, pull your elbows back and rest your forearms on the mat in front of you facing either inward with your palms pressed together in the center; or put your arms out straight ahead of you with your palms down. These are variations on the sphynx position. In this position, let your head drop down to stretch the spine and neck and release tension.

Comparable is the seal position, pressing palms flat on the mat in front, straightening the arms and arching the spine, raising the head.

These can all be done with cushions to alleviate soreness and accentuate bending angles more comfortably. Place a yoga cushion under the area of focus and achieve the position. Once there, hold the position and breathe deeply. This position can be held indefinitely, or the cushion can be moved to different spots in rotation.

Rigorous Option: Hatha Yoga; Strength & Freedom
An all-levels Hatha yoga class, this class will tone, warm, and open the body. It's a slow-moving class with long posture holds which strengthen and stretch.

Start with a standing forward bend, legs straight with body bend forward, hands touching the mat. Bow down as deep as your body will allow. Fold inward. Bring both feet together and raise into a chair pose, with knees bent and spine straight but forward-leaning, lifting your arms straight out and up over your head for balance. Reach up as far as you can. Take a deep breath and then, exhaling, clasp both hands in front of you and bring them to your heart. Lean forward, hands still clasped and knees still bent (even a bit more for balance).

Now twist to the right so that you can place your left elbow outside of your right knee. If you can't do this, place your left hand on the outside of your right knee and place your freed right hand on the small of your back.

Either way, now pull your right shoulder back. Set your hips down a bit and hold this position, breathing deeply. Now go into a forward fold, the position you started with, and do the same for the other side.

Cycle through from the chair position to bringing both hands to your heart. Lean forward, hands still clasped in front of you, knees bent a little more for balance.

Now twist to the left so that you can place your right elbow outside of your left knee. Or place your right hand on the outside of your left knee and place your freed left hand on the small of your back.

Pull your left shoulder back. Set your hips down a bit and hold this position, breathing deeply. Now go into a forward fold, the position you started with, and do the same for the other side.

Repeat as desired.

Meditative Option: Transform Tension to Vitality
This meditation is designed to be done during fasting and during periods of regular diet and weight management. It helps achieve a more restored state to help move the *prana* (life force) through the entire being. This one can be done as an adjunct to another class or on its own.

Sit in a comfortable position, lotus of possible, lying down if necessary. Start with a very deep breath. Now feel your self, your energy, lowering down through your body and into the ground, deep into the Earth. Now feel it coming up again, from the earth and into our body, through your open chest and to the crown of your head. Now exhale, feeling your energy descend back into you and travel downward back to your core. The more you exhale, the further that energy descends. Then inhale again, slowly and naturally, and feel the energy rise. It rises in conjunction with the speed and depth of the breath. The more you inhale the higher it goes, the slower you exhale you lower it descends. This unites the self with the earth below and the sky above, observing the oneness of all thing. But note that you're not controlling the breath, you're simply observing it, understanding it and yourself in a whole new way.

Day 5

Gentle Option: Yin Yoga for Energy and Clarity

Great for a depleted body or spirit, this one is great for when any faster is deep into a fast. This class's yin poses work with the body's chemical intelligence and gently detoxifying the spinal column, kidneys, and enhancing internal organ blood flow.

Begin by lying flat on your back. Pull your right leg up, knee to the chest, placing both hands on the calves just below the knee. Pull gently and breathe deeply. Let your left arm drop down to the mat. Extend your left arm out to your side while your right hand guides your left knee across your body, twisting the lower body to your right. You may have to adjust the angle of your left arm for comfort. Your weight should be on the side of your pelvis with your lower back strong and straight.

Now stretch your right arm out as well, letting your upper body stretch. Now turn your head to the left. Hold and breathe deeply, feel the effects of the twist. Hold this pose as long as you like before returning your head to look directly upward and uncrossing your left leg, once more lying flat with your arms at your sides and your legs together.

Now do the same thing with the other side. Pull your left leg up, knee to the chest, placing both hands on the calves just below the knee. Pull gently and breathe deeply. Let your right arm drop down to the mat. Extend your right arm out to your side while your left hand guides your right knee across your body, twisting the lower body to your left. You may have to adjust the angle of your right arm for comfort.

Now stretch your left arm out as well, then turn your head to the right. Hold and breathe deeply, feel the effects of the twist. Hold this pose as long as you like before returning your head to look directly upward and uncrossing your left leg, once more lying flat with your arms at your sides and your legs together. Repeat as desired.

Rigorous Option: Earth Yoga

The grounded yoga practice uses gravity to connect the self to its bodily roots and then beyond to its earthly roots. This is a moderately challenging *vinyasa* flow practice which invites balance and stability and which appreciates and honors all the different connections the Earth provides.

Start with downward-facing dog. Walk or hop both feet up to both hands, then halfway lift before going back down in a full forward fold. Rise up straight, arms reaching up, looking up, inhaling. Then exhale as you lower your arms, hands clasped (standing at attention). Release hands and raise them up along the sides and above the head, spine and arms straight.

Follow that up with a forward fold.

Halfway lift, place both hands flat on the mat and walk or hop your feel back, spine and legs straight in a plank position. Press the head back and up, spine arched and arms straight, in a tall cobra position. Inhale then exhale into a downward facing dog.

Inhale and raise the right leg up and back behind you, straight, rotating the right hip to extend the leg as high and straight as possible. Then bend the right leg at the knee, angled toward the left. Hold and breathe deeply. Then straighten the leg, square the hips, and bring the right leg down under the chest, foot on the mat. Extend the left leg, point the left foot outward, and rise up to a standing position with both feet splayed. Extend your arms to your sides, turn your head to look down your right arm to your right hand and beyond. Take your left hand and run it down the left thigh and point the right hand upward. Hold and breathe deeply. Slowly return to a standing at attention position, then lower yourself back into downward dog to repeat for the other side.

Inhale and raise the left leg up and back behind you, straight, rotating the left hip to extend the leg as high and straight as possible. Then bend the left leg at the knee, angled toward the right. Hold and breathe deeply. Then straighten the leg, square the hips, and bring the left leg down under the chest, foot on the mat. Extend the right leg, point the left foot outward, and rise up to a standing position with both feet splayed. Extend your arms to your sides, turn your head to look down your left arm to beyond your left hand. Take your right hand and run it down your right thigh and point the left hand upward. Hold and breathe deeply. Slowly return to a standing at attention position, then lower yourself back into downward dog. Repeat as desired.

Meditative Option: Morning Manifestation Meditation

This short meditation is designed to help energetically and mentally align with your goals for the upcoming day. It should help clear the clutter from your mind and connect to your best intentions and the utmost of your abilities.

Get into a comfortable position, get control of your breathing, locate your energy center and calm it so that it rests peacefully in the core of your being. Now concentrate on what follows; memorize it or have somebody read to you. Read it yourself into a voice recording app on your phone, if that helps. Then let the words pass through you and settle in your brain. Don't fight it; just do it.

Sift through the clutter in your mind. Shelve your to-dos, what's unfinished for now. Sift through the mundane and repetitive thoughts and patterns you may be stuck in so that you can reconnect with your inner intuition, your inner knowing. What emotion is in your space, mind or body or soul, that you don't need, that you want to clear away? Let it go. Acknowledge why it is there, then let it go, especially if it will not serve you today. Allow it to dissolve.

It's easy to imagine your new yoga regiment has you well on your way toward total wellness. You've achieved greater discipline and you've seen and felt the rewards. You're stronger, more capable, more well-informed, more confident. Your body and mind have been more deliberately enjoined and focused to work with one another toward the greater good.

But the journey isn't over yet. There are two crucial steps on the journey toward total wellness, greater health and awareness, and mastery of mind over body. We're reaching the superego promised when the mind/ego controls the body/id. It requires every bit of strength and knowledge this book hopes to offer, and will only encourage both to greater heights. You may already have guessed where we're going, an what we'll be doing next.

Meditation for fasting.

SECTION 7: MEDITATION FOR FASTING

CHAPTER SEVENTEEN: Meditation for Fasting

Meditation is the ancient, robust tradition of physical and mental wellness derived from the idea that a person can separate themselves from their circumstance, transcend it, and reach spiritual wholeness.

Like the other things in this book, meditation is easy to lose track of. We're barraged with bad foods, electronic lighting, unyielding stress, long hours, increased pollutants, desperate economic demands, we lose every opportunity for relaxation or resetting.

Meditation is a solid exercise in discipline, and discipline is helpful when applied to fasting, exercise, yoga, or any of the things in this book. Every facet of everything touches on every facet of everything else. It connects in a complex web of physiological and psychological wellbeing.

Meditation is good for men or women, but it is particularly effective and powerful with women. Women are four percent more likely to meditate. The 2017 National Health Interview Survey demonstrated that 16.3% of women have used meditation, compared to only 12% of men.

Here are some other meditation stats you may find interesting:

- Over 14% of US adults have tried meditation

- The number of people who meditate has tripled since 2012

- 7% of US children meditate

- Women are more likely to meditate than men

- General wellness is the most-cited reason people meditate

- Between 200 and 500 million people meditate

Meditation and Weight Loss

The body and mind are connected, and both are powerful tools. But the mind is in charge, or it should be. When the body is in charge is when bad decisions are made.

Meditation can set the mind free to better understand why the hand reaches, what it reaches for what it does, why the mind allows it. Meditation allows this. Meditation may bring the practitioner closer to core beliefs and even childhood disruptions which might be affecting adult behavior. Eating is often a response to anxiety, stress, self-esteem and body issues, depression, insecurity, and other destructive behaviors and conditions. Understanding that is the first step on the journey to controlling it. Meditation is often be the first step toward understanding.

How Meditation Works

Meditation is based on a very simple practice. One finds a relaxed physical position, sitting or lying down, standing, or even walking. Putting walking aside for the moment, imagine yourself sitting in a quiet place, physically comfortable.

The meditator focuses on one thing, something very simple. A beginning meditator often begins by focusing on their own breath. It's easily accessible and it connects the meditator to their own body. This helps achieve the closed energy cycle and strong connection of mind and body.

The practitioner focuses on the inhaling, holding the breath, then releasing. The focus isn't on accomplishing the simple act of breathing, it's on being deliberate about breathing; about intake, holding it for a regular count, deliberate about the release. It's about mindfulness of how the lungs feel as they take in the air, how the blood feels as you hold that breath, how the body feels when you release it.

Some choose to focus on their own heartbeat, or do body scan which starts at the head or feet and focuses on each part of the body between one and the other. Some choose a focal point, like a tree top in the distance or a nail hole the wall. Some people focus on a monotone which they utter, others on a repeated phrase called a *mantra*. Some people envision their ideal future, a perfect house or mate, or a family photograph. Some focus on whatever their idea of what God might look like.

Some prefer walking, though there will be no focal point, rather on the simple act of walking. The focus is drawn by a combination of surroundings, breathing, autonomous movement, and energy management. Walking is a popular form of meditation; people do it often and it takes no training. And it doesn't feel like meditation, there's no effort to it.

Another meditative technique is the cigarette break. As disgusting and dangerous as the habit is, it serves to draw the smoker's attention to breathing, to feeling the breath, savoring the exhalation. We're glad that fewer people choose this kind of meditation. We certainly don't recommend it.

Being mindful during a big dietary shift such as fasting means sticking to an eating plan. This could mean writing out a weekly menu and posting it on the refrigerator door. Support groups are helpful, especially for first-timers.

Meditation is Intermittent Fasting for the Mind

Intermittent fasting asserts mindfulness and deliberateness into our dietary lives, causing autophagy and stimulating reprograming of the body. Meditation does the same for the mind.

The body has two different nervous systems, the autonomic and the voluntary. Automatic behaviors include things like breathing. Voluntary behaviors include things like holding your breath. Breath is one of the few places where the two systems meet, making it a great way achieve a stronger connection between mind and body.

Many effective meditative techniques see a meeting of the automatic and the voluntary. Focal meditation uses the involuntary sense of sight, but used voluntarily. Hearing is an automatic sense, making hearing your own voice a meeting of voluntary and automatic nervous behaviors.

Once the body and mind are closely connected, the mind can better control the body.

Think of it in Freudian terms. Sigmund Freud proffered a theory that the human psyche is constructed of three parts; the ego, id, and the superego. The ego is the adult part of the psyche, it deals with the world with practicality, it masters social behavior. The id is the child part of the psyche, it deals with itself and its own immediate wants and desires without regard to consequence. The superego is the moral perspective attained only when the ego controls the id.

Now let's think about what we've looked at so far. For our purposes, the mind equates to the ego, dealing with the outside world. It is strategic, deliberate, practical. The body is the id of the total self, wanting immediate gratification. Complete wellness equates to the superego, the moral high ground. It works going backward too; Complete wellness can only be attained when the mind has control over the body.

And meditation is the perfect manifestation of the mind controlling the body.

Nonjudgmental Awareness

Our modern lives are demanding, hurried; five quiet minutes can be a luxury. With so much digital entertainment, even on minute of total silence is hard to find. Consider setting a certain time aside every day, perhaps first thing in the morning or maybe the last thing before bed or even tea time in the afternoon. Or do it opportunistically, whenever the moment may present itself.

Call it *nonjudgmental awareness*.

It's not truly meditating since it doesn't require focusing on a focal point bodily function or even a mantra. This is the kind of meditating you do on a walk. Instead of thinking about one thing, you think of nothing. The clarity still comes. Whether you're sitting, walking or taking a shower, you're engaged in several automatic behaviors, though when combined they're more deliberate.

This is a common trick among professionals who puzzle over tricky concepts and principles; lawyers circling a tricky problem, writers smoothing out story questions, doctors and social workers facing life-threatening questions. Concentrating too much on any problem can create a forest-for-the-tress problem. Overthinking a problem jams up the rational system. Stepping away to perform some physical chore is a great way to distract the mind. This is sometimes called *thought showering,* as showering requires fairly automatic but voluntary actions that require just enough conscious to distract the mind. This can free up the mental jam and let an answer become easier to find. Walking implements the same method of bringing mind and body together.

Nonjudgmental awareness is about not judging the things you see. It's hard to be aware and not be judgmental. We're trained to employ cognitive training and critical thinking. But people are not problems, they *have* problems. And children are not equipped to navigate the difference between understanding something and judging it. They're often not taught these differences, (too often parents don't know the differences). But there is a surprisingly big difference between any person and their opinions, actions, mistakes. The clear mind sees this, and meditation makes that clear.

Transcendental Meditation

This is the meditation we all know, focusing on breath, focal point, or a mantra. It's about quiet and stillness, focusing on one thing. It's terrific for clarity, mental sharpness, and discipline.

To the uncluttered mind, thoughts are easier to understand, answers easier to see. This can be done for just five minutes a day, or several hours at a time, or anywhere in between.

An hour per day is recommended for serious meditation.

Transcend the fear so prevalent in the modern world; terrorism, climate crises, increasing violence. Who wouldn't be afraid? Focus on a selected point; your breath, body, or mantra.

Let go of the guilt as well. Life is demanding, you have a right to take time for yourself. It's not selfishness, it's self-care. And it will make you all the more effective in dealing with the outside world. Do it for yourself, without guilt or fear. Just do it.

Once you've let go of the fears and guilts of the present, you may start to let go of the fears from the past. Meditation allows introspection and reflection and lets you transcend any emotional corruption to discover rational clarity. That clarity helps you to overcome negative feelings and lingering pains that can cause present-day self-sabotage.

Be nonjudgmental of the thoughts which your new clarity brings. Don't fight or deny them, don't try to blot them out. You don't have nothing to be fearful of or guilty over. But it won't happen overnight. Good change is gradual.

Before we move on to the program, let's review some meditation apps, which may prove helpful in your quest for total wellness by way of intermittent fasting. Some of these are free, others offer subscriptions. We suggest double-checking their prices, as these are subject to change.

Meditation Apps

Calm is considered one of the best. The app's guided meditations do more than lead you through anxiety and lack of focus. enefits include:

- Different modalities and tools

- Well-being offerings like sleep stories

- Celebrity voicings

Insight Timer offers benefits features few others can match, including:

- Over 45K free meditations

- Supportive community

- Filtering by need, goal, duration, benefit

- Seven-day free trial

- Meditation introductory course

Headspace Meditation & Sleep is great for people with sleep issues, a common problem while fasting. It offers:

- Wind-down practices

- Breathing exercises

- dim, meditation-friendly lighting

- sleep meditations

Ten Percent Happier Meditation is based on the top-selling book and offers:

- Mindful day tracking

- Short, on-the-go sessions

Unplug is great for those with little meditation time. Five minutes is enough time to unplug with this popular app. It offers:

- Ambient sounds and timers

- User self-direction

- Refocusing during stress

- 30-day challenge

Habit is best for simple use, offering:

- On-the-go meditation

- Clearly organized

- Extensive library of meditations

- Meditations for stress and panic attacks

- Offline use

Benefits of Meditation for Women

Women today often report feeling tired, stressed. Brain function is often compromised by drugs or liquor. Disorders like Alzheimer's disease, depression, ADHD, and chronic anxiety are on the rise, especially among women.

Nearly two-thirds of the over 5 million Americans with Alzheimer's are women. Roughly 12 million women in the US experience clinical depression every year. About one in every eight women will develop clinical depression. Depression occurs most frequently in women between 25 and 44 years old.

Transcendental meditation is known to improve creativity, intelligence, memory, learning ability, emotional stability, and neurological efficiency. This will keep anyone more vibrant, alert, and astute at just about all ages.

Neuroscientists found that the human brain produces high-power alpha waves during transcendental meditation. This brain pattern corresponds to relaxed inner wakefulness (expansion, serenity, and bliss). When these alpha waves become synchronized, the brain's powers of executive judgement are strengthened.

The coherent, integrated brain works better as a whole. This is the central concept of improved mental performance; increased creativity, better memory, sharper focus, and broader comprehension.

TM is the meditation technique found to produce alpha coherence consistently and throughout the entire brain. Researchers found that the experience often restores clarity of mind, inner peace, and neurological balance.

Natural Stress Relief and Aging Reversal

The peaceful and refreshing rest of Transcendental meditation in your daily routine will dissolve stress, refresh the mind, and reduce wear and tear on the body. There are over 600 research studies verify the benefits of TM, and the National Institutes of Health gave $26 million to scientists over 20 years to further the study of TM's health benefits.

Women currently comprise over half America's workforce, and many are the main caregivers of their families. This causes an accumulation of stress damaging to physical and mental health. Twice daily Transcendental meditation is often recommended for women, if possible.

Research tells us that TM has a holistic effect on the body's overall health; normalizing hormone levels, blood pressure, while generating measurable improvements in cholesterol, diabetes, brain functioning, and cardiovascular health. The body maintains a calmer, more rested, and energetic way of functioning. It is known to make women more resilient to stress outside of meditation.

Combating Stress

Stress is known major factor in how we much age, inside and out. Research proves that people practicing Transcendental meditation have a younger biological age (organ function, health of skin and hair, muscle and bone) than their chronological age (how many years they've been alive).

Transcendental meditation works to unfold the wholeness of the inner self the spiritual essence of life itself. This experience of transcendence is spiritual, because there is no external, material content necessary for that state, only a pure state of being.

Neuroscience has demystified transcendence. Studies on brain function during Transcendental meditation verify heightened awareness by its signature EEG pattern (brain wave signature): High amplitude alpha coherence.

Spiritual Growth

TM does not require forsaking involvement in the world or forgoing material comforts in the name of spiritual enrichment. Enlightenment and elevated awareness maintain serenity even amidst dynamic activity or worldly enjoyment.

Unfortunately, the goal has been mistaken for the path, and that leaves well-intentioned seekers having to strain to maintain a contrived posture of mindfulness or equanimity. These qualities are worthy of striving for, but hard to acquire. And they should be hard to acquire, that's what gives them their value and indicates their quality.

Enlightenment, or the complete awakening of human consciousness, is really every person's natural birthright. Daily TM time can bring women the spiritual growth they often crave both simply and easily.

Relieving Anxiety

Experts agree that women are more vulnerable to stress than men and that they recover more slowly, physically and emotionally. They are twice as likely to have chronic anxiety too. TM reduces anxiety as it calms the nervous system and provides profound inner peace.

TM shifts physiology into a more balanced, harmonious functionality which is the very opposite of stress. Biochemicals in the blood which are associated with anxiety and tension, like plasma lactate and cortisol, are significantly reduced, so the brain can function with greater coherence. Practitioners of TM show increased skin resistance during the practice, an electrophysiological measure of restfulness or calmness. Trait anxiety refers to how anxious a person usually is; state anxiety refers to how a person feels at the moment. A Journal of Clinical Psychology-published study shows that TM is more effective in reduction of trait anxiety than contemplation or concentration techniques. After TM, one likely feels rejuvenated and refreshed, worries are lessened. Emotions and thoughts are clearer, at ease. Life is more fulfilling.

A 2014 meta-analysis published in 2014 found that individuals with 90% or higher showed dramatic anxiety reductions (down to the 57th percentile) after regular TM. The technique has also proven effective in treating depression and insomnia.

Meditating and Mothering

Mothers work harder than just about anybody, and they're gravitating toward meditation more and more. Children are sensitive to a mother's stress, which makes meditating and its resultant calm even more important.

TM is easy and affordable to learn and practice. It can be done almost anytime and just about anywhere, which makes it popular for the average mother's busy life. It's great for orderly brain function, which a busy mother needs, and it can combat stress, anxiety, fatigue, depression, and insomnia, which the new mother is likely to suffer from. Mothers tend to work their TM schedules around those of their children; school periods, days they'll be away, so that the children do not feel ignored.

Meditation and ADHD

Girls with ADHD (attention deficit hyperactivity disorder) or ADD are under-diagnosed. This is because, rather than exhibiting the disruptive behavior often seen on boys, girls with ADHD often experience difficulty in paying attention or focusing. Adult women may also go undiagnosed and may suffer from depression, anxiety, feelings of inadequacy, and chronic disorganization.

Recent studies found students with ADHD who practiced Transcendental meditation showed a significant reduction of symptoms within just three to six months. Other relevant benefits include:

- Heightened EEG coherence

- Increased brain processing

- Increased verbal fluency

- Reduced stress and anxiety

Scientists attribute ADHD to a lagging in the human brain's natural development. TM allows the brain to create neural connections which correct that underlying problem.

And now we'll apply all this knowledge to a few real-time physical applications. Of all the things we've looked at, meditation may be the most beneficial and the most user-friendly and the most beneficial, and it ties the previous practices together.

CHAPTER EIGHTEEN: Meditation Programs for Fasting and the Immunity System

Meditation Program for Fasting

This meditation will guide your mind toward better health. First, find a comfortable position; on the mat or bed, or in a chair. Your back should be straight and upright. Be present and open-minded. Close your eyes, take a slow breath in through your nose. Breathe in and out, long and slow; the longer and slower, the better.

Your mind is cleared and your awareness is sharp. You're safe and relaxed while in this meditation. When I talk about self, when we think about self, we focus on awareness and our awareness is taking in these words, hearing and feeling them resonate through your whole body.

If you are fasting, you are already healing your body and mind. You extend your lifespan and improve your later years. Imagine your life becoming more enjoyable as you age. Cancer, obesity, heart issues; it's a long list of ailments that fasting may prevent. Eating when we are truly hungry creates self-respect. This process is essential to cleanse the body's impurities. Abstinence of food sharpens mental discipline and freedom; freedom within your physical and mental health. Fasting and eating right provide extra vitality, the very essence of life. Now you can spend more quality time with your family as a healthier and more energized person, living their best life to the fullest.

Relax your body and mind, knowing you are well on your way.

Feel what is coming in through your senses. You are not your senses, you simply use them to observe. Meditate. Be calm. Listen to the sounds in the room, even if that is nothing more than the vague sounds from outside.

Take a deep breath through your nose and release it through your mouth. Do it again. You are fasting again, getting healthier with each minute. Keep the regiment up, even though it may be difficult. The rewards are worth the effort. It's too important for you not to give up.

Visualize yourself living your best life; high in energy, free of disease. Picture yourself sharing it with those you know and love. Fasting will bring that reality to you, so let it guide you toward that ideal future and let that ideal future guide you through your fasting regiment.

Slowly return your awareness to the room and to your body. Center on your heart, slowly bring your awareness outward toward the rest of your body. Shrug your shoulders and feel that energy pass through them. Bend your spine from side to side, muscles pushing at the vertebrae and releasing excess tension.

Meditation Program for the Immune System

This meditation improves your immune system through meditation.

Be comfortable; sitting up, with your back straight, preferably leaning on a few pillows. Roll your head to loosen your neck; be relaxed and focused.

Connect to your breath by inhaling through your nose then exhaling slowly through your mouth. Do it until the mind and body are tranquil. Bring awareness to the center of your mind. Greet it, know it. Slow down and connect with your own immune system. Focus on connecting to your white blood cells, governing the immune system. Greet them. Note how it feels as you familiarize yourself with your immune system.

Even considering that the immune system strengthens the body is a form of meditation. That means you're already on your journey to tranquility and away from anxiety and stress, getting further with every breath in, every moment holding that breath, and every moment exhaling it.

Concentrate on both feet. Feel the toes, move them and flex them. Feel the bones, the tendons. Move up to the feet, arching and twisting them, rolling them on your ankles. Focus on the calves, muscles contracting and pulling and releasing. Feel the skin stretched over the muscle, the hair on the skin. Move your attention upward. Feel the thighs, your strong femur, tendons stretching from knees to hips. Feel the groin, center of your body. Be aware, the physical power of the genitals, the base of your vital organs as you feel through the digestive tract. Sense any congestion there must be.

Breathe deeply and steadily as you do this survey. Scan up to your stomach, your livers and kidneys, your spine. Be mindful of all the parts of your own body, their functions and their condition. Be mindful of your breathing while the scan goes up to your lungs as they expand and contract, heart beating steadily. Be aware of your own bones, ribs are strong and protective.

Feel your shoulders. Scan down the length of your arms, down to the elbows, the forearm, down to the wrists and hands. Feel how the tiny bones intermingle with tendons, nerves, and muscles. Think about these frail bones that do so much work in your life, doing so much heavy lifting.

Now slowly come back through the arms, back to your shoulders, your neck, your spine in this delicate area. Scan your head, the jaw and teeth, ears and face, nose and eyes. guide your focus to the top of your head, completing this full-body meditative scan.

Do it again, and you'll have familiarity with how every part of the body feels. Start with your head and work your way back down. Revisit areas you'd overlooked for too long. This second scan makes things more noticeable; little pains, stiffness, twitches or weakness become more apparent.

Now that you have scanned your body, pull back to see it, as if it were for the first time. What does it look like, smell like? Is it in its prime, or is it in decline? Make your body as aware of it as you are. Direct your body's resources to these areas with both your mind (meditation and discipline) and your body (exercise and yoga).

Picture the future version of yourself, your life. How do you feel there and then? How do you look? Let these visions replace any doubt, allow stillness and certainty to replace doubt and anxiety.

Envision yourself transforming into that person, becoming that person with every breath in and out, every new or repaired cell, with every better choice you make and with every walk you take.

Early morning walks and bike rides are nice ways to exercise your body. Be mindful not to overstress it, let its healthy functions to occur. Daily exercise is crucial to good health. There are no magic pills or short cuts. A healthy body is like a mindset, and a mindset is definitely a state of mind, which is awareness. This awareness of who we are and could be; living a peaceful, strong, contented life with everything we need or want.

Take a deep breath in through the nose to focus on your awareness before releasing with big sigh. You're making better decisions in your life, and your immune system will function better. Exercises don't have to be strenuous, heathy food is delicious. It brings energy, a longer life, greater appreciation for the quality of life. It allows us to focus our attention on internal heat and heat fosters relaxation. Imagine a sauna, relaxing and detoxifying, generating autophagy and rebirth.

Take another deep breath to bring awareness back to the shoulders. Roll your head on your shoulders to bring awareness back to the body, remain loose as you go into the rest of the day.

We have journeyed from the physical (including fasting, dieting, exercising) to the mental (including yoga and meditation). But there's one more step, one that transcends body and mind and still draws them together. It is not nutritional or dietary, and it is not recognized as a facet of mental health, psychology or psychiatry. It's the last frontier of non-traditional treatment. It has a demonstrated a history of effectiveness. There things it can cure and things it cannot. Take a look and see if it can save your life, or simply improve it. Now let's take final step toward the fully realized reunion of mind and body; total wellness.

Hypnotism.

SECTION 8: HYPNOTISM

CHAPTER NINETEEN: Hypno-fasting

Hypno-fasting sounds like a new approach. Hypnosis itself is fairly new, and there's a lot we don't quite understand it. But hypnosis and weight loss have a longstanding and well-established connection. Weight loss was one of the first maladies hypnotism was turned to. And why not? Both are widely misunderstood, and weight loss is a longstanding and tenacious problem often requiring drastic action. And it's been proven to work.

With your opened mind and opened heart, with your greater understanding of physiological actions and reactions, it's time to turn your attention to the final frontier of general wellness.

Hypnosis.

History

It seems like a post-psychoanalytic novelty, but hypnosis dates to ancient Egypt and Greece. The word *hypnos* is the name of a Greek God, it's the Greek word for *sleep*. Keep in mind that these bygone empires accomplished amazing feats of engineering with minimal tools. Today's modern computer technology can't replicate those ancient wonders such as the Pyramids of Giza the Parthenon atop the Acropolis in Athens.

If these cultures took hypnosis seriously, we should too.

Both those ancient cultures had religious centers where people went to seek consultation. Hypnosis of a kind was used to induce dreams and interpret them, to give vision oracles. Ancient writings are filled with references to them. John of Patmos' Book of Revelation is believed to have been written in a deep hypnotic state. Reading it, that's easy to believe.

The father of Chinese medicine, Wong Tai, recorded techniques including incantations in 2600 BCE. The Hindu Vedas chronicled techniques using hypnotic procedures In 1500, BCE. Druidic, shamanistic, yogic, voodoo, and other religious practices use on a trance state induced by use of some type of hypnotism.

Austrian physician Franz Mesmer (1734 – 1815) is known as the father of modern hypnosis. The word *mesmerize* comes from his name. He was maligned, and he was a genius and a pioneer. He developed the theory that diseases come from blockages of magnetic forces in the body.

Mesmer was popular embodying the image of the hypnotist; black cape, goatee, magnetic eyes. He was theatrical and rebellious, and there wouldn't be hypnosis without him.

London University professor John Elliotson (1791 – 1868) introduced the stethoscope to England and was forced to resign after championing mesmerism (not then called *hypnosis*). He then gave private demonstrations, furthering interest and literature on the subject.

James Braid (1795 – 1860), a Scottish eye doctor discovered that having a patient fixate on a particular thing (as in transcendental meditation) was a critical aspect of hypnotism. British surgeon James Esdaile (1808 – 1859) used hypnosis for pain relief and performed hundreds of surgeries using hypnotism as an anesthetic.

Frenchmen J.M. Charcot (1825 – 1893), Charles Richet (1850 – 1935), and Ambrose Liébeault (1823 – 1904), also did formidable work furthering hypnosis. Emile Coué (1857 – 1926) pioneered auto-suggestion. He coined the phrase, "Day by day in every way I am getting better and better." He suggested guiding people to self-healing, and that is where hypnosis enters our subjects of interest. He believed that all hypnosis was really just self-hypnosis.

In a sense, Coué also anticipated the placebo effect. That is treatment of no intrinsic value. Its power is in the suggestion of potency: patients are told that that they're taking a potent drug, but are given a sugar pill instead. In some cases, placebos can work better that many popular drugs.

Sigmund Freud (1856 – 1939) felt that hypnotic remedy was found only through the careful guidance of a trained professional. Milton H. Erickson, MD (1901-1980) did work which is still oft-cited in the study of hypnosis. His techniques are considered among the most effective.

What is Hypno-fasting?

Hypno-fasting, as you might have guessed, combines intermittent fasting with hypnotherapy/hypnosis for losing weight through fasting.

Intermittent fasting has beneficial effects, but it can be difficult for some people. We're raised on three meals a day, and they've gotten bigger even as they offer fewer nutrients. Physically, psychologically, and socially, we're addicted to the habit of eating, without regard to nutritional necessity. It can be hard to reverse these deeply engrained patterns.

Hypnosis may help with that, as habits are practiced bodily, but they're generated mentally. After doing the exercises and practices we've reviewed in this book, your mind is stronger and its more dominant over your body. That will help with hypnosis as you fast. Hypnosis in any case will help achieve mental mastery.

Hypnotism can be useful on the young and old. It works regardless of wealth, health, creed, race, or social strata. Fat or thin, rich or poor, hypnosis is equally effective.

Hypnosis is not magic or mind-control. A person cannot be made to do something which they don't want to do (as in the film *The Manchurian Candidate*). Hypnotic blackouts are mythological, so is the idea of getting stuck in hypnosis and not ever coming back to reality. In fact, minor states of hypnosis happen quite often without theatrics. It may happen when your mind wanders, whenever you may just get lost in your thoughts. It can happen several times a day, depending on where you are, who you are, what your mind is like.

Like other things we've studied, hypnosis can direct focus to block out distractions, which is the principle of meditation. And, like meditation, it's a conscious state. It's not a sleepwalking state of blank-slate suggestibility. It's a feeling like you've about to fall asleep; awake but relaxed until movement seems unnecessary.

Nobody is beyond hypnotism. Some may be more responsive, some more closed and resistant. If you don't want to be hypnotized, you can't be. The subject plays a part in the process, and it requires an opened heart and an opened mind.

Like intermittent fasting, hypno-fasting can be sustained and done regularly for the rest of your life. You've developed the parallel skills of self-awareness and self-discipline, both of which are excellent for focus. The more you do of both, the better you will get at them, and also at related practices we've reviewed here. Your exercising regiment aught to be enhanced by this discipline which you've learned and developed while fasting. That energy should transfer to the self-awareness which you achieve during meditation and yoga. All things work together and work off of each other.

Hypnosis cannot eradicate the hunger which a fast brings, that comes and goes. But it can help you accept it and not fight it. It can help you embrace your hunger as a part of life and growth.

Hypnosis Apps

We'll go through some hypno-fasting courses, and you'll put this fascinating concept to the test. But first, we'll do a quick survey of the latest revolution in hypnosis, the hypnosis app.

This shouldn't come as a surprise. They have apps for all kinds of things. We've already taken a look at apps for yoga and for exercise and even for fasting. And apps are a great way to partake in this practice without disrupting anybody.

Hypnobox is among the best self-hypnosis apps. It aims to achieve a deep state of relaxation, which leads to being more open to suggestion. The app can be customized to use a female or male or voice, sessions can be tailored and background music can be imported.

Relax and Sleep Well Hypnosis focuses on relaxation and offers sessions on anxiety, stress, mindfulness, and self-esteem.

Harmony Hypnosis Meditation offers mantras, music, visual images, and sound effects.

Perhaps the best app for losing weight is Lose Weight Hypnosis app. Audio sessions uses suggestions which influence behavior and mindset. The app is good for weight loss and relaxation.

Digipill is popular for relieving stress. It's a well-known health and fitness app too, using psychoacoustics and *neurolinguistic programming.* Psychoacoustics employs sound to induce psychological response. It's a method of neurolinguistic programming, postulating a connection between sensory experiences, emotions, and behaviors. The app offers programs for stress relief, weight loss, motivation, and smoking cessation.

Anxiety Free's app relieves anxiety through self-hypnosis and guides users through activities to relieve stress. One study indicates that self-hypnosis can be effective for ongoing and situational anxiety, which occurs from a specific event in the past, present or even the future.

You may be experienced in at a few practices we present in this book. Or not. You may want to read through the programs first. You may record them into a voice recorder app. Reading the material will help it to sink.

Hypnosis and Women

Studies of more than 5,600 people found that roughly 30% of men who'd been hypnotized had stopped smoking, compared to only 23% of women. This suggests that women might not be as susceptible to hypnotism as once thought (women are generally associated to being more suggestible). Scientists at the Ohio State University engaged in the study attributed the result to a female susceptibility to smoking rather than having anything to do with hypnotism.

Another study assessed the connection between age and hypnotic suggestibility. A total of 2,660 undergraduates took the Harvard Group Scale of Hypnotic Susceptibility, Form A (HGSHS:A) over seven years. It found that hypnotic suggestibility decreased from the age of 17 to about 40, and increased thereafter. Compared to males, female participants scored higher on HGSHS:A.

CHAPTER TWENTY: Hypnosis Programs

Here are six one-hour hypnosis programs, one for the things which plague women most while dieting, fasting, and aging.

The programs are designed to be spoken. Using the same devices you used before, pre-recordings or a partner, there are things to keep in mind.

Read slowly, mindful and deliberate. The words have meaning, the sounds have meaning. Let the words linger, with mindfulness of their rhythm and their importance.

Create a soothing tone. Speak in a low tone, soft, not shrill or sharp. Imbue the reading with the supportive and nurturing spirit of these sessions. Whether you are prerecording the scripts or not, you may want to include background music, of a soothing nature. Sound effects might be good too, including rain, wind, singing birds, a babbling brook, whatever feels appropriate. These programs are designed to help you. Shouldn't you have a say in the way they sound? It could make a huge difference in how they affect you. A voice recorder app may not give you much flexibility, but you can always read the script into a laptop with Garage Band or other recording program and add downloaded music and sound effects that you like. Record and add your own music if you like.

We do suggest you not skip ahead. Like everything else this book, these are sequenced to build one upon the other.

Fasting

Find a comfortable position, sitting with your back straight or laying down. You are comfortable, breathing regularly, slowly. You feel relaxed, at peace. You're in a safe place where nobody means you any harm, nobody needs you for anything which might be distracting. This is your time, a time for yourself. You've no other needs, no other desires. You are at peace and ready for a journey of discovery, into the depths of your own body and your own mind.

You can feel your own breath, filling your lungs, chest expanding, before feeling it ease out again. Breathe again, slowly, feel the breath become a part of you, inside you, before letting it go again to return to the world around you. It was a part of you briefly, giving you the very stuff of life. What did it take with it back into the world? It left you stronger, more at peace. It made you more a part of the outside world; uniting inside and outside, two worlds becoming one.

Now listen to the sound of my voice. You are open now, as you've never felt before. Your heart is open and at peace, your mind is at home and at rest. Air is inside you, all around you. You are open to the images I will suggest to you, your imagination ready to carry your soul self out of where it sits, out from the back of your skull, and into your body as you've never gone before.

I'm going to count from five down to one. As I do, your body will become heavier, your whole self sinking into a relaxed state, almost ready to fall asleep yet remaining conscious. Hear my voice as I count. Five … four … your eyes close, your ears hear only my voice. Three … two … your arms and legs are heavy, at ease, comfortable. Your breath is even, you're completely at ease. And … one.

Take a moment to relax. I'm going to be silent for a moment to let you take a moment to enjoy the feeling which is overtaking your body now. There will be nothing but stillness and quiet, perfect peace around you, inside you. Remain quiet, remain calm, and wait for my voice to return.

Your body is calm, but you feel now that there is a disturbance. You have been fasting, and I know that it has been challenging. It's unusual, sometimes uncomfortable. You feel pangs of pain and also of doubt, wondering if you are strong enough. You may feel that you cannot do it on your own.

But you do not have to go it alone, because you are not alone.

You're concerned about the strength of your own mind, wondering if you can maintain the discipline needed to go on fasting. But your mind will be your strength, your mind will be your ally, the part of you that can do what beguiles and confuses you. But there will be no more confusion, you will have total certainty about your powers, about the powers of your mind, the powers of your body.

You are fasting, and that can cause pangs of hunger. You feel your body adjusting to the changes. They're good changes, and your body knows that as well as your mind. The pangs of hunger are your body's doubt, just as your doubts are the pangs of your mind's hunger. Both work together toward the whole self, the soul self. But to do that, you must let your mind self rule and control your body self.

Your mind is strong, and it can control your body. You can feel your body, now relaxed and heavy, in a near-slumber. But your mind is something you are only now beginning to feel. You can sense it, the collection of your every thought and memory, the cradle of every inspiration. Not the brain nor the body, but the mind. It is the most powerful part of your whole self, your soul self, and now you must set it free so that it can do what it has to do to make the body whole, to make your self whole.

Find your mind, there in the back of the brain. Can you feel it? It's like a glowing spot, an orb without mass, just a bright light. Feel its warmth, feel the brightness of its shine, it's power. It is the best of what you are, the most of what you can do.

Now let your mind move, just a bit at first. Push it forward from the back, then to each side. Feel its mobility, feel your power to move it, to manipulate it. Your mind must have control over your body, your body wants that and so does your mind. But you must have control over your mind, it wants that and so do you.

Now you can feel that power, now you can sense your own strength and see even more clearly the course of action you must take, you know what you can do.

Let your mind move then, move from the brain and deliberately, mindfully into the body. Feel it shifting from the brain and let it slip into the spine, the throat. Feel it, like a glowing, pulsing sphere, displacing nothing and gently warming everything as it descends into the ribs. Feel it shed light on the heart, that knowing glow of the mind, calming its beat, slow and even. Feel your soul go lower, past your lungs as they slowly draw the air in, hold it, let it out. They're strong, getting stronger with every breath. Your whole body is getting stronger. Feel the cells in your skin, crackling with new life as old materials are drawn away and new cells rise up, strong and youthful. Feel your blood running smoothly through your veins, carrying nutrients and oxygen to every part of your body, every cell.

Feel how glad your body is to receive your mind, feel the closer connection of your mind and your heart. They have never been as close as they are now, but you can bring them together like this just by the sheer power of your greater self. Feel how welcome your mind is in your body, how comfortable your mind is. With this new movement of your mind, your brain gives up all doubts. You have taken control and doubt is the first to be riven away. There can be no more question. Your body knows it, it knows the power you command, and it is relieved that your mind has come to its rescue.

Let your soul sink deeper now, slowly, sinking down to where your stomach strains. Your body is just getting used to the change. It's grateful that you are putting it to the test, stressing it the way you are. It knows that these are the signs of positive change. But the pains are its doubts and it needs to learn from your good example. Your stomach is calling out for the solace that only your mind can bring.

In time, things will be easier for the effort. Food will be more easily and more thoroughly digested. Your body will be happier, and it knows that. Wrap your soul around your stomach to soothe it, to fill it. Let your very human mind fill your stomach. Feel it growling, first filling the bottom of your stomach, as if you've just has a satisfying snack. The pangs feel like they're receding, satisfaction runs warm in your tissues. Imagine having had a piece of mango or orange, the vitamins rushing through your blood.

Be calm and quiet for a moment. I am going to be silent and let you focus on your mind as it fills and warms your belly. Your mind is the most powerful part of your whole self, and it can well satisfy your stomach, and it will be easier than eating, easier than drinking, just as easy as taking that steady breath, in and out. It is instinctive, perfectly natural, you simply have to learn to trust those instincts; to trust in their power to guide your mind and for your mind to guide your instincts.

All things work together; the systems of the body, the parts of the whole self, the soul self. And now they all work together toward one area, where your mind is centered. Your belly feels empty, even though it is not. It feels anxious even though it should feel calm. It needs to be reminded of its place, its purpose. It needs the mind to reassure it, to support it, to fill it.

The level of mind fullness rises in your stomach as your mind gets bigger, inflating in your stomach. Little by little, feel your mind filling your stomach. Feel it pushing away the hunger, satisfying your body the way hypnosis satisfies your mind. Little by little, your stomach's pangs of doubt are pushed out as your strong mind grows stronger and bigger.

Feel your mind growing bigger still, pushing away any empty corners until your stomach is totally full. Now you feel as if you have just eaten a tremendous meal, satisfying in every way. You've had sweet and savory, and there's scarcely room for another bite.

You can hardly move for being so full. And there's no need to move. Everything is just as it should be now, your body perfectly comfortable. I'm going to remain quiet for a time now, but I won't be far off. Spend a few quiet moments feeling your body, savor this new feeling of fullness. Hunger is alien to you now, there is only complete and utter satisfaction. Relax and enjoy it, know that you can achieve this, you yourself, now that you know how. You are in complete control, now more than ever before. And that control will always be with you, always there to drive out your pangs of doubt and pain.

Your mind can rise up now, slowly up and out of your belly. You leave it completely satisfied and filled, no more pangs, no more doubts, and no more straining. Your body is at rest, you have no wants and no desires, only to remain so calm and peaceful.

Your mind rises slowly up further, under your lungs and heart, warming them as the keep air moving in and out, regularly, smoothly. Your mind fills your chest, ribs rising and falling as your mind rises into your upper chest and into your neck. Your shoulders are warm with the proximity of your mind as it rises higher. It fills your neck, your throat, before ascending even higher up into the base of your skull. It rises higher, filling your skull and warming your brain.

Your mind is now where it feels most comfortable, close to the brain. But it feels loser now, ready to leave that bony fortress to visit any part of the body. If there is pain, the mind can be brought to that area to deliver whatever remedy is necessary. You will remember it, your mind will remember, and your body will remember, when pain returns anywhere in your body at any time in your life. Your mind is strong, stronger than your body. You decide if there is or is not pain, your mind can decide this. You know now how powerful a tool it is, how much control over your body your mind can have.

But it is not the body which serves the mind, but the mind which serves the body. The mind cares for it with proper diet, with choosing to fast and seeing the fast through. It is the mind which remains in charge, a benevolent ruler of the kingdom which is your body. It can move among the various areas, each like its own miniature fiefdom. Your mind governs them all, with kindness and mercy, the ruling mind-self.

You feel whole, you feel satisfied, wanting for nothing. Everything is well with you, vitality and clarity return to your body and mind. Your arms and legs are heavy, your body ready to fall asleep. But I'm going to ask you to come back now, to full wakefulness. Your arms and legs will no longer be heavy. They will be light and strong and powerful. Your mind will be alert, sharp, and your body will be ready to press onward to the end of your fast; without food, without wanting, without pain.

I'm going to count up to five, and when I do, you will be at complete wakefulness. One … two … three … your eyes are fluttering, refocusing on the room around you. Four … your mind is more alert, your arms and legs feeling light and fluid and comfortable. And … five. You are back now, your mind and your body reunited and closer now than they have ever been before. This makes you more powerful, more ready to face any challenge. Your fast is no longer a challenge. In fact you feel lighter, more flexible, fully satisfied. Instead of breaking your fast as you were tempted to do, you consider extending it. The longer you'll fast, the better you'll feel.

Take some time to rest and reflect. You have become more mindful of your body and more deliberate with your mind. Your body and mind are more closely reunited, but so is your soul self closer to each, creating a holy triumvirate which cannot be assailed. You are the champion of your body, and its servant, and you are now better able to serve than ever, and better able to learn more.

Was this your first such experience? If it was, how did you find it? Were the visions crisp, could you envision what I was suggesting? Could you feel the warmth of your mind illuminate the different parts of your body? Did your stomach respond, do you feel full? If not, perhaps you need to spend longer with your mind in your stomach, or perhaps you should move it slower through the body. Don't be afraid to go back and try it again tomorrow, even before you move on to other sessions. Remember, this is all about you, and you should take things at your own pace.

But whatever you feel, you've got no reason to be anything other than excited. Any progress is good progress, and whatever you felt, that was progress. Even feeling nothing at all leaves you with somewhere to go. You've gotten over your initial doubts, about fasting and about hypnotism. Every journey begins with a single step, and this step could yet prove to be instrumental to your personal development. Take it, and all the steps which follow, knowing they will forever bring you closer to where you want to be.

Weight loss

Make yourself comfortable in one of your favorite spots. Sit or lay down comfortably, though be careful if you're laying down that you do not fall asleep. A comfortable recline would be best if you cannot sit up. Whatever makes you most comfortable and most open and receptive. Once you are relieved, you can begin to truly relax. Know that you are in a place of perfect privacy. You are secure where you are, with nothing to be afraid of or worried about. Your worries are outside this room, no longer part of your mind self. Your body self is comfortable and it awaits the comfort of your mind to better lead it where it needs and wants to be. Because your mind may be dominant over your body, and it should be. But the two work together as everything does, creating perfect synergy. A healthy body makes for a healthy mind as much as the other way around. Both make for a healthy soul.

Listen to the sound of my voice. I'm going to guide you through a session today, and you're going to concentrate on the sound of my voice. Your mind will be open and receptive, your body will be calm and relaxed. You're going to be able to envision the things I suggest, and you will feel and touch and taste the things I describe. It will be as if you're in a different place entirely.

I'm going to count backward from five, and when I'm done, you'll be in a perfect place to begin your journey today. Listen to my voice as I count. Five … your eyes close, your world is a vast darkness, limitless. Four … your arms and legs are heavier, hard to lift. But you have no need to lift them, nothing to lift or reach for and nowhere to walk or run to. You've no needs at all as I count three … two … one.

You're now in a place of perfect relaxation, ready to go where your soul wants to go, where your body wants to be. You've no doubts about how to do this, as you've done it before. You're no stranger to the world of the soul self, the imagined place where your mind creates and your body responds.

Your body is not at peace as it should be, your mind and your body both know it. You've been fasting and dieting, but you still feel weighed down. There are unwanted pounds clinging to the territory which is your body. Your healthy cells and organs what to be rid of it, and you have exercised and fasted and you still have this unwanted, even unhealthy fat.

Your soul self embraces your body and its imperfections, that is true. Your mind self knows that bodily perfection is not your true goal, but something to strive for. Better health is your goal. You love yourself, every part of it.

Think of yourself as the soul queen of the kingdom which is your whole self. You may travel with your mind through the fiefdoms of your body; your stomach, your heart and lungs, any part of the kingdom is accessible to the queen. And the subjects are grateful for their merciful and mindful sovereign.

But you've had to recognize that you are under siege by outsiders who are robbing your kingdom of its worth, its resources, slowly destroying it. And now you are being called to marshal your forces against this enemy.

The enemies are bad fats and bad cholesterol. You've come to know them well, and you know you have the knowledge and the power to vanquish those enemies once and for all and restore peace to your kingdom.

You can feel your healthy cells proliferating through autophagy. You can feel your fat stores beginning to loosen as they are being drained, little by little. You can feel our bile carrying toxins out of the body, proteins burning the fat cells one by one. In the various quadrants of your kingdom, the forces of biological order and wellness driving the enemy back.

You can already feel the victory that awaits you. You can sense the systems of your body finally working together in a coordinated way, deliberate and mindful as you have instructed it to be. Your previous efforts are slowly coming to fruition. You cannot see the with the eyes of your head, but the eyes of your mind can envision those battles raging, the enemy being driven off of your body, cells being captured and deconstructed and carried away, never to be seen again.

But the war is ongoing, and you have given orders and fortified your troops. You know it will be a long fight, but one that you will win. Good change is gradual, and a certain victory is earned before it is won. You've given your body the tools it needs to succeed, and your continued efforts will be required. But you're not troubled. You lead your forces with courage and conviction, convinced that you will ultimately prevail. But like all good leaders, you know you must rely upon your troops, your battles, giving you the war at long last.

But it won't be immediate, it can't be. You're committed to leading these battles as long as you must, confident in your own leadership and in the power of your biological armies. You've reset them for battle against this enemy, armed them with the best nutrients and supplements, fortified them with exercise and yoga and even meditation.

And for now you seek solace and peace above the mayhem of the battles going on throughout your biological kingdom. You need to rise above your kingdom, elevate yourself above the fray and find true peace.

Picture yourself climbing into a hot air balloon, lined with sandbags around the rim of the basket. The silk balloon is brightly colored, strips of red, blue, yellow, purple, white. The basket is sturdy, a bright flame shooting up from the engine into the balloon. You drop one sand bag and the balloon starts to rise. Look out over the terrain that is your body. Mountains of muscle rise, rivers of blood flowing evenly in your veins, pockets of fat encroaching on the paradise of your kingdom.

The balloon rises slowly, a blue sky stretching out above. The worries of the world, the strain of combat for control of your kingdom, sink away beneath you. Thinks seek calmer as you rise. You release another sandbag and the balloon rises just a bit higher. You look around at the blue sky above and around, clouds getting closer as birds fly past. Feel the breeze blowing a bit harder, feel the warmth of the sun.

Look down at your own body beneath you, laying naked. Skin is thick with fat in some parts, the molecular battles no longer visible. All seems calm, at peace and at rest. The balloon floats easier, moving you a bit faster as you ascend. Breathe in and take a big, deep breath of that crisp, fresh air.

The sun is warm on your face, welcoming, as the balloon rises. There is nothing to fear, no forces working against you. Gravity and atmospheric pressure play their parts together to hold everything in place, just as everything else in your world now works together in perfect harmony, a natural cycle which propels you higher than you'd ever imagined you could go.

You release another sandbag and the balloon goes even higher. You look down and your body is small beneath you, hovering in the vacuous blue like the Earth itself. Your body is the Earth, your balloon is the mind as it lets go of its doubts and worries, as it literally rises above its conflicts and challenges.

Below, the molecular battles go on, though they are far from your concern. Your perspective is enlightened and lifted. You can see the wholeness of your body, the gradual change that is happening over time. Around you, the clear blue sky of possibility stretches out, the balloon of your mind rising higher as you let go of another sandbag.

You sail upward toward the sun, your body even smaller beneath you. But you realize as you drop another sandbag that the balloon is your body, and what you've left behind was your previous vision of your body. You were seeing it as you always had. But now you see things differently. Now you can see that your body can be whatever you envision it to be in the world of the mind, of the whole self. All are just parts of the soul, the place you now traverse. The sun shines above, warming and nurturing. Nothing remains below but the tops of clouds and the backs of birds as they fly past, singing.

You drop another sandbag, knowing that the sandbags are the pound of extra weight. As you discard them, your body flies higher. It's lighter than air, able to ride the currents free of any encumbrance. And it's just as easy as unhooking the bags and letting them fall away. Release the weights, cast aside that which is not needed. Feel how light your body feels now, how it sails upward and away from all the conflicts and stresses that were weighing it down. Your body has never felt so free, your mind has never felt so free, and you gently spiral upward toward that bright, beautiful sun. It is the father of all life on Earth, nourishing and warming, giving sight and strength. The earth evolves around the Sun just as the body evolves around the mind. Your body balloon is drawn to the sun mind for another reunion. All things are part of your soul self in this place, and all things are coming to a perfect union.

You are warmer as you approach the sun above and just to the side. It's light begins to blot out the blue, the glare of its yellow shine filling your eyes, surrounding the balloon.

Finally, you are reunited in meeting of body and mind, the sun surrounding the balloon on every side. The balloon and the sun become one, the body and mind conjoined. The light becomes so bright that it blots out everything around you until there nothing around you. The balloon is gone now, your mind self floating effortlessly in the heat and warmth as the essence of life surrounds you. The light is so bright that it becomes darkness again and you are once again floating, body heavy and tired.

You are once more in that place of perfect calm and darkness, your body motionless. You are where you began, knowing that every part of your ascent was simply a passage through your own world, your own self. You stepped out of and returned to your own body, seeing it for what it truly is, not just for what it seems. It is your transport through life, your mind can control its shape and size and motion. Your whole self depends on both working together.

You know now that you will prevail, that you can always rise above and jettison that which your body and your mind do not need. You can vanquish any foe and reign over a peaceful and happy kingdom.

For now, all is well. The battles will go on, but you know now that you needn't let them dominate your attention. You have loyal servants fighting the battle by your command, freeing you to find the spiritual wholeness you seek. You won't be able to wait until you've lost every extra pound. You must unite your future, lean self with your current, heavier self. Only then can one truly become the other. And you've learned how to make your body whatever you want it to be; a battlefield, a bright balloon, a clear sky, or a bright sun.

You are in your body once more, safe in a room of your own selection. There is no harm or judgment where you are, no doubts or concerns. All is well, and time will tell. Good change is gradual.

Take a moment to relax. You won't hear my voice, but you won't be alone and you won't be afraid. I will soon guide you back to the world of the physical self, the room you started in, the life you lead. The realm of the soul self will always be there, waiting for your return. In a way, you're not truly leaving it, because it is you and you are it. You are all things in that world.

It's all about you.

You feel heavy, tired, but as you listen to the sound of my voice, you will return to full wakefulness and complete alertness. You will feel relaxed and contented, you will feel comfortable in your own body, knowing that beneath the surface good things are happening and progress is being made, even if you can't see it.

One … two … your arms and legs are a bit lighter now, your heart and lungs regular and strong. Three … your eyes are fluttering, eyes refocusing on the light. Two … one … now you are aware of where you are, and you feel refreshed and capable and in full and complete control of your body, your mind, your life, your whole self.

Take a moment to relax and reflect. How did it feel to be embroiled in the stress of constant battle? Did it seem like the life you've led for so long? How did it feel to know your body is fighting for your even as you are fighting for your body? How did it feel to rise above, to see your body from a different perspective, as a different thing, as all things? Your body became the Earth, the balloon, the sun, both your point of origin and your destination. It relies upon you as you rely upon it. Perhaps you know now that your body is constantly at war on your behalf, protecting you. You are the champion of your body, but your body is also your kingdom with its own army of protectors. Enable them, feed them properly, instruct them on what to do and they will be fighting your battles on a small scale until the war itself is finally won.

You've become even closer to your own body and mind, all things working in even greater conjunction. You are even more comfortable traveling into the realm of the soul self. You know your place at the source of power. You have a new appreciation for what your body does all day and all night, and how big a part you must play in its victory. You must decide to cut loose the extra weight and fly high, but this is a journey that will only bring you back to your true self, your best self, your soul self.

Now you're better prepared to move forward and use these techniques again to advance your progress toward your best life, the one you envisioned in your meditation. You can get there, but you'll have to know what you can do and what you have to allow to happen. You'll know what to get rid of and what to hold dear, as these are the keys to a longer, happier, healthier life.

Self-image

You're in a calm place. There are no distractions around you, nothing to divert your attention from the sound of my voice. You are comfortable, resting on a recline or sitting with your back straight. Your blood is circulating freely, you're muscles aren't constricted, your breathing is deep and easy. Breathe in and out now, holding it in for just a moment or two. Feel the air in your lungs, feel the nutrients flowing in your blood, feel your cells reproducing, healthy and happy.

You're preparing for another experience in the realm of the soul self, the world which you inhabit, which inhabits you. My voice will guide you, and you will be open and receptive to the things I am saying. Your body will be relaxed, your mind will be sharp and your visions will be clear. Your senses will be heightened, your understanding made deeper.

For now, listen to the sound of my voice as you close your eyes and relax your body with another deep breath. I am going to count downward from five, and when I am done, you will be in a place of total and complete relaxation.

Five … four … your world is dark, calm, still. You can hear my voice, you can feel your own heartbeat. Three … two … your arms and legs are heavy, your whole body feeling as if you ae ready to fall asleep. And … one. You are now in a state of perfect calm, body heavy, eyes closed and too heavy to open. You're in that place between sleep and wakefulness, when your mind is especially clear and strong, your body especially docile and compliant. You are now perfectly suited to go to that place of your self soul, to transcend the body with the mind.

You feel good, safe, at peace. Your worries and stresses are behind you, in another place now. Feel the space all around you, the tiny atmospheric particles which surround you, too small to feel. But you can feel them, because everything here is a part of you, you are a part of everything. Feel the billions of tiny molecules touching your skin, your face, the spaces between your fingers, as if you were underwater and you could not see it and could still breathe freely. Take a deep breath and feel those countless molecules flow through your nostrils and into your lungs, filling them before you release and exhale. You realize there are molecules everywhere, filling every seemingly empty space.

And so it is with your body, every part of it dense with tissue and activity. Blood flows, cells break down and reproduce. Fasting has reset your body, and a better diet has nourished it properly. Exercise and yoga have made your body stronger, supplements have helped control your hormones.

All is well in your biological kingdom, and you are the reigning monarch, the queen of all you survey. But heavy is the head which wears the crown, and you know this too well. You are not a happy monarch. You have been wrestling with the way the world sees you and your kingdom. You look at yourself and seem to see something quite different than what others see. You see a different you, an uglier you. You see only your faults, a shambling echo of what you might have been.

You see parts of the whole to be exaggerated, one part too big for the others, until it is not a person you're seeing at all, but a collection of disfigured parts to comprise one monstrous whole.

But you are not a monster to be shackled in the queen's dungeon. In this place, you are the queen. You are the ruler over all you survey. You are the champion here, and nothing is beyond your power to rule with confidence and mercy.

Imagine your doubts and insecurities as angry peasants, in distemper and seething with righteous fury. They know this creature well, for it is their own creation. It is the result of years of isolation which these parts of your psyche has had to endure. But you needn't harbor these insecurities, these rebels to your lightened spirit and enlightened mind. But they are strong in number, and their throngs collect outside the castle walls.

They have been hunting the wretch across the countryside for years, ever since that twisted image became too great for your insecurities to manage. It has run rampant over you're the terrain of your mind self for years, disrupting the peace in your kingdom.

But this beastly apparition, created by your insecurities and now hounded by them, is their greatest enemy. This is what riles them to rebellion. It is their cause to destroy that which they have created.

Indeed, the queen knows this wretch, and for years you have let it prowl the shadows of your kingdom. It has compromised your reign for years, and now is the day that you will rise up and put an end to the disruptions in your kingdom, to end this ongoing battle between body and mind. The two must be at peace for the whole self to prosper, but this wretched visage represents the very chasm between the two. It is the way the mind perceives the body. But you now have greater powers of the mind, and you are ready to use them to bring peace back to your soul self.

Imagine yourself in your chamber. You glance a mirror and see the queen that you are, beautiful and confident, radiant of strength and confidence. You are lovelier than you realize, lovelier than you've ever been before.

The rowdy throngs are collected below, torches and pitchforks rising with their shouted cries. "Death to the wretch! Give the beast up to us, Your Majesty!" You are in the calm of your bedroom, a canopy over the bed, silk sheets and other finery. But you stand and walk out to a grand balcony, the breeze in your face. But all is not well, the streets are filled with angry peasants, clamoring against you. "Give us the wretch, Majesty, that we may kill it and be rid of it once and for all."

They shout, the fools. There is no peace in their souls. There is no happiness for them. They are insecurities, fears, doubts. The thing they see does not exist, the thing they hate is themselves and they are too blind to see it. They cannot see what is there, and see only what is not there.

They clamor below, but you are calm. You are the sovereign of this place, and nothing is beyond the scope of your control. You could wash them from the streets with a sudden flood were you only to imagine it. But you know they would return, forever chasing their embattled ghost. You know that you cannot deny insecurities, they will only thrive in isolation. Only reason, only the power of the mind, can settle their rebellion and open their eyes to the light that inside you and all around you.

You raise your hand and the countless throngs of rebels goes quiet. Their mumbling and murmuring come to an end, all eyes looking up in silent expectation.

"You've come for the wretch, all that is ugly in our kingdom." The cheer, raising their pitchforks and torches. With your words, they quiet again. "But don't you see that it will only return? You cannot destroy that which does not exist." Silent confusion surrounds them. But you are no longer confused, nor beguiled by the wretch. You know these insecurities all too well.

"As long as you are here, the wretch will always be here. For it is not the ugliness of the kingdom, you are!" The crowd screams and shouts, but you are not intimidated. You know these insecurities cannot truly hurt you so long as you take command of them and maintain calm and reasonable rule. For insecurities are unreasonable, they cannot sustain plain and simple truth. But they will always try to find a way around it.

"Give up the wretch," one rebellious peasant shouts, the others cheering.

You call down, "You shout, you fools. There is no peace in your souls! There is no happiness for you. You are insecurities, fears, doubts. The thing you see does not exist, the thing you hate is you yourselves and you are too blind to see it. You cannot see what is there, and see only what is not there!"

They stare up at you, their strength already beginning to ebb as your dominance rises. "You are the blind leading the blind, and you shall all fall into the pit! You think yourselves grand? You, insecurities, you are the lowest of the low. You defile the streets of this place, you corrupt my happy kingdom. You rebel against truth, against beauty. You do not seek to rid out the ugliness, you need it to survive. You need to remain what you are. You will seek it out so that you may continue to thrive."

They know you are right, and you know they do because they are a part of you. Like all things in the realm of the soul self, you are in control of every facet, every turn. And insecurities are the hardest things in the realm of the soul self to control, to contain. But you have the power, you know the truth, and only truth can defeat insecurity. The beast they pursue is illusion, delusion, and they need it to survive.

"You seek the wretch," you proclaim from your place of power, elevated above your insecurities. "Here is your wretch, your very queen! Am I not the same creature, one and the same? All things which are here are me, within me. This wretch exists only in your minds, but it is I you see when you envision this ugly creature. Look again! Do you see ugliness or beauty? Do you see a creature cowering in the shadows, or one who stands before you, proud in the bright sun of her own reign? Do you find me grotesque, monstrous? Tell it to me plainly."

You know they cannot. You know you are their queen, and that your beauty radiates through that place. It is a place where they are not welcome, a place they do not want to be. Your light shines out, from your face and body, your castle a fond of bright light. There is no ugliness in our castle, only strong walls and colorful banners. But insecurities cannot abide the light, they need the shadow to survive.

They turn to shuffle away, retreating their assault.

But you know they will only return if you allow them to survive. For the good of the kingdom, these insecurities must be wiped out forever. For it is they who created the wretch which haunts the kingdom, they themselves are that wretch. The kingdom rumbles, but you stand calmly at the balcony.

The rebels cry and break to run, but torrents of floodwater pour in from every angle, driving them into a heaving crowd in front of the castle. They cry out, they beg for mercy. They promise loyalty in favor of mercy. And you are a benevolent ruler, after all.

But insecurities lie, this is their reason for being. They have no true contrition, they only seek to manipulate, to pollute the kingdom. They will always return, stronger than before. The floodwaters rage, waves high as they splash against the little shops and cobblestone streets of your kingdom. They are your cleansing powers, waiting for your command.

You give it; without a word, without a stroke of your hand. But the waters know your will, and they rush in like an avenging army to fill the streets, plowing down the hordes of your insecurities. They scream as the waters flood them, knocking them over and consuming them. Their screams are muffled and silenced until only the sound of the waters remains, splashing and frothing in a cleansing churn of your power.

You stand there, your insecurities helpless before you, obliterated.

Now the waters recede, by your silent command. You stand as the levels lower and the waters pull back further, finally out of sight. The water leaves your streets clean, puddles are languid, water drips somewhere in the background. But there is no sign of even the slightest insecurity, not a single one. The birds sing in the trees, shop doors open for business, and peace returns to your kingdom. The rebellion, the doubt, the insecurities are gone, and with them is the illusionary creature they created. In truth, it only existed because they existed. Without the insecurities, the wretch could not survive. Without their illusion, the insecurities themselves could simply be washed away.

You turn and step back into your bedroom, silk and finery and the light of royal calm all around you. You see yourself in that same mirror, beautiful and regal, strong, untouchable in your place of power. You are the queen of all you survey, and you are well able to protect that place of your soul self against even the most insidious insecurity.

All is well now, and you can move forward knowing the folly of those insecurities, the folly of their illusion. You won't be beguiled again, those insecurities and their imaginary creature will never plague your kingdom again. And if they do, you'll know just how to recognize them and just how to deal with them.

Now, with peace restored, it is time for you to return to the realm of the physical self. As you listen to my voice, you will return to full wakefulness, your mind will be sharp and clear. One … two … your arms and legs aren't so heavy now, your breathing still regular and calm. Three … four … your eyes are opening, adjusting to the light, refocusing on the room around you. And … one.

You are calm, you are safe, you are at peace, all is well. Your body is refreshed, your mind is alert. Breathe deeply and hold it, then exhale. Breathe again, easing your way back into the realm of the physical self.

Now take some time to relax and reflect. Do you feel cleansed, do you feel rid of the insecurities which corrupted your self-image? When you imagine your face, do you see the grotesque, the wretch, disfigured? Or do you see the face you saw in the mirror in your royal bedroom, radiant and beautiful? Did you feel empowered, ridding the realm of your soul self of those dangerous insecurities? Do you think they might come back in some other form? If so, are you confident that you will be able to recognize them and repel them again?

You should be, and if you must face them again, that will only increase your confidence and your power. You brought in the floodwaters like God saving Moses. For in that place you are more than just a queen, you have the powers of a god. And you are learning how to use those powers for good and not ill, to keep the peace in your kingdom and not let your insecurities run wild.

Be confident that you can move forward into an even brighter and better reign, that your soul self is stronger, that your mind and body are once more firmly reunited.

Sleep

You are in a comfortable place, reclining or seated with your back straight. There are no kinks in your muscles, nothing to restrain your relaxation or comfort. You are in a place where you know you are safe, that you are protected and secure. There is only calmness around you, nothing to distract or deter you from another journey into the realm of the soul self, where your mind is in total control and your mind vision is clear and bright.

But first, take a deep breath and hold it, feel it in your lungs before you release it, also slowly. Take in another breath, feel your body absorb nutrients, oxygen, before returning that air into the atmosphere. It is a vital part of life, necessary constantly, yet it is effortless most of the time. But this time, you are mindful and deliberate of your breath, as you are of all things increasingly. You know more, about what you do and what you think and how you feel. You have greater insight, thanks to your meditation and yoga, clearer thinking thanks to better diet, supplements, and the natural process of autophagy. Your mind and body are united, working together toward the whole of your soul self, made manifest in your general health and wellbeing.

I'm going to guide you through your journey, so listen to the sound of my voice, feel it resonate in your ears, your brain, your heart, your soul. Make them a part of yourself and of your self, your soul self. Make them part of the journey, part of the self.

I want you to relax, take a deep breath, and listen to the sound of my voice. I'm going to count down from five, and when I finish you will feel completely relaxed and at easy, a point of near sleep, barely awake. But your mind will be alert and sharp. Five … close your eyes, blot out any thoughts or worries, they're all behind you now. Four … breathe deeply, in and out. Three … your arms and legs are heavy, laying comfortably where they are, no reason to lift them, nothing to carry and nowhere to go. Two … you're barely awake now, your body completely at rest. But your mind is alert and ready. And … one. You are now in a state of complete comfort and relaxation. You are receptive to the images I will share with you, your senses are alert to smells, tastes, everything I will describe. Your mind is strong in the place of the soul self, and you have the knowledge, experience, and power to rule over everything which occurs here. But this isn't so in the realm of the physical self. There, you have trouble sleeping, falling or staying asleep. The anxieties and stresses, worries either real or imagined, plague you and keep you from getting the sleep you need. These are the worries of the real world, and even sleep offers you no respite.

You know how important sleep is to your whole self, your soul self. Sleep gives the body a chance to practice autophagy, to fast for a time and reset the bodily functions. Sleep gives the brain the chance to do the same. And since the brain is where the mind typically resides, a healthier brain means healthier brain activity, and that means a healthy mind. And since the mind is or should be in control of the body, the mind must be strong and healthy. For this, you know it needs and wants adequate sleep.

Now imagine yourself in your bed, in the realm of the physical self. You're warm and cozy in your bed, pulling the sheets up, your head sinking into the pillow. Feel how comforting it is, how welcoming, a warm embrace. Take a moment to savor that feeling, to recall the sense of security from childhood, knowing everything was being taken care of for you; no real worries, no true concerns.

Now imagine your worries, like flying insects hovering around your head. They buzz up to your ears and eyes, trying to get into your nose and mouth. They sit on your skin, they constantly annoy you. You try to swat them off, but they come right back. They're numerous and tenacious. You swat them away again, but again they return.

Use the power of your mind against them. Because unlike real insects, which seek your blood or tears or something physical, these pests feed off your mind. They are mental pests, after all, not physical. No physical remedy, from alcohol to drugs, will get rid of them.

So imagine a bubble around you, growing from inside and then pushing outward through your skin. Imagine that bubble stretching out around you, pushing the annoying disruptions and distractions further away from you. Imagine them as little black bugs, banging against the bubble from the outside, trying to get in. But the bubble is strong, and the little bugs have no chance of getting in.

Now you can breathe easily and not worry about those invasive little rascals. Now you know you are isolated from them, protected from them. I'm going to be silent for a moment or two now and let you enjoy the feeling of being completely isolated from those outside distractions or concerns. You won't hear my voice, but I will return shortly and we will move onward in our journey into the realm of the soul self. I am back, and you are still in your bubble, surrounding you and your bed, protecting you from all distraction. It's perfectly clear and durable. Nothing can get in to distract or harm you. You are completely protected by the power of the bubble, by the power of your own mind.

Now feel that bubble rising up, lifting out of your bedroom. You pass through to the night around your home. See the stars in the dark-blue sky, a full moon bright and round above you. It is perfectly tranquil, the world and all its distractions sinking away beneath you. Nobody there can reach you. None of your stresses or anxieties are anywhere near you. You have elevated yourself above them, so far above and so strong in your bubble that you are out of their reach.

Around you now, all is dark and calm and relaxed. You're in a bubble floating above the world, drifting easily into space. And you have no fear, no concern. Your bubble can withstand anything. Even without it, you are in control of this realm, all of it serves you to the smallest whim. Anything you can imagine is made real.

Take a deep breath now and relax, stretch out and feel your muscles tighten and then release and you exhale. Look at the stars twinkling around you, the moon getting closer as you ascend even higher. The moon seems to be calling to you, the bubble rising toward it. It is as it should be, the gravitational pull of two bodies toward each other to become one.

The sky is dark and tranquil around you. You lay back in bed, as much a passenger as the captain of that mind vessel as it carries you upward. For all your power and control, you are able to lay back and trust your instincts, trust yourself. For all things here are born of you, of your soul self. You have no insecurities here, you have no anxieties or stresses. This is the place of transformative sleep, of total relaxation. Take a moment to lay back and feel how tranquil it is, how calm. You are near to sleep, almost impossible to stay awake now. But your mind is alert, seeing with clarity the things I'm suggesting, feeling the tiredness and the heaviness and the readiness for sleep.

The bubble ascends toward the moon. Nearer, nearer, the moon is huge above you. The light is bright, all encompassing, digesting the bubble with you inside it until you are consumed by the moon itself. Now the bubble and the moon are one, you are safe at the center.

But your consciousness stretches out, no longer a body on a bed but a spark of light free to move freely and in any direction. It is the light of your soul, your soul self incarnate. You are freed of the distractions and anxieties, you are free of any human encumbrance. You swirl around the inside of the moon, the bubble replaced by the heavy rock of the moon as your soul self flies up through a dark cavern and up through a cave opening in the bottom of a mountain range. You fly over the surface of the moon, free of any weight or burden. Craters and mountains glide by beneath you as you fly freely, surveying the lunar landscape.

Look at how calm the moon is, how still and tranquil the moon is. See how it lacks any of the scuttle and scurry of Earth, no insects to disrupt a night's sleep, no honking horns or air pollution. It is pristine, it is entirely quiet and still. Nothing moves here, nothing lives here.

Nothing lives here. But you are a creature of life; you *are* life. You are a creature of Earth; you *are* Earth. Here you are all things, here all things are you.

As you fly, imagine the vaguely familiar terrain begins to transform beneath you. Imagine the sharp, gray rocks transforming to the lush rain greens and blues of the Amazon rain forest. Imagine the gray crags becoming gorgeous beaches, snow-covered mountain peaks. No longer the moon, you fly over Earth, transformed by the power of your mind. You can fly anywhere, do anything.

Look at the beautiful and fragile Earth beneath you. The lighted cities are clusters of bright color, the stretches of dark are the expansive seas. The minutia of human life is still too far below you to notice. You see only the tranquil and fragile glory of that spinning blue ball held delicately in place by forces even the greatest minds still don't quite understand.

But you understand all in this realm, there is no place for doubt which you cannot reach and cleanse. There is no weakness or vulnerability for you, only limitless power as you'd never have in the realm of the physical self.

You fly over the planet, closer and closer, unphased by worry. You're close and fast, seeing things you've recognized all your life, mountains and buildings and canyons which are fabled in the human experience. You fly over your own country, familiar landmarks rising up. You approach your own neighborhood, slowing down and descending as you approach your own home from the outside. Glide further, closer, sinking in through the roof and ceiling and back into your own bedroom.

See yourself laying in your bed, fast asleep. See the satisfied smile on your face, the sheets pulled up comfortably around you, your body still and your mind at peace. You're dreaming even then of flying over the moon, drifting in your bubble, safe and secure. Sink back into your physical self, your body and mind once again reunited and allied. Your soul self is likewise satisfied, and you are in a state of complete and whole wellness. You are sleeping peacefully, and you will wake up the next morning happy, relaxed, and refreshed.

But for now, you are not asleep. You are still in a state of near wakefulness. And as I count back up from one to five, you are going to return to complete wakefulness. Your mind will be sharp, your body will be strong and vital. One … two … your eyes are fluttering open now, blinking to help refocus. Three … your arms and legs feel a bit lighter now, your breath is regular. Two … your strength is coming back, focus is sharpening. And … one. You are now in a state of complete wakefulness, you are not sleepy. But you know that the next time you have trouble sleeping, you will be able to apply this technique to rise above your stresses and anxieties and find the peace you need, the peace you can always access, to get the sleep your body needs.

Now let's take a minute to relax and reflect.

How easy was it to create the bubble to protect you from the distractions of the realm of the physical world? Did you feel secure in it? Did you enjoy flying over the moon? Did you have trouble imagining the transformation from moonscape to Earth? What was it like seeing your own sleeping physical self? Was it hard to rejoin that self or did you feel locked outside of your own physical body?

If it was, you needn't worry. You are already getting better with your experience. You are familiar with the realm of the soul self now, and you are gaining confidence in your ability to control it, to control yourself. Your whole self is coming together with more power and control than you've ever had before. And you know you'll go on to have more control in the future. The next time you use this technique, which you can use by memory whenever you are struggling to fall asleep, you will do it with greater power and effectuality. Think of this as a practice run, an exercise in finding some calm in your day and a way to strengthen your mind's muscles to rule that realm of the soul self.

Relax with a few deep breaths and prepare to move on with your day. If you are doing this at night and are about to fall asleep, do so with confidence, with relish. Look forward to a restful night's sleep without distraction, without disruption. Go on with your life and your travels, go on in your journey with confidence. You are the center of your own whole person, and you can take command over petty distractions, over nagging insecurities, over anything which challenges your general wellness and overall good health. You are increasingly strong and capable, and your levels of comfort and relaxation are growing as the rest of your health prospers. Every day, in every way, you're getting better and better.

Household & Social Stresses

You are in a comfortable place, free of distraction or worry. Nobody has a need of you now, your time is your own. You don't have to worry about anyone other than yourself. You do so free of worry and fee of guilt. You give all that you have, and now you have to give to yourself.

For now, be mindful and deliberate of your surroundings. Make sure your body is comfortable, either laying down on a recline or sitting comfortably. Your muscles are free of tension or tangles or knots. Your limbs hang easily, without strain or restraint. Whatever your position, your back should be straight and your chest open so that you can breathe openly. You want an opened heart center and an open mind. Both will work together toward the shared goal of your total wellness and good health.

Once you are quiet, breathe in and out a bit, feeling the air come in, stay, then leave. It's a fleeting relationship, yet one which never ends during your lifetime. It's one we rarely think about, one we take for granted. But for now, you are mindful, deliberate of your breathing.

Take a moment to appreciate your body, how it works to turn this simple act into a life-sustaining act. It controls itself, needless of the mind. There is one level where the body is the most powerful engine of the total self, the soul self.

But you are here to let your mind take control, so appreciate the body for what it can do, uniquely, and what it cannot do; what the mind must do for it.

I'm going to count down from five, and when I'm done you're going to be in a deep state of relaxation. You will be nearly asleep, but you will not be asleep. Your mind will be alert, open to my suggestions. Your mind's eye will be able to envision what the eyes of your head cannot see. It will seem real and, in that sense, it will be real. What will be real for your mind will be real for your body, because your body and mind will be as one, perfectly united as they should be.

One … your body turns itself over to your mind self, becoming heavy as your eyes close. Two … three … your limbs are getting heavy, your breath is easy and regular. Two … your world is dark and quiet, a soothing bath for your soul self. And … one.

You are now in a blissful state, not asleep nor completely awake. Your body is relaxed and your mind is alert and ready to take another journey. Let my voice be your guide, trust in my and in our own instincts and experience to help you navigate this place where mind, body, and soul converge.

You are in a place of perfect peace and of your own control, and this is not always the way of the realm of the physical self. There, you are constantly under pressure; to act, to react, to think, to feel; all things at all times. Social demands compete with professional, worlds seem to collide.

The modern woman faces demands on every level at every moment of the day. Family demands can dominate, and professional interests may complicate. Add to the responsibilities of being an equal in the workplace and a leader in the household, women are often required to be living fantasies in the bedroom, socialites with their friends. Women are asked to be all things to all people at all times. These demands are raining, they rob a woman of her clearer view of herself. That may lead to visions of a grotesque self-image, fostering dangerous insecurities.

But you are a woman of power, a benevolent ruler, a traveler in time and space. Daily challenges may overwhelm others, but you have a unity of body and mind and a breadth of knowledge which enable you to go where few can go, and do for yourself what nobody else can do for you.

You have learned to escape the into a good night's rest, and this is now within your power as the ruler of the kingdom which is your soul realm. You are a powerful leader who protects her domain, even as she sleeps.

But these pressures are common to your sleeping hours as they are to those of wakefulness, because of their deliberate and mindful awareness of your wakeful attention. You face daily stresses and demands that seem beyond your scope, reaching for goals and dreaming dreams which seem to be beyond your grasp.

But you will be able to prevail against them in the realm of the physical self once you have contained them in the realm of the soul self. You've have done as much with your insecurities, with our sleeping hours. It will be more of a challenge during the day, when the ongoing demands arise again and again, matters of routine and of sudden urgency. But once you know your mind can control your body, that they are one, you will see that your mind can control your body's circumstance, as they are also one.

Your waking life may take place on land, but it is much like being on an ocean. So imagine yourself once again in your safe place, your bubble rising up from the center of your body, radiating outward until it expands through the skin and encases you, transparent and durable. Imagine the bubble getting bigger around you, expanding to give you plenty of space to breathe and to drift in its center. You are fully supported in the center of that bubble, both the captain and the passenger. You've piloted this bubble before, and you know it is a place of safety, security, your transport to lands unknown.

Now take it across the land, out of your neighborhood and over the city, over the mountains or forests or deserts, whatever surrounds where you live. You're leaving that place, leaving the distractions of your daily world. You're deep in the realm of the soul self now, where your mind is the most powerful tool, in the firm and skilled hand of your soul's free will.

Pass now to a great ocean. See it stretching out before you, all around you. Your bubble glides quickly and easily. You turn to see the land fading fast behind you. No matter. You turn and look forward, where you know you are going; where you know you need to go.

The sun is bright in the sky above, glare bouncing off the bubble wall. You can smell the sea breeze, salty and fresh. You glide out further, until you know you are out in the middle of the ocean. You don't need to look back to know that you're nowhere near land. Everything is tranquil, calm, far from the disruptions and chaos and stress of daily life.

I'm going to be quiet for a moment and let you enjoy your place hovering above the calm ocean. Waves lap, dolphin jump not far off, the sun reflects silver off the chop, seabirds call in the distance.

Now, imagine that the waves are growing choppier beneath your bubble. Crests go higher and crash down harder, white water frothing. The wind blows harder, whistling as it passes over and around your bubble. But you're not fearful, you know you cannot be harmed. Instead, you marvel at the display of nature; in this case human nature. Because this storm is of your own making, a reflection of your waking world, the realm of the physical self.

The waves rise up from the turbulent ocean, splashing up against the bottom of the bubble, water dripping from the clear, plastic sides. The wind howls, pushing the bubble to the side and another great wave rises up and smashes into the bubble. Still, you're not afraid. You marvel at what you're seeing. It is the rise of the storm of your physical life, made manifest by the power of your mind in the realm of the soul self. You can see how these storms arise from the tranquility of life, how frightening and overwhelming they can seem. Looking around to see no land, you know how isolated any person might feel, how lonely all that chaos might make someone feel.

But you don't feel that way. You're calm and you're grateful for a chance to see things as they truly are. Seas will rise, chaos will come. But there is still safety, refuge, and there is always a way to take control of even the most chaotic experience.

The sea rages beneath and around the bubble, one wave so great that it rises up on the side of the bubble. It blocks out the sun as it looms over the bubble. You have no fear as the wave crashes down on your bubble, sending it deep into the water.

You are surrounded by dark green brine, fishes scurrying in the new tumult. The currents are strong and another surge soon sends your bubble bursting up out of the water and through the surface. You hover, but another wave crashes into the bubble from the side, sending the bubble rolling.

But you are not afraid. These waves are a part of this ocean, which is a part of this world. And this world is a part of you. All things work together. Even out to see, this is part of your kingdom, and you reign supreme and all-powerful. Look down at the churning sea beneath you. It seems ominous, dangerous, deadly. But it is only the rising of the waves. It is the same ocean which is often calm and will be calm again. Nothing has changed, and you can sense that. You know that because here, in this realm, you know all. You are all.

You float in the center of your bubble, hovering above the stormy sea which mirror, illustrates the storms in your life on land, in the realm of your physical self. Each can be calm and can be stormy, and each can be calmed again.

You hold your hand out, palm flat to the waves beneath you. You close your eyes and concentrate. Feel the waves in your belly. They're already a part of you, a collision of body and mind. Soothe their collision, suppress their rage and bring inner peace to the storm inside and watch the waves recede. These are not forces working against you from without, they are forces which you can control from within.

Watch the wave calming now, beneath you just as they are within you. All things work together.

The waves are slowed and small now, the wind quieted. The birds are calling in the distance, the sun warmed above you. Your inner calm has effected the outer chaos. And as it is in the realm of the soul self, so can it be in the realm of the physical self. Your bubble begins to bring you back to land, the calm sea stretched out beneath you as shore appears small in the distance.

I will be silent for a time now to let you enjoy the journey back to wakefulness, to the realm of the physical self. Look out over the sea, calm and beautiful. Appreciate your new skills in being able to control such a thing. Be grateful that it is part of your realm, your kingdom. Affirm your commitment to keeping it healthy and vibrant.

Now your bubble passes over the familiar terrain until your arrive back at your country, your city, your house. Your bubble transports you into this room, your body, this time which we are spending together.

I'm going to count from one to five now, and when I'm done, you're going to be back to total wakefulness. Your mind will be sharp, your body will be relaxed, your soul will be refreshed. One … your limbs are lighter now, heart beating steadily. Two … three … your eyes are fluttering open, refocusing now … four … your limbs are ready to move, your heart beating strong and steady. And … five. You are now returned to complete wakefulness and awareness, your body is strong and ready, your mind crisp and powerful.

You are imbued with confidence, with the knowledge that you can calm any storm, within or without. Your inner peace will bring outer peace.

Let's take a moment to pause and reflect. Do you recall the biblical passage of Jesus calming the waters? Do you understand now that we all live on stormy seas, but that faith and inner peace can calm the fear those storms generate? Do you see now that, in the realm of the soul self, you have the powers of even the most revered of saviors? You are, in fact, more than your body's champion, more than queen of your kingdom, but savior of our own kind, the populace of your soul realm.

And you can carry that into the turbulent realm of your physical self. The demands which push against you from every angle can be managed if your mind self can be managed. You know now that the only sense of control over the seemingly uncontrollable is to have self-control. When you can control yourself, nothing else can control you. When you cannot control yourself, everything else can control you.

So be glad for your new sense of control. Be reassured that you are making good progress. Your journeys are reaping great benefits for you, building one upon the other. You are uniting the disparate systems to work toward the shared goal of your idealized self, your best possible life. Rejoice, because even now you are assembling that life block by block, brick by brick. You are forging the road which is taking you were you want to go, wherever that may be.

You're calm and you're grateful for a chance to see things as they truly are. Seas will rise, chaos will come. But there is still safety, refuge, and there is always a way to take control of even the most chaotic experience.

You will take that lesson with you, back into the chaos of the real of the physical self. The demands of family, profession, and social circles will not seem so overwhelming when they come across your calmed state of mind. The force of your will can calm them. When they rise, you can calm them again. The cycles of the seas are to rise and fall, so it is not a crisis, merely the give and take of life. Knowing this, you are better able to endure and reduce any storm which arises in your life.

Menopause Symptoms

You're in a safe, comfortable place. You're in control of your environment, your body, your time. You've set this time aside for yourself, with no guilt for it and not hesitation. Your other chores are done, there is nobody who needs you. There is nobody to distract you, no demands to encroach upon your personal time. All your efforts have led you to where you are now, in your journey and in your life. You have been through your reproductive years, and you are now entering a different phase in your life. But it is still your life, and as such it is up to you to control it.

This is not unfamiliar to you, thanks to your practices and better diet, your greater understanding of your body and your mind and how they work together. You know how to control your soul realm, your mind self in firmly in control. And will have to be for what is next, on your journey and in your life.

You're in a calm place. There are no distractions around you, nothing to divert your attention from the sound of my voice. You are comfortable, resting on a recline or sitting with your back straight. Your blood is circulating freely, you're muscles aren't constricted, your breathing is deep and easy. Breathe in and out now, holding it in for just a moment or two. Feel the air in your lungs, feel the nutrients flowing in your blood, feel your cells reproducing, healthy and happy.

You're preparing for another experience in the realm of the soul self, the world which you inhabit, which inhabits you. My voice will guide you, and you will be open and receptive to the things I am saying. Your body will be relaxed, your mind will be sharp and your visions will be clear. Your senses will be heightened, your understanding made deeper.

For now, listen to the sound of my voice as you close your eyes and relax your body with another deep breath. I am going to count downward from five, and when I am done, you will be in a place of total and complete relaxation.

Five … four … your world is dark, calm, still. You can hear my voice, you can feel your own heartbeat. Three … two … your arms and legs are heavy, your whole body feeling as if you ae ready to fall asleep. And … one. You are now in a state of perfect calm, body heavy, eyes closed and too heavy to open. You're in that place between sleep and wakefulness, when your mind is especially clear and strong, your body especially docile and compliant. You are now perfectly suited to go to that place of your self soul, to transcend the body with the mind.

You feel good, safe, at peace. Your worries and stresses are behind you, in another place now.

But you're here to find the answer to a symptom of your body's midlife change. You are besieged with hot flashes, they're almost insufferable. You are suddenly hot, sweat collecting along the back of your neck, seeming to hover around and inside you like a cloud you can't escape. They seem to come out of nowhere, and at times when you can't simply jump into a cold shower. You know why they happen, and you know what they mean. They're symptoms of a hormonal imbalance due to a change of life. Menopause is a transitional time, and it can be difficult to get through.

You've tried diet and yoga, even meditation. Now you must stand at the helm of your soul realm and fight the battle on a purely and supremely mental level. Draw upon your experience, your confidence. Look back to past successes and to upcoming challenges and know that this is one almost every woman has to face. But this is a challenge you are uniquely prepared to fight and to win. And you will do it with the powers of the mind, which is the greatest weapon of your will.

For this campaign, instead of encircling yourself in a bubble and travelling outward into the inward, you must go straight into the center of your body. But your hormones are generated from all over, and those hot flashes course through your entire body. You cannot disengage your mind to flow to that part of the body to calm and soothe it.

This is like nothing you've faced before. You cannot reason with heat, you cannot flood it away with an inundation of water or of will. It is all around, an invisible enemy which is part of who and what you are. This time it is your hormones which are storming and raving and rebelling, but they are too wild to collect before the castle. Some of these hormones are older than the queen, they were inherited from previous kingdoms and they simply cannot be forced to obey. You have quelled them with the techniques in this book, but you know they are the cause of this unrelenting heat. Still, it surrounds every other force, every other thing in the kingdom, threatening the entire community, feeling like it is going to burn down the entire kingdom.

Despite your better diet, despite your efforts, your hormones are dancing to the tune of change, and that is one tune the queen cannot call. Her own body must dance to it as well, but in this realm, the queen must reign supreme. Her people rely upon it, others in neighboring kingdoms expect it, and the desperation of the situation demands it.

None of the queen's horses and none of the queen's men can fight those waves of hormonal heat which sweep across the land, parching the soil. It makes the people angry, interfering with national relations. Descend into that inner kingdom which is the realm of your soul self. You are the ruler here, your powerful mind the tool you use to govern, your body the width and breadth of your kingdom.

But the heat pours over the land, hot rains and dried seas give the place a parched feel, as if nothing will ever grow here again.

Word has come in; your crops are drying up. Wells are dry, food my run out. The aged in your populace worry for their lives. Children huddle in their mothers' arms. Men cannot work, the entire kingdom seems to be grinding to a halt. This heat threatens the sanctity of your rule.

Imagine that you are in your royal bedroom of your castle. Outside, in your Capital city, there are no rampaging riotous rebels. But the good people are parched, barely alive, the merciless sun beating down on them and on you. Even the queen of this realm is not relieved of this misery. And it pesters, makes the royal robes cling and stick, discomfort with every turn. It makes the queen irritable with others, and that disrupts her royal court. She owes it to them to present a royal presence, but the challenge to remain sunny under such heat is more than even a queen can often manage.

And she above anyone is poised to do something about it.

You are poised to do something about it.

It is not the first challenge the queen must face, and it will not be the last. This is a ruler of legend, her achievements storied among the people of her kingdom. You are ready to conjure another stunning victory for your people.

You look out over the withering town. You look up at the clear sky, white with the sun's glare. But by the sheer power of your imagination, you conjure a bank of clouds drifting in to cast shade over the town and the townspeople alike. The temperature dips a bit, even the mighty sun blocked out, its harmful rays nullified.

The people look up in hope, eyes wide, lips quivering. You stand above them on your balcony, the breeze blowing through your hair as the first flecks of rain fall. They hit your cheeks, so small they can only barely be felt. First a few fall, and then others. The shade becomes darker and the breeze is just a little lighter as your clouds take their position to block the sun. The rainfall starts lightly at first over the townspeople. They look up at the clouds, reaching to touch the raindrops. Their tongues reach out with eager wonder, grateful as the rain falls harder.

You let more rain fall, splashing down to coat the streets to a wet sheen. Little puddles form and children stomp their feet to splash, smiling in their youthful glee. Old folks cling to one another, hugging and crying with relief for the new, refreshing rain.

You lean back with your arms out, the water soaking your royal robe. The breeze cools you, your hair plastered against your face, your back as you stretch your arms out to bid the rain to fall even harder. Raindrops patter against the window panes, the rooftops, underscoring the cheers of the weary townsfolk. They raise a weary cheer of relief, the rain falling harder to save them from the terrible heat.

The wind blows cooler, pushing folds of your wet robe behind you. You stand in the glory of your victory over the sun itself. Here, nothing is beyond your control, not even the sun itself.

Your own body heat cools too, though you show nothing of your discomfort. It was for the commoners to moan and complain and be led by the strength and confidence of their monarch. You have once again risen to the occasion and championed your kingdom, your body.

The rain comes down harder, fresh and cool. The breeze is cooler too, refreshing against your face. The heat is gone and the people rejoice. You yourself feel cooler, more vital, wet with cool rained and chilled by a fall breeze. The heat is gone, the people are contented, the queen is happy again.

You will not hear my voice for a time, but I will still be here, giving you time to savor the coolness of the feeling, the refreshing coolness and dampness, the heat riven away by the shadowy shelter of the clouds. Enjoy the feeling of ultimate power and ultimate refreshment. No need to rush. This is a moment of truth, a moment of victory.

Retire back into your royal bedroom and sit at your dressing table, the mirror in front of you. The rain has washed away your makeup, leaving your naked face; true, natural, your real face. Little by little, the old version of your face is replaced by the new. You have wrinkles you didn't have as a young woman. You've had experiences you could hardly have imagined as a little girl. You've had a life and you still have one. You have experiences waiting for you which require your wisdom, your joy of life. You have good times and new people and wonderful memories ahead. The seasons change, sometimes hot for a time and then cool once more. All things work together, everything in its season.

Every day, in every way, you're getting better and better.

Lay back on the royal bed and take a deep breath, savoring the feeling of being in your body. True, you are older, a bit slower. Things are changing which you can see but which you cannot fail. This is the way of life, nature preparing you for a time of leisure, a time to enjoy all that you have created.

And when you do so, you will do it with relish, with verve. You will be ever mindful and deliberate about every day of your life, through hot or cold. You can always whether the change of seasons. Yours is a kingdom meant to last for many, many seasons. You are a queen for generations.

Long live the queen!

Lean back and enjoy the feeling of being in your body, one you are making better and stronger every day. Along with a sharper mind and a better union between the two, you are well-equipped to lead your kingdom through any change of season, from one into the next.

It is now time for you to return to the realm of the physical self. As you hear my voice, you will return to full wakefulness, your mind will be sharp and clear. One … two … your arms and legs aren't so heavy now, your breathing still regular and calm. Three … four … your eyes are opening, adjusting to the light, refocusing on the room around you. And … one.

You are calm, you are safe, you are at peace, all is well. Your body is refreshed, your mind is alert. Breathe deeply and hold it, then exhale. Breathe again, easing your way back into the realm of the physical self.

Now take some time to relax and reflect. You have mastered the power of the elements, outwitted an invisible enemy and once more restored peace to kingdom of your life. Your reign is once again peaceful and quiet and happy. You know now that not even the most complex hormonal storm can undo you, no weapon forged against you shall prosper. Your people are happy, you are happy and comfortable once more.

How did that rain feel on your face, cooling and soothing? How did the cheers of your townsfolk feel? Was it even more rewarding to refresh them than to refresh yourself? Were you refreshed when they were? They were you, after all, and you they. You were the rain, you were and remain everything which is found in the realm of the self.

Do you look forward to going back? Do you relish the idea of ruling a place of goodness and virtue. That is the place you envision as your best body, your best life. It may not be the place you first though of, but now all things are coming together, one thing fostering another. Your inner vision is clearer, your understanding greater. You know more about your body and your mind than you ever did, and you've only just begun to reign over a new era of calm and peace and tranquility. All will be happy, none will rebel, everything will be right with your world.

And if crises should arise, if waves should rise up around you, if heat should bare down on you, you will be more than ready to handle them, to handle anything which disrupts or distracts you.

Go back to your day now, confident in your royal power, knowing you are well on your way to living your best life, being your best you, achieving all that you want to achieve; knowing and loving all those whom you wish to go on knowing and loving.

Go and lead by example, confident that you can share anything you've learned with anyone who wants to know. Because their happiness is your happiness. All things work together.

Long live the queen!

CONCLUSION

Congratulations! You began this journey with a desire for change and a hunger for the knowledge of how to make that change. We promised if you retained only one significant lesson from the ones we present, it could change your life. Retaining all oof them could be a revolution not only for yourself but for every willing and interested person you know. Which lessons did you learn the most from? Which was more intriguing, that fats can be both good and bad, and that they come from different foods? Did you know how important hormones are to good health and overall wellness? Did you know you could manipulate your hormone level to prevent an hormonal imbalance? If you did, did you know about the hereditary aspects of hormonal function? Or was it the differences between the various kinds of cholesterol? Which type of fasting did you try, if any? If more than one, which worked best? Had you ever heard of autophagy? Have you practiced yoga? Did you do it this time, or just read the book through before applying it? Do you feel excited and ready? What about the exercises and meditations?

Keep asking those questions. This book intended to ignite a curiosity which is meant to take you further on the journey. Whether you use other books from our extensive library or pursue your interests elsewhere, the important thing is that you do pursue it. Keep asking new questions and keep finding new answers, keep putting them into practice. We've tried to be comprehensive, but no single book can give you every bit of information you'll need or want. Keep in in mind that, though these are ancient practices and time-tested truths, new data will come up, new diet fads and new nutritional information to keep you guessing. It will always be best to scrutinize new fad diets. Always come back to the hard data in this book and others and avoid sham practitioners who flog one crazy approach or the other. Use common sense and use what you know about nutrition. If there's something you don't know, find it and learn it and know it, then pass it on.

Because like everything in all our books, this information is meant to be shared. The statistics are that you and many of the people you know and love almost certainly are facing some of the health conditions addressed in this and our other books. You owe it to them to offer them the same information we have offered you. It's for their overall good health and for the greater good.

With hypnosis, the sky is the limit. You've learned to control your body with your mind, and we've offered you insight into different ways to control your mind. You can always look into new ways of thinking and being. And, as we've said, you'll probably want to come back to this book for reference and refreshing. We all need that, and this book and our others are designed to make it both easy and convenient to come back again and again.

But don't let this book be the only one you read. Check out our other books on communications and leadership skills, mental disorders at home and in the workplace, an expanding catalogue of the latest theories, insights, and cutting-edge tech to make yourself a better person and your world a better place. Whole wellness is a journey without an end, and there will always be another avenue to follow. Good, look for them and follow them.

If you read without applying any of the exercises or practices, that's fine. You now have a working understanding of autophagy, nutrition, diet exercise, as well as physical and mental unity. They should all be even easier and more natural knowing what you know. And if you don't remember it all, just go back for quick reference!

Or you might not have waited. If so, take a moment now to reflect on your accomplishment. You've already done things most people never do, tried things most people have never heard of. Keep doing that. Remember that it's about you, not them. Go where you want to go, no matter if they would or wouldn't, can or cannot.

How did the practices and exercises make you feel? Physically and mentally stronger? By how much? Have you lost weight? How much? Savor your accomplishments, reward yourself by achieving even more! Be mindful and deliberate when you do, knowing that you are in control, that you are your body's champion and the author of your own fate.

If you're a woman, did you learn anything new about your body? Were you surprised about the special challenges women face, particularly as they age?

Also remember or caveats: Good change is gradual. Make sure to transition into and out of dietary or exercise applications, big and small. Consult a physician before starting any new dietary or exercise protocol. Keep in touch with your doctor to note changes and be sure no damage is done. Don't overstress your mind or your body. Stress can be good, as it challenges and instigates change. Too much is harmful and can damage bone, muscle, and organ function. You're on a journey, so every seeming destination always leads to something over the horizon, something bigger and better perhaps than you can even imagine.

Every journey is unique to the traveler. Every discovery reveals new challenges, every destination points to another. Along the way, you'll travel with more energy and strength, with more people following. Ultimately, you'll find that idealized self and perfect life you're working for. Once you've achieved that you'll want to move forward, improving things as you do. There's always room for improvement; and we'll be there with you wherever your journey takes you.

Let's keep going!

RESOURCES

https://getkion.com/blogs/all/intermittent-fasting-weight-loss

https://getkion.com/blogs/all/how-to-fast

https://getkion.com/blogs/all/breaking-a-fast-mindfully

https://intermittentdieter.com/best-foods-to-break-a-fast/

https://www.healthline.com/health/autophagy

https://www.medicalnewstoday.com/articles/autophagy#health-effects

https://www.whitneyerd.com/2020/01/the-truth-about-autophagy.html

https://paleoleap.com/long-fasts/

https://www.healthline.com/nutrition/6-ways-to-do-intermittent-fasting

https://www.jagranjosh.com/general-knowledge/list-of-important-hormones-and-their-functions-1516176713-1

https://www.hormone.org/your-health-and-hormones/glands-and-hormones-a-to-z

https://www.healthline.com/health/hormonal-imbalance#hair-loss

https://www.healthline.com/health/hormonal-imbalance#other-complications

https://www.ncbi.nlm.nih.gov/pmc/articles/PMC4445642/

https://www.arbor-health.com/blog/estrogen-dominance

https://www.uclahealth.org/endocrine-center/genetic-syndromes

https://health.clevelandclinic.org/are-you-planning-a-cleanse-or-detox-read-this-first/

https://www.healthline.com/nutrition/how-to-detox-your-body#The-Bottom-Line

https://skinkraft.com/blogs/articles/toxic-chemicals-in-cosmetics

https://thefoxandshe.com/skincare-ingredients-to-avoid/

https://experiencelife.lifetime.life/article/8-hidden-toxins-whats-lurking-in-your-cleaning-products/

https://www.lovense.com/bdsm-blog/enema-solutions

https://draxe.com/health/coffee-enema/

https://www.everydayhealth.com/diet-and-nutrition/diet/detox-cleanses-most-popular-types-what-know/

https://www.byrdie.com/best-juice-cleanses-4800007

https://www.cookinglight.com/eating-smart/clean-eating/3-cleanses-you-should-never-do-and-3-worth-trying

https://www.gaiam.com/blogs/discover/10-ways-to-detoxify-your-body

https://www.healthline.com/health/type-2-diabetes-ketogenic-diet

https://intermittentdieter.com/best-foods-to-break-a-fast/

https://www.mayoclinic.org/healthy-lifestyle/nutrition-and-healthy-eating/in-depth/paleo-diet/art-20111182

https://www.medicalnewstoday.com/articles/324405

https://www.webmd.com/diet/atkins-diet-what-you-can-eat#3

https://www.atkins.com/how-it-works/library/articles/7-day-keto-meal-plan

https://www.mayoclinic.org/diseases-conditions/diabetes/in-depth/diabetes-diet/art-20044295

https://www.marksdailyapple.com/how-to-exercise-while-fasting/

https://www.menshealth.com/fitness/a30300614/intermittent-fasting-working-out/

https://www.webmd.com/diet/a-z/hormone-diet

https://www.eatingwell.com/article/7805452/hormone-balancing-foods-how-diet-can-help/

https://www.health.harvard.edu/staying-healthy/the-truth-about-fats-bad-and-good

https://www.heart.org/en/healthy-living/healthy-eating/eat-smart/fats/dietary-fats

https://health.clevelandclinic.org/where-does-body-fat-go-when-you-lose-weight/

https://www.prevention.com/fitness/g20459708/best-workouts-to-target-belly-fat/

https://www.keckmedicine.org/what-is-the-difference-between-good-and-bad-cholesterol/

https://yogasynergy.com/article-on-fasting-and-yoga-by-john-mcwhorter/
https://dailycup.yoga/2019/11/10/why-you-should-consider-fasting-4-tips-to-prepare-for-your-first-fast/
https://www.chandriniyoga.com/blog/2018/4/29/the-practice-of-yoga-while-fasting
https://www.juruyoga.com/the-practice-of-yoga-while-fasting/
https://www.yogadownload.com/Utilities/ProgramDisplay/tabid/359/prodid/13004#.YH0Alz9lBPY
https://glennfay.medium.com/intermittent-fasting-and-meditation-remedies-for-weight-management-acdbf53ba76c
https://medium.com/the-ascent/meditation-intermittent-fasting-for-the-mind-7ab6a98cdb23
https://ourworldindata.org/obesity#what-are-the-drivers-of-obesity
https://www.ncbi.nlm.nih.gov/pmc/articles/PMC6347410/
https://www.healthline.com/nutrition/top-13-evidence-based-health-benefits-of-coffee#TOC_TITLE_HDR_5
https://courses.lumenlearning.com/introchem/chapter/hydrogenation/
https://booksy.com/blog/us/what-is-holistic-medicine-and-why-should-i-care/
https://www.nhs.uk/live-well/exercise/exercise-health-benefits/
https://www.hypno-fasting.com/faq
https://hypnotc.com/hypnotherapy-fasting-weight-loss/
https://www.verywellmind.com/best-hypnosis-apps-4800547
https://www.hypnotherapy-london.info/the-history-of-hypnosis/
https://www.spaceotechnologies.com/best-intermittent-fasting-apps/
https://www.tomsguide.com/best-picks/best-workout-apps
https://www.verywellfit.com/best-yoga-apps-4176689
https://www.nhs.uk/live-well/exercise/exercise-health-benefits/
https://www.hypnoticworld.com/hypnosis-scripts/
https://www.mayoclinic.org/healthy-lifestyle/nutrition-and-healthy-eating/in-depth/vegetarian-diet/art-20046446
https://www.tasteofhome.com/collection/vegetarian-meal-plan/
https://www.everydayhealth.com/diet-nutrition/ketogenic-diet/comprehensive-ketogenic-diet-food-list-follow/
https://www.tasteofhome.com/collection/7-day-mediterranean-meal-plan/
https://www.healthtoempower.com/the-real-truth-behind-autophagy-inducing-fasts/
https://draxe.com/nutrition/intermittent-fasting-women/
https://www.precisionnutrition.com/intermittent-fasting-women
https://www.msn.com/en-us/lifestyle/rf-buying-guides/best-detox-for-women-reviews
https://www.dishfordiet.com/best-diets-that-work-for-women-after-50/
https://www.healthline.com/nutrition/best-diet-for-women-over-50
https://top5diet.com/top-diet-programs/?msclkid=4c8115f86bfc10f0c7c67574ae59ed96
https://www.mybeautygym.com/22-yoga-benefits-for-women-health/
https://www.youtube.com/watch?v=l0Ebi54JjUA
https://tm-women.org/benefits-mind-healthy-brain/
https://tm-women.org/stress-relief/
https://tm-women.org/spiritual-growth/
https://tm-women.org/relieving-anxiety/
https://tm-women.org/meditating-moms/
https://tm-women.org/reducing-symptoms-of-adhd/
https://www.crunch.com.au/perspire/best-workout-tips-for-female-beginners/
http://www.hypnoforwomen.com/
http://news.bbc.co.uk/2/hi/health/3933279.stm

https://www.researchgate.net/publication/6385117_An_Update_on_Age_Hypnotic_Suggestibility_and_Gender_A_Brief_Report

https://www.hopkinsmedicine.org/health/wellness-and-prevention/why-cholesterol-matters-for-women

https://www.who.int/gho/urban_health/physiological-risk-factors/women_obesity/en/

https://womenshealth.obgyn.msu.edu/blog/global-obesity-rates-higher-women

https://www.mayoclinic.org/diseases-conditions/pcos/symptoms-causes/syc-20353439

https://healthcareers.co/yoga-statistics/

https://www.cdc.gov/arthritis/data_statistics/national-statistics.html

https://www.thegoodbody.com/meditation-statistics/

https://www.alz.org/blog/alz/february_2016/why_does_alzheimer_s_disease_affect_more_women_tha

https://www.mhanational.org/depression-women

https://www.pewresearch.org/fact-tank/2016/03/23/qa-why-are-women-generally-more-religious-than-men/

https://www.cdc.gov/nchs/fastats/womens-health.htm

Intermittent Fasting & Autophagy For Beginners: Detox Your Body, Burn Fat Rapidly, Promote Longevity& Improve Hormonal Health For Men& Women + 5 Extreme Weight Loss Hypnosis

TABLE OF CONTENTS

INTRODUCTION

The World Health Organization estimates that 700 million adults are obese. It's linked to roughly five million deaths around the world yearly, roughly eight percent of global deaths per year. Thirteen percent of adults worldwide are obese and thirty-nine percent are overweight. One in five children and adolescents are overweight all over the world.

Experts estimate that over 34 million people (over ten percent of the population of the United States, have diabetes. Roughly 26.8 million people (also over ten percent of the population) had diagnosed diabetes and over seven million people have the disease but have not been diagnosed.

Hormonal imbalances strike both men and women (women at a whopping 80%).

There's no doubt that our fast-paced, nutrient-deficient world has wrought havoc on our bodies. Pollutants corrupt and weaken our immune systems, our cells cannot engage in the necessary process of autophagy, which recycles usable cellular materials and discards toxins and unusable cellular waste. This affects everything else in the body and in the mind, creating downward spirals which can take your entire future with it, swirling down the drain like a tubful of dirty water.

On the other hand, there are ways to combat and even reverse the corrosive effects of having a toxified body and mind. It's widely known in the medical field that people who engage in regular physical exercise have:

A 30% lower risk of early death

- Roughly 50% lowered risk of type 2 diabetes

- Roughly 35% lowered risk of stroke and coronary disease

- Roughly 50% lowered risk of colon cancer

- Roughly 20% lowered risk of breast cancer

Fasting is also a powerful weapon for weight loss and overall good health. A review study illustrated that people who participated in intermittent fasting cut between four and seven percent from their waist measurements over a period of six months.

So there little doubt that there are a number of natural remedies for these life-threatening conditions. This book is your guide to these and other remedies for these and other conditions! This book will give you the history, the latest information and the results of the most cutting-edge studies and experiments. You'll learn everything you need to know (and you do need to know it) about autophagy, fasting and hormonal imbalances. You'll put into practice the leading methods of weight loss and general good health; cleansing and detox, dieting, exercise, yoga, meditation, and even hypnotism. You will obtain a working knowledge of good health from the molecular level all the way to full-body longevity. You'll learn what to eat and what not to eat, and why! You'll learn how your body works, how your mind works, and how they work together. But you'll do more than learn, you'll *do*, putting these concepts into real action which will change your body, your mind, your entire life.

These exercises come from the leading experts in their field, the programs chosen specifically to address the maladies this book is written to address. So you don't have to sift through information which may be valuable but not precisely relevant. The data comes from the world's most trusted sources (The World Health Organization, for one). This book, like all our books, is held to the highest standard of excellence and integrity, making complex medical information easy to understand and making complex concepts easy to ingest. We've helped countless readers improve their lives, shedding light on everything from true leadership skills to various mental disorders and much, much more. Readers come to us time and again to help them remedy the things which plague their lives, the things which plague so many lives. This book addresses the discrepancy between body and soul, between temporary satisfaction and true happiness.

But the benefits are a lot more specific than that. Sure, we can promise you long-lasting good health and mental stability, but the question of how to achieve them will also be answered. It's not just about what, but how, and this book will walk you, step-by-step, through processes you'll come across. Wellness is the destination at the end of your journey, and we'll take that journey with you and be with you every step of the way.

The statistics prove that these approaches work. Generations of longevity demonstrate the fact. New technology now illuminates what was once misunderstood or even unknown to modern science. But these things have finally caught up with the advancing technologies which create processed foods, electronic light, a barrage of media, Now you'll have a fighting chance against industrial superpowers who make fortunes from shortening the lives of people like you and me.

In fact, there's so much diverse information here, just one lesson well-learned could change your entire life. If you read and understand the chapter on fats and cholesterol alone, you'll have learned the difference between good cholesterol and bad (a difference which even now may be taking you by surprise). That alone could make the difference between your life and your death. Even understanding what autophagy is and how it works is worth the price of entry, as it will change the way you look at your body and your life. It's your body, shouldn't you know how it works? It's your mind, shouldn't you know how to use it? Instinctively, you know these things to be true. It's why you're reading this introduction and deciding whether or not to buy and read this book. But even deeper down, you realize you haven't got a choice. If you're looking for a remedy, that means the problem has been going on for some time now. Even as you read this, your blood may be thickening while your bones become hollow and brittle. You're eating things you want but don't need, and every heartbeat could be your last. You may be living on the precipice of a heart attack or stroke. Or you may simply be looking at the slow decline which will rob you of the idealized life you've worked so hard for. Don't let that dream die, don't let your body die. Your health is in your hands, both figuratively and literally. If you don't do it now, when will you? It's easy to procrastinate, to think nothing will work (we have a book about that too). But it's vital that you take the crucial next step. You've already taken the first step, and that's to seek help. The next step is to accept that help, and the other steps are delineated in this book. Follow them, but don't follow them blindly. As we point out in this book, this is a guide. But you'll still want to follow your doctor's recommendations, do other research. Questions will arise, and no book can anticipate every question you may have. So take the hunger to learn which this book will help you develop and let that carry over to other research, other forms of due diligence. It's your overall wellbeing, and you are responsible for it. But again, you won't have to do it alone. We're here for you as long as you are there for yourself.

And it's not just about you. Because chances are that, even if you are in constant control and perfect health, you know somebody who isn't. The statistics bare this out. So if you're concerned about someone else, the information in this book is even more vital. You may already be convinced that there's a problem. But all too often those who have these problems are in denial. This book is designed to turn them around, to change their outlooks and set them on the journey toward a better and longer and healthier life.

But will they do as they're told? Not likely. You have to lead by example. So consider adopting some of these practices even if your weight and muscular integrity are in fine shape. You can always do better. Stress always comes up in life, and that can cause inflammation and related diseases. Good health is a matter of mindfulness and deliberate action. We can all always be more mindful, more deliberate, and be in even better mental or physical health, no matter where we are on the spectrum of good health. All we need is information, inspiration, and dedication.

So just do it. Don't waste another second. Read this book, do these exercises, engage in these practices, Share it with your friends. They'll all want to know what you're doing once you turn up leaner and happier and healthier, with clear skin and a vibrant glow. They'll beg to know your secrets, and you'll be well-prepared to share them. You're about to lead them down a road to wellness you or they may never have known existed. But now you hold the roadmap. Look down; your feet already taking the first few steps. Now you take the rest; we'll take them together.

Now let's get started!

SECTION 1: AUTOPHAGY AND FASTING

CHAPTER ONE: Autophagy

Autophagy is the human body's method of flushing out damaged cells, so as to regenerate new, healthy cells. It's easier to remember than you may think; *auto* refers to *self*, such as in *automatic*, and *phagy*, meaning *to eat*. Some people even think of autophagy as *self-devouring*, and we'll soon see why that's actually highly beneficial and even essential to good health.

Not only does autophagy remove dysfunctional cells, it can recycle some parts of those cells and use them for cellular cleaning and repair by use of organelles called *autophagosomes*. This process binds unwanted cellular matter with other cellular components called lysosomes. A lysosome releases acidic enzymes which break the material down, allowing some materials to be reused while others are discarded.

Autophagy Genes

The pathway of lysosomal autophagy degradation clearly plays a huge role in organismal, tissue, and cellular homeostasis. It's mediated by certain genes called autophagy-related (ATG) genes. There are definitive etiological links between mutations in the genes which control autophagy and also human disease, particularly cancer, and certain genomic, cardiovascular, neurodegenerative and inflammatory disorders. Autophagy targets dysfunctional organelles, pathogenic proteins, and intracellular microbes. ATG genes have many roles of considerable physiological importance. It also plays vital roles in other membrane trafficking and in signaling critical lysosomal pathways.

There are actually least three distinct types of autophagy, including chaperone-mediated, microautophagy, and macroautophagy. They differ as the mode of delivery of the rejected cargo to the lysosome. Macroautophagy is the primary mechanism which is used by eukaryotic cells in order to maintain nutrient homeostasis and organellar quality control.

Benefits of Autophagy

Autophagy was only discovered as recently as the 1960s, in human liver cells, and has been associated with a variety of other organs and tissues as well.

One of the first and most evident benefits of autophagy manifest in what seem to be anti-aging effects. This is so because autophagy helps replace old cells with new ones, maintaining the body's youthful functioning and appearance.

Autophagy also removes toxic cellular proteins which are associated with Alzheimer's and Parkinson's diseases and other neurodegenerative diseases.

Autophagy also recycles these residual proteins to provide energy and other options for cellular repair, as well as prompting the regeneration of healthy cells.

Autophagy is on the frontline of cancer research and treatment. This only makes perfect sense, as cancer is basically the uncontrolled reproduction of dysfunctional cells, and autophagy is the process of flushing out and recycling damaged cells to prevent their proliferation. Autophagy seems to slow down as we age; likewise, the likelihood of cancer increases as we age. The connection between autophagy and cancer is theoretical at the moment, with little hard evidence to back it up.

In fact, a study in 2019 found that autophagy can stall cancer cell development, it may promote their growth as well. This appears contingent on the stage of the tumor.

A 2020 review article suggests that autophagy may help protect liver cells from alcohol- and drug-induced injury to the liver. It may also prevent or limit the progression of several dangerous liver conditions, such as Wilson's disease, nonalcoholic fatty liver, chronic alcohol abuse-related liver disease.

Autophagy may also play a vital role in the human immune system as it cleans out infectious agents and toxins. It may also control inflammation, which may help manage cells with neurodegenerative or infectious diseases and protect them from incoming microbes.

When cells are stressed, autophagy increases, allowing the body to survive and even to thrive. Starvation is just one of these stresses, and it apparently encourages autophagy, according to experts. And this only makes sense; when the body has nothing else to eat, it eats itself. This is how stores of body fat are burned for useful energy. Cells are recycled and reused when necessary, and in basically the same way. It's not a sustainable survival method, but it can be life-saving in times of crisis.

Diet and Autophagy

Autophagy is unquestionably related to diet. And it's not just about what you eat and when, but if you eat at all.

And better diet and weight control are more necessary now than ever. Obesity affected 13% of adults globally in 2016.

Obesity is often the catalyst of metabolic syndrome which is a cluster of metabolic abnormalities. These include high blood pressure, type 2 diabetes, high blood pressure, and low HDL (good) cholesterol. We've already seen the terrifying statistics on global obesity.

So weight management and loss are important to good health, and autophagy is crucial to weight management and loss. That brings us to the dietary specifics of autophagy.

The first dietary change associated with autophagy is intermittent fasting. Having nothing else to eat, the body will recycle stored fats, proteins, and cellular nutrients. Again, this isn't a sustainable way of survival, but it does kickstart the process of autophagy. We'll take a closer look at fasting in a moment.

Ketosis, or the keto diet, is a diet often associated with autophagy. Because it restricts caloric intake of carbohydrates, it stimulates the body's use of reserves to burn energy. In the keto diet, roughly 75% of the body's calories come from fat and only five to ten percent from carbohydrates. This shift causes the body to change certain metabolic pathways. The body then begins to use fat for fuel rather than the glucose which is derived from carbohydrates. This shift in metabolism is what is known as ketosis.

Given the limitation of carbs, the body produces ketone bodies which provide a variety of benefits, such as breaking up fats.

The keto diet and intermittent fasting are both associated with low glucose levels, low insulin levels, and high glucagon levels. It's the glucagon level which is of interest here, as this initiates autophagy. Low sugar levels cause the kind of positive stress which triggers autophagy.

Exercise also plays a key role in triggering autophagy. And this only makes good sense. Exercise burns calories and causes the body to devour its resources, especially given a restriction of new carbohydrates. Autography from physical exercise is prevalent in organs which play a part in the metabolic processes, such as the pancreas, liver, muscles, and adipose tissue (body fat).

Curcumin, found in the turmeric root, is a popular spice in foods around the world and is often found in East Indian foods. Curcumin is associated with good health and long life.

A study using animals found a link between autophagy with a heavy reliance on curcumin may prevent diabetic cardiomyopathy, which is a heart muscle disorder affecting sufferers of diabetes. A different study using mice suggests that curcumin was useful in helping fight the cognitive impairment resultant from chemotherapy. It does this by inducing autophagy in specific brain regions.

But scientists stop short of asserting that increasing one's curcumin intake has a direct connection to inducing autophagy in the human body.

Studies have also shown that insulin, unsurprisingly, prevents autophagy. Insulin is released in response to food intake, and since fasting induces autophagy, eating and insulin release would be expected to hinder it. IGF-1 (or insulin-like growth factor) which increases with overall protein intake, also seems to inhibit autophagy.

A moderate amount of coffee is associated with the reduced risk of several diseases and chronic conditions. It may help prevent type 2 diabetes, protect against dementia. It carries essential nutrients like:

- Pantothenic acid (vitamin B5), providing 6% reference daily intake (RDI)

- Riboflavin (vitamin B2), providing 11% RDI

- Magnesium and niacin (vitamin B3), providing 2% RDI

- Manganese and potassium, providing 3% RDI

Coffee has an unusual effect on autophagy. In a study done on mice, coffee increased restorative activity during fasting. On the one hand, fasting invokes repair and rest. But coffee activates the liver. Many experts agree that coffee should not be ingested during a water fast.

It's important to note here that any major change in diet should be preceded by a consultation with a physician. Pregnancy, heart conditions, diabetes, or hereditary traits should all be taken in to consideration before any significant change in a diet or exercise regiment.

Side Effects and Risks of Autophagy

We've taken a look at the benefits of autophagy. But even that has brushed us up against some of the unknown qualities and quantities of the process, including the promotion of cancerous tumor cells. So let's take a closer look at the other risks and possible side effects of autophagy.

The first thing it's important to note is the difference between the risks associated with the actual process of autophagy on one hand, and the risks involved with an individual's efforts to induce the process of autophagy.

First, the risks of autophagy itself are considerable. Studies have shown that autophagy in excess may damage heart cells. Links have been established between various heart problems and excessive autophagy. As we looked at briefly, autophagy and cancer are closely associated. And while there may be anti-cancer benefits to limited autophagy, studies using mice showed that inhibiting autophagy limited tumor growth. This suggests that autophagy may contribute to tumor growth.

Fasting and Autophagy

How long should a person fast to achieve the so-called *autophagic flux*, the shift occurring in autophagy? Experts suggest between three and five days but not longer.

Studies done on mice show that fasting can result in autophagy in various organs, including the heart, the liver, and the brain. Mice who fasted for 24 hours showed neuronal autophagy, and it only increased after a total of 48 hours. Another study with mice showed that 18 of fasting resulted in autophagic structures in liver cells.

One human study demonstrated a 30% increase in LC3-II, an autophagic marker, after 72 hours of fasting. It also increased p62, another autophagy marker of autophagy, p62. A different study demonstrated that human volunteers who fasted for four days had increases in autophagic activity the most abundant human white blood cells, called *neutrophils*. But other types of white blood cells did not show similarly increased activity.

That's a good rundown of autophagy. It's important to know because it's at the heart of everything we're going to look at from this point forward. It is at the very center of what we're doing it, how we're doing it, and why. It's the body's natural mechanism of renewal. It's the cornerstone of what we're building, a tower of good mental and physical health. But for now, let's take an even closer look at fasting, long-term and short-term, the benefits and the drawbacks.

CHAPTER TWO: Fasting

Fasting is an ancient practice of self-denial. It's often spiritual and sometimes political, but for our purposes it's mostly dietary. That doesn't mean the psychological aspect isn't important, in fact its crucial. Fasting is where body and mind will meet, as we'll see soon enough. But for now lets look at the particular parts and then pull back to see how they all work together. First up was autophagy. We now know how important it is to good health. Fasting is one of the very best ways of instigating autophagy, which puts it next on our list.

Some of the benefits of fasting include:

- Gut health

- Heart health

- Brain health

- Body composition

- Energy levels

- Immune system health

- Appetite regulation

- Anti-aging and longevity

- Willpower, self-control, and relationship with food

There are different types of fasts for different results, and these depend largely on the maladies a person might be suffering, from obesity to toxicity. Different fasts can have different results.

If your goal is general digestive health: caloric liquid fasting (CLF) is best. This intermediate-level practice requires the faster to consume low-calorie liquids only (bone broth, low-sugar juices, water, unsweetened coffee and tea). These fasts may last been one and five days and may have potent effects on the strength of digestion and flora in the gut.

If you're fasting for longevity, a non-caloric liquid fast is an advanced fast which allows only non-caloric beverages (unsweetened coffee, tea, and water). One can go on with a fast like this for between one and seven days, but no more. The cellular cleanse of this approach is ideal for autophagy. We'll talk more about these in a moment.

For body composition, intermittent fasting is probably best. Which we'll now discuss in far greater detail. We basically break up fasting into two cycles; intermittent or short-term fasting, and long-term fasting, and there are a few variations on both of those. Our focus in this book is intermittent fasting, so we'll take a look at that first.

Note: Whatever fast you choose, precede a fast with a period of light eating. Let the transition period be half of the anticipated fasting period. If you're planning a one-day fast, eat light the half-day before. Preceded a week-long fast with three-and-a-half days of light eating. The body will be prepared for the drop-off, which will not seem as steep and hard to manage.

Intermittent Fasting

We've already seen some of the benefits of autophagy, and they're closely related to the same benefits of intermittent fasting. They include weight loss (belly fat), improved organ health, muscle strength, improved metabolism, and overall longevity.

A 2014 review study showed that intermittent fasting may generate three to eight percent weight loss over three to 24 weeks. Similar studies show the same thing, but to lesser degrees. Intermittent fasting is known to boost norepinephrine, which elevates the metabolic rate, from roughly four percent to roughly 14%.

Intermittent fasting is also known to increase Human Growth Hormone (HGH). This hormone (and we'll take a closer look at them later) helps prevent muscle loss which happens during weight loss. It also boosts insulin levels, increasing availability of body fat as fuel. This is key to ketosis, the center of the ketogenic diet, which we'll also look at in greater detail. It's one of the premiere diets for before and after fasts and cleansing.

Intermittent Fasting and Weight Loss

Intermittent fasting has a demonstrable effect on weight loss, as we've seen. And while intermittent fasting has many other benefits to the human body, weight loss is certainly one of them.

Before we go much further, it's important to note that fasting of any sort is not recommended for women who are pregnant, anyone under the age of 18, sufferers of diabetes or low blood pressure, or who may have an eating disorder or a history of the same.

Losing weight is basically about burning more calories than you consume. To do this, one generally changes their diet to reduce caloric intake while changing their exercise regiment to burn more calories. There's no particular mystery to that.

But the body isn't that simple, as we've seen with just a cursory look at autophagy, and as we'll see in much greater detail later in this book. For now, let's agree that there's a bit more to losing weight than caloric balance. There's also more to intermittent fasting than just losing weight. We've already taken a brief look at how intermittent fasting triggers autophagy, keeping organs healthy and encouraging longevity.

But there is still the matter of weight loss and intermittent fasting.

First of all, it's important to understand what factors may affect weight loss. They include:

- Sleep

- Age

- Gender

- Stress

- Genetics

- Medication

- Hormones

- Microbiome

- Metabolic rate

- Health status

- Food quality

These things affect satiety, appetite, and energy levels, which determine calorie intake and processing.

Intermittent fasting (sometimes called time-restricted feeding), is more an eating schedule than a classic diet. It's less about *what* you eat, but *when* you eat … and when you *don't.*

As an example, the 16/8 intermittent fast requires 16 hours of fasting followed by an eight-hour eating window. period during which you consume all of your daily calories. Other popular variations include 13/11, 18/16, and 20/4. We'll take a closer look at these and other shortly.

It's important to note that, while intermittent fasting is a powerful weight-loss tool, there are no studies which show that it is more effective than other weight-loss regiments. We'll take a look at other potent and popular diet regiments later in this book.

For now, let's keep our focus on intermittent fasting and its effects on weight loss. Some of the benefits of intermittent fasting for weight loss include:

- Easy: As you'll see, it's easier to follow than counting calories

- Flexible: Different methods of intermittent fasting (IF) can be made to fit any lifestyle

- Self-awareness: Learning the difference between physiological and psychological hunger

- Self-control: Limiting eating windows requires and encourages discipline

What about the drawbacks of intermittent fasting? Not everybody loses weight with intermittent fasting. Why is that?

Premenopausal women may or may not lose weight with intermittent fasting, and it can even be detrimental to some. It's for this reason we don't recommend it for premenopausal women. We have another book like this one, focusing on fasting for women, and it has more in-depth information.

Overeating during the eating windows is another reason some people fail to lose weight. It's important not to eat too much, and to eat food which is as healthy as possible. Limiting alcohol intake is also crucial to weight loss with intermittent fasting and is recommended for organ health.

Insufficient exercise may limit weight loss during an intermittent fast. While we'll explain later how vigorous exercise can be detrimental to the body during fasts. But some exercise (walking, for example) can be beneficial and will prevent muscle atrophy.

Different Methods of Intermittent Fasting

There are several popular ways of short-term fasting. One popular way to do is known as *the 16/8 method.* Also known as *the Leangains protocol,* this method is simple to follow: Daily fasting for between 14 and 16 hours with an 8- to 10-hour eating window. The eating window may allow for two or more meals of healthy foods low in carbohydrates.

It may sound like a lot of math (or maths, if you like) but it's really not far from the average dietary cycle. For example, if your eating window opens at 8 am, it closes at 6 pm. That's really just a matter of eating an early dinner and cutting out the midnight snacks. For some reason, women seem to do better with a shorter fasting block and longer eating window, of between 14 and 15 hours.

Water, coffee, and drinks with zero-calories can be consumed during the fasting blocks.

Variations on this approach include 13/11 (13 hours fasting with an 11-hour eating window), 18/16 (18 hours fasting with a 16-hour eating window) and 20/4 (20 hours fasting with a four-hour eating window). These seem increasingly complex, and they can be harder to follow that the first approach. In point of fact, they're really not. Look at them this way: The 13-hour fasting approach may begin at noon and end at one in the morning. That offers an 11-hour eating window which lasts until noon the next day. It's basically a breakfast-and-early-lunch cycle, that's not so hard to follow. The 20/4 approach give the faster a regular eating window for whatever their preferred meal; a long breakfast, lunch, or dinner period. Work schedules may make the dinner hours the best for the 20/4 approach. The 18/16 approach is tricker because it's not a straight 24-hour cycle. This approach staggers the schedule, so you're basically having breakfast one day, lunch the next day, dinner the next day. Once the faster falls into that regular schedule, it's still easier to remember than more complex diet plans, which we'll look at later in this book.

Another method of short-term fasting is *the 5/2 diet*. This method divides the week into two blocks of five days and two days. Dieters eat they normally would, but then severely restrict their caloric intake for the other two days.

Keep in mind that the two days do not have to be sequential, though they may be. A dieter may choose to separate them, often on Mondays and Thursdays, for example. Many dieters appreciate the weekends as times to celebrate and eat normally and find weekdays better days to sacrifice comfort foods. Those two days might include two small meals of 250-300 calories each (men are recommended to intake just a bit more calories than women).

There is also the *Eat Stop Eat* method. This is basically the habit of fasting for 24 hours on a periodic basis. Dieters may eat at 6 pm on one day, then fast until dinner the next night. It's little more than skipping breakfast and lunch for one day, maybe once or twice week. If a dieter prefers breakfast, they can eat a big breakfast and then fast until the next morning and eat a reasonable breakfast along with other meals latter that day. Water and coffee and zero-calorie beverages are allowed during fasting times, but naturally no solid food.

Eating regularly during non-fasting days is important. Don't double-up on regular days to make up for fasting. The whole idea is to limit caloric intake and encourage the body to draw on its resources, not add to the stored energy.

Note that 24 hours can be a long time for a lot of novice dieters. Newbies might try a 16-hour fast at first and then expand that block as they become more comfortable.

Alternate-day fasting is just what it sounds; one day of regular eating followed by one day of fasting (or very limited intake, 500-600 calories max). As a lot of people prefer a week-long cycle, a lot of alternate-day fasters both start and end the week on regular eating days, comprising a total of four regular days and three fasting days in the week, with Sunday and Monday being two regular eating days in a row.

This can be a punishing regiment for beginners and is recommended for advanced dieters.

The Warrior Diet made popular by fitness guru Ori Hofmekler, finds the dieter eating small portions of raw vegetables and fruits throughout the day and then one big meal at night. This allows for a four-hour eating window at the end of the day, preferably not too late. This is one of the most popular types of intermittent fasting.

Spontaneous meal-skipping is one of the most forgiving types of intermittent fasting. It involves the dieter occasionally skipping meals. It's a myth that the human being needs to eat every couple of hours. So the dieter skips a meal irregularly. Let your daily schedule dictate what to skip. Interruptions and crises will arise, so take care of them and let that midday meal slide past. It won't kill you … in fact, it just might save your life.

The health risks and drawbacks to short-term fasting seem limited, temporary, and manageable. They may include dizziness or lightheadedness, distractedness, inability to concentrate, and nausea.

Long-term Fasting

While short-term fasting often includes a full day without eating (but not without drinking some beverages), long-term fasting may go on for two days or more.

A *dry fast* is the most extreme type of long-term fasting, wherein the dieter consumes no food or beverage of any kind, including water. We don't recommend this, as it can have terrible effects on the body, including liver and kidney damage, skin damage, tooth loss, and heart problems. Twenty-four hours is as long as anyone should go without drinking something.

Water fasting is like dry fasting but with water. No calories are ingested in this type of long-term fasting. Water fasting means drinking only water, but consuming no calories during the fast.

A comparable technique is juice fasting wherein only fruit or vegetable juices are consumed. A variation on this technique is the broth fast, which provides liquid and minimal caloric intake. But neither juice fasting nor broth fasting are true fasting. Keep in mind that intermittent fasting isn't strictly fasting either if you're drinking coffee during your fasting periods.

But protein has to be accompanied by some fat to help break it down for our human digestive systems. Native Americans used to cook and eat rabbits whole, eating the eyes, the brains, any source of fat the animal could offer.

Let's turn our attention to water fasting, which is common and effective in a lot of ways.

Weight loss is among the most prominent effects of water fasting. One day of fasting uses the liver's storage of glycogen, and the body turns to reserves after that; either fat or protein.

Fasters may lose one to two pounds per day of water weight. Proteins are used by the body first, but this can mean a breakdown in muscles before the fat reserved is tapped. Fat is the preferred fuel for this reason.

Once the excess proteins are used, the body draws on fat reserves and converts that to energy. Fat is more energy-dense than protein, so weight loss slows as the fat is being burned off, at a rate of roughly one pound every two days.

While long-term fasting is a powerful tool for weight loss, it's important to note that the weight often returns after the fast. This happens because the dieter often returns to bad eating habits, too many carbs and sugars to create glutenous fat. So once the body is in a state of ketosis, looking to fat as a fuel, it's important to keep it up and not revert to old ways of eating.

A study of obese patients who reported weight loss during two weeks' fasting found that half of the patients either failed to return a follow-up call, indicating that they'd put the weight back on, or that they'd put the weight back on within two years.

Long-term fasts have other benefits too. Like intermittent fasting, long-term fasting promotes autophagy, which we already know has multiple health benefits.

One study found benefits to sufferers of hypertension of extended fasts (an average of ten days) and of cancer patients undergoing chemotherapy (an average of five days).

Long-term fasting may also allow a dieter to reset their relationship with their favorite foods. Once physically away from the comforting crutches of sugar snacks and massive meals, the dieter my find that they find solace in other, healthier ways.

The dangers and risks of long-term fasting are more drastic than those related to short-term fasting. One of the most considerable risks of long-term fasting, it should surprise nobody, is starving to death. It's unusual unless deliberate, as in a hunger strike, which can last between 46 and 73 days.

Short of that, there still serious risks. Fasting stresses the heart by cannibalizing cardiac muscles for fuel. Muscle is the first sacrifice of fasting until the body shifts to ketosis. Heart failure may occur in extreme cases, and long-term damage to the heart muscles becomes increasingly likely as long-term fasting continues.

But long-term fasting and heart damage has a second, and dangerous aspect. The body uses its store of potassium and magnesium. When combined with muscular compromise, these mineral deficiencies can be fatal.

Infectious diseases can also be a threat to long-term fasters, as they lack the nutrition for a strong immune system.

Less dangerous risks include low energy, mood swings, irritability, and an increase in cortisol and norepinephrine, stress hormones. This can cause a fasting high, encouraging more (and more dangerous) fasting.

Another drawback to long-term fasting is the rate the body detoxifies. Fat stores toxins, and fasting releases these toxins into the blood, causing nausea and sickness. The more rapid the detox, the more dangerous it can be.

One study followed a monk's 40-day fast, consuming roughly 60 calories per day from communion. After 36 days, the man had lost just short of 40 pounds, developed hypotension (low blood pressure). He had no significant changes in serum magnesium, potassium, phosphorous, or calcium, but did show a slight bump in serum zinc and uric acid, which stabilized in the third week and then normalized.

Intermittent fasting as certain advantages, including practicality, sociability, personal comfort. It forgoes the drawbacks of muscle loss, malnutrition, infectious diseases, and heart failure.

The long-term fast can have radical effects on the faster's perspective about food, ending lifelong cycles of malnutrition and bad diet, eating disorders, and food-related conditions like obesity and type-2 diabetes. It also leads the faster to confront the emotional causes of eating disorders.

Still-growing children should not fast; they need constant nutrition to healthy development. The elderly should also not fast, as they're likely to have inadequate stores of energy or may have advanced heart conditions which would put them at risk of heart failure. Sufferers of chronic problems with the heart or kidneys should not fast, nor should pregnant women or women trying to get pregnant.

If you're going to engage in a long-term fast, here are some tips:

- Talk to your doctor first about your goals and timeline.

- Explain to your friends and family to help socialize you so you don't have to be isolated.

- Get a fasting counselor or coach, or look into fasting groups.

- Integrate yoga and meditation.

- Integrate supplements of potassium, sodium, phosphate, calcium, and magnesium.

- Forgo vigorous exercise during fasting periods.

Fasting Apps

There are lots of fasting apps, and we don't have the time to run through them all. We're setting some which are designed specifically for women for our book on fasting for women, but there are plenty which are good for both men and women, and each has its benefits. All are free to download for Windows or IOs.

Zero is a popular app with a variety of valuable benefits:

- Easy customization of your fast

- Easy tracking of fasting progress and goals

- Easy journal entry for the completion of fasts

- Easy integrate with smart devices and wearables such as Apple Watch to monitor heart rate, weight, resting, and sleep

Fasting Tracker also has a number of handy benefits, including:

- Easy adjustment of fasting duration

- Easy logging of waist size, weight, ketones and glucose

- All access to in-app community for support

- Articles and videos

BodyFast offers some unique features, including:

- Fasting timer

- Fasting coach

- Weight tracker

- Statistics

- No advertisements

- Notification alerts

- Sharing progress

- Staying accountable to friends on various popular social platforms

Vora offers:
- Daily fast tracking

- Diet plan

- Tracking others' progress for inspiration

- Export data to CVS

  Fastient offers:
- Ways to visualize fasting progress

- Ways to journal about your fasting progress and experience

- Ways to check fasting history

- Ways to import previous fasts from comparable apps

- Emojis

- Quick-tag

- Progress pictures

- Dark mode

FastHabit allows the users to:
- Stop, restart, or even to adjust fast

- Visualize progress in percentages

- Keep records of weight log

- Set fasting reminders and then get notified

Well, that was quite a bit of information, wasn't it? We've learned about autophagy, and the various ways of fasting in order to instigate and maintain it. You should have a greater working understanding of fasting than you had before, more than others around you have. Now you must start putting it to use. You may already have decided what kind of fasting is best for you, or you may not have made up your mind. Either way, that's great! Knowing what you want and need will help you to set the goal and achieve it. If you're not sure yet, it means you're on the journey to discovery. This book will give you all the information you need to make the right choice at the right time. And, as you'll see, it's a choice you can always adjust at any time, and go on adjusting as your understanding and as your needs change.

But whatever type of fasting you choose, you'll have to break that fast sometime, and that brings us to our next chapter; breaking a fast.

CHAPTER THREE: Breaking a Fast

When you're ready to break your fast, you have to be careful. Too much food too soon can lead to refeeding syndrome. If your body undertakes the shift from ketosis to carbohydrate-based foods cause the body to release insulin for digestion, a process that requires phosphate, magnesium, calcium, potassium, and a variety of essential vitamins, particularly B1. Severe deficiencies can lead to heart failure and hypotension, sometimes leading to sudden death.

When refeeding, your body stimulates stem cell regeneration, as well as boosting hormones, immune system cells, and metabolic activity.

Here are some verified guidelines on avoiding refeeding syndrome when breaking a fast:

Start off by eating no more than ten calories per kilogram (daily) of body weight or less for breaking longer fasts.

Supplement with vitamins and minerals as described and take them a half-hour before breaking your fast.

Eat bone broth or pure fruit juice to break the fast. Follow up with pureed soups, avocados, well-cooked vegetables. Avoid fruits, as the fructose could be punishing on an empty stomach.

Eat smaller portions but more often, and eat slowly.

Those are the simplest guidelines. But fasting and then breaking that fast is about more than eating or not eating. It's about resetting your body, even on a molecular level. But it's also about resetting your relationship with food. As we've touched on (and will again), there is psychological eating and there is physiological eating, and the differences are plain.

Physiological eating is:

- Necessary

- Healthy

- Deliberate

- Motivated by physical need for food

While psychological eating is:

- Unnecessary

- Unhealthy

- Habitual

- Motivated by psychological need for comfort or distraction

So when breaking a fast, keep in mind that your relationship with food should fundamentally change from a psychological relationship to a physiological relationship.

In order to gain and secure over your eating habits and redefine your relationship with food, consider asking yourself these four questions:

His method involves asking yourself the following four questions:

1. Why? Why are you eating? If you're at the end of a feeding window and think of packing in a few extra mouthfuls simply because it's allowed, you may be eating for the wrong reason. Holidays, celebrations, and vacations are classic excuses to overeat, but that rarely makes any of those occasions more enjoyable and it certainly doesn't do anything to maintain proper bodily metabolism or healthy autophagy.

Other bad reasons for eating include boredom, sadness, tiredness, and even thirst (often mistaken for hunger).

Consider alternatives to eating in these instances, including taking a walk or spending time with friends and family. Call them on the phone, there's an old-fashioned thought.

2. What? What are you eating? Because of the new stem cells being created after a fast, it's important to break a fast with the right foods. Some prefer organic foods, some may adhere to a food regiment like the ketogenic diet. But don't break your fast with junk food, no matter how much you think you may deserve it. In fact, you deserve better. Garbage in, garbage out; that's more important after a fast or cleanse than at any other time.

Remember your goals and let what you eat support those goals. If your goal was ketosis, don't load up on carbs. If weight loss is your goal, don't load up on fats unless you're on the ketogenic diet. Be mindful and deliberate of what you eat, don't just fall into old habits.

3. How? How are you eating? As we pointed out briefly before, eating slowly is important. It gives your body to digest at its own pace and not be overwhelmed. Also, eating slowly is likely to create the feeling of being full without eating as great a quantity of food. This is more difficult and more important than ever in our fast-paced world of drive-thru convenience that delivers the most unhealthy foods right into our hands with limited time to consume them. The whole idea of a drive-thru is to eat on-the-go, but this is not how your body usually feeds and digests. The human body prefers a parasympathetic state. It would rather rest and digest in body and mind.

So be mindful of, well, your state of mind when you're eating, and the state of your body too. You might think of restricting your eating windows to the healthiest times, limiting late-night snacking. Eating in the morning, midday, or early evening is best. And when you are eating, try not to do other things. Avoid watching TV or working at a computer. These distractions interrupt mindful eating, and that's what this is all about. Know what you're eating, why, when, and (as we'll soon see) how. These distractions will not help you reestablish a new relationship with food, it will only confirm the old relationship (as chances are this is an old habit). You want to be deliberate, not habitual; mindful, not mindless.

4. How? How are you engaging with your food and to the experience of eating? It's not such a silly question. Some people eat to become full or satisfied. But some savor the pleasures of eating, the intermingling of flavors, textures and colors. One may think it's a cultural thing (the French and the Italians in particular are known for the culinary pride), this isn't true. Every culture has important ties to their food. Any American may have the same savory appreciation for a good hamburger that any Frenchman does for a plate of escargot. Food is as central to various Asian cultures as to various Latin cultures, where the creation of the food is as central to family unity as the eating of the meal itself.

And for a lot of cultures, food is part of the celebration of life.

Is food a celebration, something to be savored in your life, or is it simply a matter of utility?

These two questions address your physical and emotional relationship with your food. Getting in touch with how your food makes you feel can help you tailor your diet to help you optimize your fasts, and thrive in this life.

And whatever you're eating, ask yourself what physiological relationship you have to the food. What reaction does it inspire? A rush of satisfaction and pleasure? Does the food energize, does it leave a bloated or lethargic feeling afterward? What emotional feelings do you have after eating? Satisfaction or guilt? Those are things to keep in mind when understanding and recalibrating your relationship with food.

Mindful Eating Exercises

Here are some exercises to help you recalibrate and reset your relationship with food. These exercises will increase your mindfulness about food and about yourself.

1. The *raisin meditation* is generally done using a raisin, though it can be done with any type of food. You'll soon see why a raisin will work better than, say, a bowl of oatmeal or a plate of spaghetti and meat sauce. This practice seeks to bring complete sensory consciousness of what you're eating. This consciousness extends from the first touch to the aftermath of the last swallow. Though not classically a

kind of meditation, it does use the pillars of meditation, which are to focus on one particular thing and blot out thought and feelings about anything else.

This practice is especially potent if you do it while first breaking your fast. Your senses will be at a peak, and you'll be particularly appreciative of what you're focusing on.

First, use your senses to understand the food (here's were a raisin beats spaghetti). Touch the raisin, hold it, pick it up and consider its weight, color, texture. Think about the process it underwent to go from grape to raisin. Think about the crevices in its raisin form, and imagine the smoothness of its grape form. Smell it and consider the smell, it's likely very mild but still familiar, probably from childhood. Note how the smell affects your other senses; does it make you salivate in anticipation? Touch the raisin, consider its density and firmness.

Slowly put the raisin in your mouth. Feel it on your tongue. Test it between your teeth. Bite into it slowly and note the release of flavors, the change in texture. Chew it slowly, concentrate on the rise and fall of the flavor, the deterioration of the grape between your teeth, how little pressure is required.

Swallow with intention and focus, feel the contractions in your throat as the swallowing reflex begins. Follow the raison as it slides down your throat. Feel the rush of chemicals as your body reacts to the new input. It will be subtle, but it will be there. Look for it, note the sensations.

2. When eating, rest your fork between bites. This is a mindfulness exercise which allows you to focus on the food in your mouth instead of the food on your plate. You can focus on the mouthful you're chewing instead of the next one you're about to chew. This encourages the kind of culinary meditation we just looked at, a chance to feel the food in your mouth, note the sensory reactions and the chemical reactions with each bite. Take a moment to note how the flavors are intermingling.

This will also help you to eat slower, which encourages more thorough digestion and continued good health.

This process does make a meal a bit longer in duration, and it may not be practical in social situations. Or it may. If you eat smaller portions (and we all should be) then eating them slower won't leave you lagging behind others with bigger portions and faster eating habits.

You can, however, cultivate generally slower eating habits that force you to pay more attention to your eating patterns.

Best Foods for Breaking a Fast

We've already seen that it's important to eat the right foods, and how to safely break a fast. Now let's look at which healthy foods are best for breaking a fast … and why. Remember that you're resetting your system, and your new cells will be informed by the newest fuels, or the last things you put into your system. That's why it's important to break your fast with the right foods.

Keep in mind that this is all the more important when breaking long-term fasts. When intermittent fasting, it's less crucial. Though it's still important eat right during intermittent fasting.

Here's a reliable recipe for breaking a fast. Start with a glass of apple cider vinegar and water, and have it before you eat. This stimulates the digestive process. Then have bowl of bone broth, two hard-boiled eggs, iron-rich greens like kale or spinach Try to keep the meal under 500 calories.

But that's a pretty limited choice, and in fact there are a variety of good foods to eat when breaking a fast. I'm not suggesting you feast on a combination of all of them, of course. Use common sense and moderation when breaking your fast.

1. Apple cider vinegar (ACV) is new to the selfcare scene, though it's a remedy which dates back to ancient cultures. ACV's benefits include:

- Levels alkaline PH levels: Though ACV is acidic, it becomes alkaline when consumed

- Kills bad gut bacteria gut: Still, ACV is helpful to good bacteria in the gut

- Stabilizes blood sugar: ACV lowers insulin levels too, and creates a feeling of fullness

- Stimulates digestion
- Improves first-meal digestion

Here's a popular recipe for an ACV drink to enjoy while fasting (not for breaking a fast).

- 10 to 12oz of water
- 2 tablespoons of ACV
- 1/2 teaspoon of Pink Himalayan Salt
- 1/2 teaspoon of cream of tartar
- 2 tablespoons of bottled lime juice or the juice of 1 whole lime
- Stevia to taste

ACV capsules are also available.

2. Bone broth is popular for its hearty flavor, but that's just the beginning of its benefits, including being:

- Rich in electrolytes (minerals which are dissolved in bodily fluids, creating electrically-charged ions.
- Rich in essential minerals (potassium, magnesium, sodium, and calcium)
- Rich in collagen for healthy bones, nails, and teeth
- Rich in glycine for better sleep, especially during fasting
- Rich in many anti-inflammatory amino acids
- Low in carbohydrates

Bone broth comes as a liquid or powder, both are mixed with a water base.

3. Kale and spinach have come up before, and for good reason. They're rich in essential vitamins and nutrients which are often depleted during fasting, including:

- Vitamin B2, B6
- Vitamin C
- Vitamin A
- Vitamin E
- Vitamin K
- Folate
- Manganese
- Magnesium
- Copper
- Iron
- Potassium
- Calcium

Kale and spinach are good raw, cooked, or whipped in a fruit or veggie smoothie. Either way, the benefits of either one include:

- Helping digestion

- Preventing constipation

- Maintaining blood sugar

4. Eggs are a terrific delivery system for a lot of protein with comparatively little food mass. That protein prevents muscle loss, making it a good way to break a fast. They're also rich in leucine, an amino acid closely related to muscle development. Eggs are also easily digested and rich in protein and can curb the appetite (particularly when hard-boiled).

5. Nuts, chia seeds and others, like flax and helm seeds, pecan and almond. Nuts are popular these days for their potent delivery of essential fats, proteins, nutrients, minerals, and fibers. Chia seeds alone are rich in:

- Phosphorus

- Manganese

- Calcium

- Copper

- Selenium

- Iron

6. Fish and fish broth are great for breaking a fast (the broth especially). But even fish meat will be a forgiving first meal, and will be a terrific source of unsaturated fat (the healthy kind) with omega 3, vitamin D, and various proteins.

7. Broccoli, cauliflower, and brussels sprouts are cruciferous vegetables, which are rich in nutrients, fiber, and vitamins. Broccoli is the most digestible of these cruciferous vegetables, which are also filled with:

- Vitamin A

- Vitamin C

- Vitamin K

- Vitamin B2

- Vitamin B5

- Vitamin B6

- Vitamin B9

- Iron

- Manganese

- Magnesium

8. Watermelon is rich in fiber, and only a semi-solid food (91% water), both of which make it very easy to digest and which recommend it for breaking a fast.

9. Bananas are filled with healthy carbs (good if you're not doing a keto plan) and are also rich in fiber, potassium, vitamins B6 and C, and can boost blood sugar.

10. Unsweetened Yogurt, Sauerkraut, Kimchi are fermented foods, which are great for good gut bacteria and enzymes lost during a fast. Avoid spicy kimchi recipes.

11. Avocado is the fattiest fruit in the world (the avocado is really just a large berry). It's ideal for breaking a fast because it's low in calories, rich in omega-3 and omega-6 fat, filled with minerals, antioxidants, and vitamins, including:

- Potassium
- Copper
- Folate
- Vitamin B6
- Vitamin K
- Vitamin C
- Vitamin E
- Antothenic acid, which maximizes the use of the others

Note that some people find avocado hard to digest.

Breaking a fast improperly can wreak havoc on the digestive system. When coming off a long-term fast, spend seven days eating these foods before you return to a normal, daily diet. To make that transition easier, eat the ones you enjoy most and can tolerate the easiest. Keep your first post-fast first meal around 500 calories. For the next week, consider your circumstances. If you're more active, consider eggs instead of broth for better muscle growth.

Observing the importance of breaking a fast brings something else to mind, a recurring theme of our practices here, and that's transition. Good change comes gradually, not quickly. If you're fasting long-term or short, if you're exercising or practicing yoga or meditation, for one session or for a whole new lifestyle, transition into and out of these practices slowly. You must precede a fast with a period of light eating (half the duration of the fast) and observe a similar pattern after the fast. Warm up to your exercises and wind down when you're done, same thing with your yoga and meditative practices. And of course, always consult your doctor before engaging in any change in diet or exercise.

And speaking of diet and exercise, this brings us to the elephant in the room, if you'll pardon that turn of phrase. We're talking about fat and cholesterol, the leading reasons for fasting and the maladies fasting seeks to remedy. But any good dietician, yogi, lawyer, football coach, or anyone in a professional capacity will swear by these words: Know your enemy. But is fat really an enemy? Is it the enemy? What about cholesterol? How much do you really know about these things, which course through your body every second of your life? If the answer is not much or not enough, fear not and read on. You're about to know everything you need to move ahead on your journey to physical (and yes, psychological) wellness.

CHAPTER FOUR: Fats and Cholesterol

Cholesterol

Cholesterol is a waxy substance which collects in the arteries. It is often mistaken for detrimental, but some cholesterol is crucial to good health.

There are two different types of cholesterol; low-density lipoprotein (LDL) and high-density lipoprotein (HDL). LDL is considered the bad cholesterol, HDL is considered the good cholesterol. The reason for this is that HDL carries cholesterol directly to the liver. There is is removed from the bloodstream so it cannot build up in the arteries. LDL delivers cholesterol straight to the arteries. The result may be plaque buildup called atherosclerosis which may cause stroke or heart attack.

Triglycerides are the third major cholesterol component. They are unused calories which the human body stores in the blood as fat. Excessive caloric intake (taking in more calories than you burn) allows triglycerides to collect in the bloodstream, raising the risk of heart attack.

It's important to understand your cholesterol numbers. Over thirty percent of Americans have high LDL (over 100). HDLs, on the other hand, should number no fewer than 40 (for men) or 50 (for women). Healthy triglyceride numbers are 150 or less. Your total cholesterol numbers shouldn't exceed 200.

Fats

Good fats include monounsaturated and polyunsaturated fats. Bad ones include industrial-made trans fats. Saturated fats fall somewhere in the middle. What's the difference? On a chemical level, all fats are structured as a chain of carbon atoms which are bonded to hydrogen atoms. The shape and length of the chain and amount of hydrogen atoms connected are what differentiates one fat molecule from another. Good fats have fewer hydrogen atoms than saturated fats. They're liquid at room temperature, not solid. So what makes a good fat good and a bad fat bad? Some of the benefits of good, unsaturated fats, acceptable saturated fats, and bad trans fats? Let's take a look at what's good about good fats. The benefits of good (unsaturated) fats include:

- Major source of energy

- Aids vitamin and mineral absorption

- Necessary to building cell membranes

- Essential for muscle movement

- Necessary for blood clotting

- Essential for necessary inflammation

Unsaturated fats

Unsaturated fats are liquid at room temperature. They're beneficial fats which ease inflammation, improve blood cholesterol levels, stabilize the heart rhythms, and which play a number of beneficial roles for the human body. Unsaturated fats are found mostly in plant-based foods like nuts, seeds, and vegetable oils. There are good fats, which are beneficial to the body, and bad fats, which are detrimental to the body. The two types of "good" unsaturated fats are monounsaturated and Polyunsaturated fats.

The monounsaturated fat came to the fore of dietary studies in the 1960s, revealing how heart rates in the Mediterranean, despite a high-fat diet. This was because the main fat in their diets was olive oil, not saturated animal fat. This is the origin of the Mediterranean diet, which we'll look at in greater detail later in this book.

The Institute of Medicine's recommendations are to use these good fats to replace saturated and trans fats whenever possible. Monounsaturated fats have single carbon-to-carbon double bonds with fewer hydrogen atoms than saturated fat. Foods rich in monounsaturated fats include:

- Nuts (hazelnuts, almonds, and pecans)

- Seeds (sesame and pumpkin seeds)

- Canola oil

- Peanut oil

- Olive oil

- Avocados

- Safflower oil

- Sunflower oil

Polyunsaturated fats are essential fats found in cooking oils. Being essential means they're necessary for normal body function, but they're not made by the body doesn't make them. Polyunsaturated fats are crucial to:

- Build cell membranes

- Covering nerves

- Muscle movement

- Blood clotting

- Necessary internal inflammation

A polyunsaturated fat's carbon chain has two or sometimes more double bonds. Omega-3 fatty acids and omega-6 fatty acids are the two types of polyunsaturated fat. The numbers 3 and 6 refer to the distance between the carbon chain's beginning and the chain's first double bond.

The benefits of omega-3 fatty acids include:

- Possible prevention of stroke and heart disease

- Reduction of blood pressure

- Raising HDL

- Lowering triglycerides

- Control lethal heart rhythms

- Reduction of corticosteroid medications for rheumatoid arthritis

- Reduction of risk of dementia

Omega-6 fatty acids may protect against heart disease and can be found in vegetable oils (safflower, sunflower, soybean, corn, walnut).

Polyunsaturated fats are found in rich supply in:

- Sunflower, soybean, corn, and flaxseed oils

- Flax seeds

- Fish

- Walnut

- Canola oil (for the polyunsaturated fat)

Omega-3 fats are crucial polyunsaturated fats. They have to be introduced into the system, as the human body cannot manufacture or synthesize them. Eating fish two to three times per week is more than sufficient. If you can't stand fish, try these plant-based alternatives: Walnuts, flax seeds, canola and soybean oil. Higher omega-3 levels in the blood are closely associated with a lower risk of death among older adults.

The general population don't get enough unsaturated fats. The recommendation of the American Heart Association is eight to ten percent of a person's daily calories should derive from polyunsaturated fats.

Most people don't eat enough healthful unsaturated fats. The American Heart Association suggests that 8-10 percent of daily calories should come from polyunsaturated fats, and evidence suggests that an increase of up to 15 percent (replacing saturated fat) may lower the risk of heart disease.

Sixty trials conducted by Dutch researchers found that when monounsaturated and polyunsaturated fats replaced carbohydrates, those good fats lowered harmful LDL levels and increased beneficial HDL levels. Another trial proved that swapping carbs for unsaturated (mostly monosaturated) fats lowered blood pressure, improved lipid level, and reduced risk of cardiovascular disease.

Saturated Fats

Saturated refers to the molecular makeup of the fat; the quantity of hydrogen atoms which surround every carbon atom. This chain holds as many as possible, and so it is saturated with hydrogens.

Almost two dozen studies suggest that there is insufficient evidence to prove a connection between saturated fats and heart disease, but there is a connection between polyunsaturated fat and heart disease. Two major studies concluded that replacing saturated fats with polyunsaturated fats such as high-fiber carbs or vegetable oils is the preferred method for reducing heart disease risk, while replacing saturated fat with any highly processed carbohydrate produced the opposite effect.

Plenty of healthy foods (like nuts and chicken) have some saturated fat. But some, less healthy foods (like cheese, beef, and ice cream) have much more saturated fat. It's found principally in animal food products, but some plant-based foods have a lot of saturated fats as well (oils derived from coconut, palm and palm kernel).

While saturated fat is better for you than unsaturated fats, it can still be harmful in excess. Experts suggest less saturated fat should account for no more than ten percent of daily caloric intake. The American Heart Association recommends no more than seven percent.

But replacing saturated fats is one thing, the question is what to replace it with. Refined carbohydrates may lower bad cholesterol (low-density lipoprotein or LDL), but it also lowers good cholesterol (high-density lipoprotein or HDL). It also increases triglycerides, also bad for the heart. We'll talk more about these things in greater detail shortly.

The biggest sources of saturated fat in the United States diet are:

- Whole- or reduced-fat butter, milk, and dairy desserts

- Pizza and cheese

- Some meats (bacon, sausage, hamburgers, beef)

- Cookies (grain-based sweets)

- Fast-food

Recent studies have disproven the old notions that saturated fat is harmful. Other extensive studies showed no connection between saturated fat intake and either cardiovascular or coronary heart disease. Replacing bad fasts with good can help to prevent the body's resistance to insulin, which is a precursor to diabetes.

Trans Fats

Trans fatty acids (also known as *trans fats*) are created by the process hydrogenation (heating liquid vegetable oils near hydrogen gas). By partially hydrogenating these vegetable oils, the oils become more stable and more likely to resist becoming rancid. The same process may harden the vegetable oil into a solid (shortening and margarine). These partially hydrogenated oils withstand repeated cooling and heating, which makes them perfect for frying.

The trans fat offers no health benefits and there is no recommended safe consumption level. And they're officially banned from use in the United States and other countries. And there is no safe level of consumption.

Trans fats are found in dairy fat and beef fat, but in smaller amounts. They're the worst fat for the blood vessels, heart, and other parts of the body. Other risks of consuming too many trans fats include:

- Elevated bad LDL rates, lowered good HDL rates

- Increased inflammation, implicated in stroke, heart disease, diabetes, various chronic conditions

- Increased insulin resistance

Later in this book, we'll look into exercises and diets, some specific to burning fat. There are yoga practices in this book with the same goal in mind. So let's stay in the laboratory, as it were, before we take all these things out into the field. We've learned a lot, but it's like Albert Einstein said: "The more we learn, the more we realize we do not know." And there's still another big field of study we have to go into. But think of everything you've learned about the different fats and types of cholesterol. Think of the confidence it gives you to prevail over it. Think of how good it feels to use your intellect, the one advantage the human being has over most other animals and even over its own body. The more you learn, the better able you'll be to conquer these once-mystical things. So let's prepare to conquer one of natures great mysteries and one of full-body wellnesses greatest necessities, the keys to the Fountain of Youth. Hormones.

SECTION 2:
HORMONES AND HORMONAL IMBALANCE

CHAPTER FIVE: Hormones

Hormones are an essential part of the body's chemical system. They travel like messengers through the bloodstream as help organs or tissues function at their best. Where they go and what they do depend on what type of hormones are being generated, and that is decided by the trouble spot in the body. Different hormones provide different functions for different parts of the body.

Several endocrine glands secret these hormones, which are necessary for healthy development, growth, reproduction, and other bodily functions. Here's a handy list and rundown of your top ten essential hormones.

The hormones of thyroid, Triiodothyronine (T3) and Thyroxine (T4), are released by the thyroid gland. These hormones help maintain the body's metabolism, regulate weight, determine energy levels, regulates internal temperature, determined hair and skin health, among others.

Insulin is released by the pancreas, from the abdominal cavity, just behind the stomach. Insulin allows the body to use sugar (or glucose) from carbs for energy to use or store. Insulin helps keep blood sugar levels from getting either too low (hypoglycemia) or too high (hyperglycemia).

Estrogen is a female sexual hormone which is released by the ovaries and is responsible for menstruation, reproduction, and menopause. Too much estrogen is known to increase the risks of uterine and breast cancer, moodiness, depression, and other conditions. Too little estrogen can lead to skin lesions, acne, hair loss, thinning skin, weak fingernails, and other symptoms.

Produced in the ovaries, progesterone is produced in the placenta (when a woman is pregnant) in the ovaries and the adrenal glands. Progesterone regulates and stimulates various female bodily functions, including pregnancy maintenance. Progesterone helps the female body prepare for conception and pregnancy, as well as regulating the monthly menstrual cycle. Progesterone levels drop when a lack of pregnancy initiates the menstrual cycle. Progesterone plays a big role in human sexual desire.

Prolactin is released by the pituitary gland. It's released after childbirth and it enable a female to lactate and breastfeed. Prolactin levels rise during pregnancy and can boost fertility.

Testosterone is a male sexual hormone. This anabolic (muscle-building) steroid helps build muscle. Testosterone is also key to developing reproductive tissues in the male body, the testes and the prostate. Testosterone also promotes increased muscle mass, bodily hair and other secondary sexual characteristics. Testosterone deficiency may cause frailty and bone loss in men.

Serotonin is a hormone known for rejuvenation, and it's closely associated with memory and learning, sleep and mood regulation, digestion, and muscular development. Serotonin deficiency is associated with migraines, depression, insomnia, weight gain, carbohydrate craving. Too much serotonin may cause agitation, sedation, and confusion.

The adrenal gland produces Cortisol, the hormone which maintains overall good health and energy. Cortisol controls psychological and physical stress. In times of stress, cortisol increases blood pressure, heart rate, and respiration. But consistently high cortisol levels may cause high blood pressure, ulcer, anxiety, high cholesterol levels. Cortisol deficiency is known to cause alcoholism, chronic fatigue syndrome, and other conditions.

The adrenal gland secretes adrenaline, known as an emergency hormone. Adrenaline is released to counter stress. It dilates blood vessels to the brain and heart.

Somatotropin is also called the growth hormone. Somatotropin is a protein hormone which has 190 amino acids that are synthesized by celled known as *somatotrophs*. Somatotropin stimulates growth, cell regeneration and reproduction, and boosts metabolism.

Here's a supplementary list of other hormones and what they do for your body.

Adrenocorticotropic hormone (ACTH) stimulates cortisol production.

Aldosterone is central to sound cardiovascular health, and it may be a cause of endocrine hypertension.

Angiotensin is a common name for four hormones and play an important role in blood pressure regulation. Learn how this hormone affects many aspects of your health and how to keep it in balance.

Angiotensin is actually the common name for four different hormones. It plays a crucial role in regulating blood pressure.

Anti-Müllerian Hormone (AMH) aids in fertility and reproductive health in human females.

Calcitonin, among the body's most critical hormones, controls potassium and calcium levels.

Cholecystokinin is a hormone best known for helping to improve digestion.

Dehydroepiandrosterone (DHEA) is a precursor hormone with little biological efficacy until converted into other hormones and used for human reproduction.

Dihydrotestosterone stimulates development of various male physical characteristics. Dihydrotestosterone levels are contingent on testosterone levels.

Erythropoietin is a hormone which supports red blood cell production.

The strongest of the three estrogens, Estradiol is important to the female reproductive system. It's the most common type of estrogen for women who are of childbearing age.

Estriol, by comparison, is a minor estrogen hormone which promotes uterus growth. Estriol prepares a human female for giving birth.

Estrone is the third type of estrogen and it's the only estrogen made by the body makes after menstrual periods stop (menopause).

The hormone gastrin governs gastric acid release. Gastrin breaks proteins.

Ghrelin is a digestive hormone which controls appetite.

The pancreas produces the peptide hormone glucagon in order to regulate glucose in the bloodstream.

That's not to be confused with the glucagon-like peptide 1 (GLP-1). This hormone, produced in the small intestine, prevents glucagon production, resulting in lower blood sugar levels. GLP-1 also stimulates insulin production.

Gonadotrophin-releasing hormone (GnRH) secretes reproductive hormones including follicle-stimulating hormone (FSH) and luteinizing hormone (LH).

The human chorionic gonadotropin (HcG) hormone is crucial to the early stages of pregnancy.

Made in the hypothalamus, the hormone kisspeptin initiates the release of other hormones.

Leptin helps control weight and appetite.

Luteinizing hormone (LH) controls female and male reproductive systems.

Melanocyte-stimulating hormone (MSH) protects skin from ultraviolet rays, promotes pigmentation development, and controls appetite.

Melatonin regulates the wake and sleep cycle and has become popular as a sleep aid.

The hormone and neurotransmitter norepinephrine breaks down fat, increases heart rate and blood pressure, and more.

Oxytocin is vital for labor and childbirth, breastfeeding, social behaviors, and bonding.

The parathyroid hormone affects calcium levels in the intestines, kidney, and naturally in the bones.

Peptide YY is produced to signal that you're full and have eaten enough. It's produced in the small intestine.

Prostaglandins aid in healing tissue damage or fighting infection.

Relaxin is produced in the female body when she prepares to deliver a newborn.

Somatostatin (SST), a growth hormone, inhibits the secretion of various other hormones.

Thyroxine aids heart and muscle functioning, digestion, bone maintenance, and brain development, and bone maintenance.

Vitamin D is a hormone which promotes bone growth and calcium absorption and bone growth.

Well, now you've met the rogue's gallery of hormones. Some are lusty rascals, some are young pup eager to grow. They're not easy to control, but you cannot (and probably wouldn't want to) live without them. But knowing, in this case, is only half the battle. Like a crowd of ill-tempered children, they have to be nurtured and looked after. They can quickly become imbalanced, and that can wreak absolute havoc. There are ways they can do this, and ways to regain control and re-achieve a lost balance. It's not that hard, but it takes mindfulness and deliberate action, as you'll see.

CHAPTER SIX: Hormonal Imbalance

This is where hormones go from the being the body's best friends to its worst enemies. Hormonal imbalance can change the whole chemical balance of the body and instigate all manner of dangerous conditions. But how do you know if you have a hormonal imbalance? And if you do, how do you know how to correct it?

Why, you read on, of course.

Signs or Symptoms of a Hormonal Imbalance

We've already seen how hormones play a crucial part in the overall health of the human body. But there's a variety of hormones which perform a variety of functions, as we've already seen. So naturally there are a variety of symptoms and signs of hormonal imbalance.

Some of the most common hormonal imbalances which affect both women and men may cause any of these symptoms or signs:

- Fatty hump on the back between the shoulder blades

- weight gain

- sudden, unexplained weight loss

- muscle weakness

- fatigue

- stiffness, swelling, or pain in the joint

- muscle aches, tenderness, and stiffness

- sweating

- increased or decreased heart rate

- greater sensitivity to heat or cold

- frequent urination

- constipation or more frequent bowel movements

- increased hunger

- increased thirst

- depression

- decreased sex drive

- blurred vision

- nervousness, irritability, or anxiety

- Thinning or brittle hair

- Infertility

- Sleeplessness

- Stress

- Dry skin

- Puffy or rounded face

- purple or pink stretch marks

Signs or Symptoms in Females

Reproductive-age females often endure polycystic ovary syndrome (PCOS), a common hormonal imbalance. The normal female hormonal cycle also changes naturally according to these states of life:

- puberty

- pregnancy

- breastfeeding

- menopause

Symptoms of hormonal imbalance which are specific to females include:

- heavy or irregular periods (including stopped or missed or frequent periods)

- hirsutism (excessive hair on the chin, face, chest, or other parts of the body)

- acne on the chest, upper back, or face, chest, or upper back

- skin tags

- hair loss

- skin darkening (along neck creases, under the breasts, in the groin)

- vaginal atrophy

- vaginal dryness

- night sweats

- pain during sex

- headaches

- Menstruation won't begin

- Breast tissue won't develop

- Growth rate remains static

Symptoms and Signs in Males

Hormonal imbalance can be just as complicated and varied for men as for women. Insufficient testosterone and other imbalances can have a variety of symptoms and signs, including:

- Breast tenderness

- Gynecomastia (development of breast tissue)

- Erectile dysfunction (ED)

- Loss of muscle mass

- decrease in bodily and facial hair growth

- Loss of bone mass (osteoporosis)

- Hot flashes

- difficulty concentrating

Boys with hormonal imbalance may experience:
- High-pitched voice

- Lack of muscle mass development

- Sparse bodily hair growth

- Impaired testicular or penile growth

- Excessive growth of legs and arms, relative to the torso

- Gynecomastia

Causes of Hormonal Imbalance

With the wide variety of hormones and functions, their causes are also widely varied, including:
- Prescription medications

- Hormone therapy

- Cancer treatments (like chemotherapy)

- Benign or cancerous tumors

- Eating disorders

- Pituitary tumors

- Stress

- Trauma or injury

The following conditions may originate with hormonal imbalances and may lead to other imbalances.
- Diabetes insipidus

- Diabetes (type 1 and type 2)

- Hyperthyroidism (overactive thyroid)

- Hypothyroidism (an underactive thyroid)

- hyperthyroidism, or an overactive thyroid

- hyperfunctioning thyroid nodules

- Hypogonadism

- Thyroiditis

- Congenital adrenal hyperplasia (causing low levels of aldosterone and cortisol)

- Cushing syndrome (or high levels of cortisol)

- Addison's disease

Causes Which are Unique to Women

A lot of causes of female hormonal imbalance relate to the reproductive hormones, and the common causes are:

- Premature menopause (primary ovarian insufficiency)

- Menopause

- Pregnancy

- PCOS

- Breastfeeding

- Birth control pills

Tests for Hormonal Imbalance

Because the variety of hormonal functions is so wide, there's no single test for hormonal imbalance. But a trip to your physician is a good place to start. Be prepared with a list of symptoms and a timeline and any external factors like stress, medications, or supplements you may be taking. Be prepared to answer the following questions:

- How often do symptoms occur?

- How do you relieve symptoms?

- Have you gained or lost weight recently?

- Is there more stress in your life?

- Are you trying to get pregnant?

- Was your last period regular and on time?

- Do you have ED?

- Do you experience vaginal pain or dryness during sex?

Expect a blood test to check thyroid health and levels of testosterone, cortisol, and/or estrogen.

A pelvic exam and pap smear may be recommended for female patients to check for unusual cysts, tumors, or lumps. For men, the scrotum may be observed for abnormalities or lumps.

An ultrasound test uses sonic waves to retrieve images of ovaries, the uterus, testicles, pituitary gland, or thyroid. uses sound waves to look inside your body.

You may also try a variety of at-home testing kids, available for a wide spectrum of conditions. These tests use blood or saliva to measure key thyroid hormones, sex hormones like testosterone and progesterone, and cortisol.

Some of these tests require the user to send a sample away in the mail. Results are often returned between five and ten days. Most, but not all, of these tests are FDA-approved.

Treatments for Hormonal Imbalance

As you might have guessed, treatments for hormonal imbalance are as varied as the causes of those imbalances. Here are few common treatment options!

Estrogen therapy is popular for hot flashes and other symptoms of menopause. This treatment employs small supplemental doses of estrogen. This kind of hormone replacement therapy (HRT) should be discussed with a medical professional.

Vaginal estrogen may be applied as a cream, administered in a tablet or in an insertable ring in the case of pain or dryness during sex. This local treatment sidesteps the risks of systemic estrogen, which travels through the bloodstream to its target organ.

Hormonal birth control works by helping to regulate the menstrual cycle. Types of hormonal birth control include:

- Birth control patch

- Birth control shot

- Birth control pill

- Intrauterine device (IUD)

- Vaginal ring

It may also help improve acne and reduce extra hair on the face and body.

Anti-androgen medications are often effective. Androgens, male sex hormones, are present in women as well as men. Women with high levels of androgens may prefer medication to block the androgens' effects, which may include:

- Facial hair growth

- Hair loss

- Acne

Testosterone theory introduces supplements to reduce symptoms of low testosterone in males. This type of therapy, available in a patch, a gel, or by injection, is popular in cases of delayed puberty.

Thyroid hormone therapy introduces supplements of a synthetic thyroid hormone called levothyroxine (comprised of Unithroid, Synthroid, and Levoxyl) may achieve hormonal balance.

Metformin is a medication for type 2 diabetes which has been helpful for some women presenting symptoms of PCOS. The FDA-unapproved treatment may encourage ovulation and lower androgen levels.

Addyi (flibanserin) and Vyleesi (bremelanotide) are the only FDA-approved medications for low sexual desire in women who are premenopausal. Vyleesi is a self-administered injectable. Addyi comes in a pill form.

Those drugs are associated with side effects like blood pressure changes and severe nausea. in blood pressure.

Vaniqa (eflornithine) is a cream prescribed for excessive female facial hair. It slows new growth but does not remove existing hair.

Natural Supplements and Remedies

There are no natural supplements proven to treat menopause or the hormonal imbalance that goes along with it. But there are supplements for the various symptoms. Melatonin may help with sleep, Coenzyme

Q-10 (CoQ-10) and glutathione are excellent cellular supplements. Resveratrol and the previously mentioned curcumin are powerful anti-inflammatories.

A lot of supplements have plant-based hormones which chemically resemble a human body's hormones. Whether these are more effective than direct hormone replacement theory isn't well-known.

Yoga and meditation are two ways a lot of people approach their hormonal imbalances, and we'll take a closer look at them a little later in this book.

Lifestyle Changes for Hormone Management

Other holistic, non-pharmaceutical approaches to hormonal imbalances include changes in lifestyle:

Lose weight. Sources report that a ten-percent reduction in total body weight may help make menstrual periods more regular and it may also increase the chances of getting pregnant. In men, weight loss can improve proper erectile function.

Eat well. A balanced diet is important to overall good health.

Decrease vaginal discomfort by using moisturizers and lubes which are free of glycerin, parabens, and/or petroleum.

Avoid hot flashes by identifying common triggers, such as spicy foods, warm temperatures, or hot beverages.

Remove unwanted or excess body or facial hair. Laser hair removal, electrolysis, or hair removal creams are popular.

Other Hormonal Imbalances

Acne is associated with hormonal imbalance as well, which creates excessive oil production.

Hormonal imbalance and weight gain are closely associated, as hormones play such an integral role in metabolism. Cushing syndrome and other hormone disorders often cause weight gain and even obesity thanks to the elevated levels of cortisol in the blood. Increased appetite and fat storage are the natura results of high cortisol levels. Severe hypothyroidism may likewise lead to weight gain.

Diet and exercise remain the best way to deal with weight, but intermittent fasting is a powerful tool as well, as we've seen.

So there are ways to control and rebalance certain hormones. Exercises and yoga practices we'll look at do the same, and we'll go through them in considerable detail. For now, let's take a closer look at hormones, because they have a strong grounding in heredity. Hormones are not strictly a matter of age, diet, or environment. They're as much about the past, even the distant past, as they are about the present or the future. And if you're going to truly be in the optimal control of your hormones, it's important to know when and if you can't control them at all; and if you can, how.

CHAPTER SEVEN: Hormones and Heredity

The word *hormone* derives from the Ancient Greek word for *impetus*. And that only makes sense, as hormones are the driving force of growth and chemical behavior, mood changing, mating, eating, drinking, fleeing and fighting.

And while there are numerous connections between hormonal imbalance and lifestyle influences, including medicinal and dietary. We've looked at some ways to treat these imbalances, many behavioral and chemical. But it's not all about lifestyle or intake. There are strong connections to heredity, and this must be considered when dealing with hormonal imbalances and how to deal with them.

Let's look at this fairly complex medical web of nature and nurture in a fairly straightforward way. Genes code for hormones and hormone receptors as well as hormone precursors. Genes also contain the necessary codes for hormonal synthesis, bodily transport and, finally, elimination. Science has already identified a lot of these specific genes as they relate to hormonal signaling.

The CRH gene, for example, codes for the corticotrophin-releasing hormone, in this case in the service of cortisol release in response to stress.

For depression and cognitive ability, genetic differences play a big part. We're not sure precisely how, other than allowing for intergenerational temperamental tendencies. Likewise, we know hormones operate on a genetic basis, but we can't say exactly how we can manipulate those genes to prevent the concurrent hormonal imbalances.

Is there a connection between hormone-related genes and related behaviors? Recent studies on alcohol use indicate that a specific gene, Srd5a1, contributes to the synthesis of a neuroactive steroid. Other papers used family designed in examining links between genetic (though latent) risks for psychopathology and hormonal processes. For example, biological mothers reporting substance abuse were linked with their children's cortisol levels early in the day. Another published paper investigated the connection between genetic risk for substance abuse in adolescence and certain genetic influences on healthy pubertal development.

And it's not just a one-way street. Genes do code for hormones, and hormones, in return, regulate genes. Steroid hormones (estradiol, cortisol, testosterone, and progesterone) ahdere to intracellular receptors which regulate the gene's expression.

It leads one to ask whether hormonal changes (such as in puberty or menopause) can suppress or activate genetic influences on a behavioral phenotype. The second question is whether changes in gene expression is involved with that influence. Which is in charge, genetics or behavior?

In short, hormones and genetics simply interact around these forces, each playing their part as required. It's more of an interplay than a cause/effect relationship.

Genetic Syndromes / Endocrine Diseases

Genetic syndromes are not necessarily connected to hormonal disorders. They are medical conditions which are caused by genetically inherited gene mutations. They are passed down from generation to generation. It's very rare that these are related to endocrine organs, occurring only once for every half-million to million cases.

For example, the majority of parathyroid and thyroid diseases have no genetic component. Patients are asked, but report no family history of the diseases.

On the other hand, roughly 33% of diagnosed pheochromocytoma (tumor of the adrenal medulla) cases are currently believed to be genetic and inherited. The most commonly associated genetic conditions include:

- Multiple endocrine neoplasia (MEN) type 2

- von Hippel-Lindau syndrome

- Neurofibromatosis type 1

- Familial paraganglioma syndrome

Multiple Endocrine Neoplasia (MEN) Syndromes

Multiple Endocrine Neoplasia (MEN) syndromes are inherited. A mutated gene creates malignant and benign neuroendocrine tumors. Since it is the endocrine glands which can overproduce hormones and present as symptoms. Early diagnosis and quick treatment always recommended to treat MEN syndromes. To better understand these syndromes, let's take a closer look at the variants: MEN-I, MEN-IIA, MEN-IIB, familial medullary thyroid cancer (itself a variant of MEN-IIA) and MEN-IV.

MEN-I: In multiple endocrine neoplasia (MEN) I, one or more glands develop adenoma (tumor) or excess normal tissue (hyperplasia). MEN-I generally strikes the pancreas, the parathyroid, and the pituitary, glands. It sometimes strikes the thyroid and adrenal glands. These endocrine glands produce and secrete hormones into the lymph or blood systems.

Symptoms of this syndrome include:

- Peptic ulcer disease

- Symptoms of high serum calcium or kidney stones

- Symptoms of pituitary difficulties, including headaches

- Low blood sugar

- Hypoglycemia

- Hypercalcemia (pituitary dysfunction)

- Abdominal pain

- Aching, burning, hunger discomfort in the lower chest or upper abdomen which is relieved by milk, food, or antacids.

- Black stools

- Vomiting and nausea

- Feeling bloated after meals

- Headache

- Weakness

- Anxiety

- Lack of coordination

- Vision problems

- Confusion or mental changes

- Coma from untreated hypoglycemia

- Muscle pain

- Loss of appetite

- Sensitivity to cold

- Fatigue

- Low blood pressure

- Unintentional weight loss

- Loss of pubic and bodily hair

- Infertility, cessation of menses, failure to lactate in women

- Loss of facial or body hair, decreased sexual interest in men

Treatment depends upon which glands are affected. Surgical removal of the gland is often the favored treatment. A bromocriptine may be recommended in the case of a pituitary adenoma. Hormone replacement therapy is often recommended after a gland has been removed.

As to a prognosis, every case has to be taken on its own. Parathyroid and pituitary tumors are often benign, though malignancies do occur. It's easier to treat the symptoms, such as those of peptic ulcer, hypercalcemia, hypoglycemia, and pituitary dysfunction.

MEN-II: Multiple endocrine neoplasia II (MEN II) presents as a thyroid cancer type and is accompanied by a recurring cancer striking the adrenal glands.

MEN-II is caused by a mutation in the gene RET. It presents as multiple tumors which do not necessarily appear at the same time. It affects women and men equally and may strike at any age. There are actually two variants of MEN-II, designated A and B. MEN-IIA may cause hyperparathyroidism, medullary thyroid cancer, and pheochromocytoma. MEN-IIB is more closely associated with neuromas (bumps on the tongue and lips), but also causes medullary thyroid cancer and pheochromocytoma.

Common symptoms of MEN-II include:

- Heart palpitations

- Severe headache

- Rapid heart rate

- Chest pain

- Sweating

- Abdominal pain

- Irritability

- Nervousness

- Weight loss

- Cough

- Cough with blood

- Diarrhea

- Back pain

- Fatigue

- Increased thirst

- Increased urinary output

- Nausea

- Loss of appetite

- Depression

- Muscular weakness

- Personality changes

Treatments for sufferers of MEN-II include surgery, needed to remove the pheochromocytoma and the medullary carcinoma of the thyroid. Treating medullary carcinoma must include the removal of the thyroid gland and (surrounding) lymph nodes. After surgery, hormone replacement therapy is often suggested.

As this is also an inherited disease, family members should be screened for the related RET mutation.

The prognosis, once again, must be mixed. Pheochromocytoma is often benign. The accompanying medullary carcinoma of the thyroid, however, and which characterizes this condition, is a very aggressive malignant cancer. Early diagnosis and successful surgery often leads to cure.

MEN-IV: Multiple endocrine neoplasia type 4 (MEN4) is a very rare form of the syndrome, characterized by anterior pituitary and parathyroid tumors. MEN-IV may be associated with renal, adrenal, and reproductive organ tumors.

Succinate Dehydrogenase (SDH) syndromes: The SDH is a gene which helps to suppress tumor growth. A mutation in this gene means a greater likelihood of pheochromocytomas and paragangliomas (a tumor which forms near nerves and blood vessels outside the adrenal glands). Tumors may cause anxiety, stress, and a fight-or-flight response.

Von Hippel-Lindau syndrome is caused by a mutated VHL gene which prevents tumor growth. Roughly 10-34% of VHL syndrome patients may develop paragangliomas or pheochromocytomas, but they may also develop hemoangioblastomas (benign tumors in the linings of certain blood vessels), retinal angiomas (benign lesions with visual and systemic implications), neuroendocrine tumors of the pancreas and renal cell cancers.

Neurofibromatosis type I is resultant of a mutated NF1 gene, which inhibits tumor growth. Patients may develop numerous benign tumors of the skin and nerves and abnormal patches of skin pigmentation. Cognitive abnormalities are common among sufferers, who are at risk for soft tissue sarcomas and other certain cancers. Over five percent of NF-1 sufferers also develop paragangliomas and pheochromocytomas.

And that brings us to the end of our studious investigation of the biology, chemistry, historical, and even psychological aspects of optimal autophagy and total wellness. Armed with this information, you're now ready to play a more physical role and put your new knowledge into effect. You've got the data, now it's time to use it.

So prepare yourself for the next stage in your journey to total wellness. It's already been a challenge, introducing words and concepts which were no doubt intimidating. You have reread passages or chapters, or you may reread them in the future. Good, that's how this book is meant to be used. What lay ahead are also things which are meant to be revisited; exercises, yoga practices, meditations, and of course diets and detoxing.

The first step is detoxing, cleaning out the system before and as you rebuild a healthier one by the process of autophagy.

SECTION 3: DETOXING

CHAPTER EIGHT: Cleanses and Other Detox Programs

The most popular (not-fasting) way to detox is a cleanse, and there are a variety of ways to do that. But before we get into cleanses a bit more deeply, let's take a quick look at some of the more drastic alternatives.

Flushing

Flushing has become a popular way of cleansing the system. But instead of doing so gradually, by means of a fast or even a cleanse, some choose to flush their bodies out. This has benefits and drawbacks and a variety of in-home and clinical applications.

Enemas are a common, inexpensive, and do-it-yourself, at-home way to cleanse your bowel and gut. Kits can be bought at virtually any pharmacy or drug store or even major grocery store.

There are a variety of different enema approaches. The main difference comes down to the solution which is used in the process. The solution will depend on the particular malady which creates the need for the enema in the first place. These may include:

- Water (general blockage)

- Saltwater (constipation)

- Coffee (use only mold-free and organic beans)

- Garlic (parasites and candida)

- Chamomile (cleansing and healing)

- Apple cider vinegar (healing)

- Probiotics (inflammation of the gut)

- Lemon juice (pH balance)

- Mineral oil (constipation)

- Soap (constipation)

Caveats of Enemas

At-home enemas do have some benefits; affordability, convenience, privacy. But there are possible drawbacks.

Coffee and lemon juice are highly acidic. They can damage intestinal lining. Tools which aren't sufficiently cleaned may cause bowel infections. Enemas eliminate good bacteria along with the bad, which leads to further digestive disruptions. Using too much solution can cause stretching and tearing of the bowel. Nausea and vomiting are common during or after a cleanse. Overuse of enemas may weaken the bowel muscles and disrupt natural bowel movements, creating a dependence.

The Coffee Enema

As long as we're going deep into this subject (don't judge me), let's take a look at one of the most popular at-home enemas, the coffee enema.

Drinking coffee remains a controversial practice. While done in various corners of the world, the benefits and drawbacks remain in question. It almost seems to go in and out of style depending on the most recent studies. Because it's so popular and widely consumed, it gets studied a lot. Over the years, coffee has been blamed for liver damage and praised for it benefits to the liver. It's been chastised as a drug and lauded as a alternative beverage to a number of other, more addictive substances like alcohol. It's known to be a powerful antioxidant.

And injecting a coffee solution into your colon has been called a great way to cleanse the lower intestines. Coffee enemas sound like some new(ish) fad, but they've been in use since the turn of the Twentieth century. At the time they were useful to speed healing after surgeries and to combat accidental poisoning. By the 1950s, coffee enemas became standard practice in cancer treatments. Only now are they returning to popularity for a variety of ailments which do not respond properly to prescription medications or traditional treatments.

Coffee's properties as an antioxidant makes it a good choice for a cleanse, as do other beneficial compounds such as palmitate, cafestol theobromine, kahweol, theophylline, and of course caffeine. They're also known to have positive effects on internal inflammation, often a digestive problem requiring an enema.

Coffee enemas have been shown to have these benefits:

- Flushing out heavy metals, bacteria, yeast, fungus from the digestive system
- Cleansing the colon and the liver
- Lowering inflammation
- Restore bowel function
- Relax bowel muscles
- Opens blood vessels
- Opens bile ducts
- Increase bile production
- Increase energy levels of bowel function
- Healing bowel disorders
- Stimulates glutathione S-transferase in the liver
- Repair digestive tissue
- Cleanse the liver
- Improving blood circulation
- Increasing immunity
- Clean out diverticulitis
- Help cellular regeneration
- Relieve digestive issues (bloating, constipation, nausea, and cramping)
- Improve gut health
- Improve moods and energy levels and moods

And so, they're often used to help manage such conditions as:

- Parasites

- Cancer

- Overdoses

- Liver dysfunction

- Candida virus

- Constipation

- IBS (irritable bowel syndrome)

- Various digestive disorders

As with any enema, it's recommended to perform it immediately after a bowel movement. Some recommend an activated carbon charcoal binder both before and after the enema to bind the toxins before release for more efficient elimination.

Enemas are recommended once weekly. Patients healing from digestive disorders may do one per day. Very ill patients, such as those recovering from cancer, may have several per day.

Coffee Enema Dangers and Side Effects

Studies haven't shown too many verified ill-effects of coffee enemas. But their effectiveness will vary from person to person and from case to case. All enemas do carry some risk, as we've discussed: colon tearing, dehydration, electrolyte imbalance, dizziness, and weakness. They're not recommended for children or pregnant women nor for anybody who is allergic to coffee or caffeine.

Clinical Colon Therapy

Besides at-home enemas, there are clinical approaches, including a variety of colon therapy clinics. Some are smaller, meant for quick visits. Others have more of a spa atmosphere, and include baths, massages, and appropriate nourishment. More elaborate overnight colon spas are around too, which provide a two-day cleanse with a (sometimes) private room overnight. My brother used to go to such a place quite often; I used to call it *Flushing Meadows*.

Cleanses

Cleanses are just about the most popular method of detoxing at home. And once detoxes became so widespread, they also became varied, with different new trends and discoveries creating new cleansing recipes and techniques. Some make wild claims, some can actually make good on those promises. So let's take a look at the spectrum of detox regiments, including diets, drinks, and powders … oh my!

It's important to note that these cleanses are so new and inventive, many have not been clinically tested. There may be anecdotal evidence (informally reported), but there is little in the way of clinical trials. And these are regiments, not copyrighted formulas, so they don't get or seek FDA (Food & Drug Administration) approval. So take these regiments with a grain of salt.

The reputed benefits of detoxification include weight loss, improved energy, relief from headaches and muscle aches, fatigue and constipation.

On the other hand, the human body has ways of detoxifying itself, including urinating, defecating, sweating. The digestive tract, liver and kidneys, all break down toxins and prepare them to be eliminated.

But proponents of these cleanses will tell you that the body's natural processes are no longer sufficient to keep up with our modern world and the considerable uptick in toxins we now have to endure. Our bodies haven't changed much since the paleolithic era. But in the last century or so, the industrial age brought pollution like the world as we knew it had never seen. The atomic and nuclear ages brought even more toxicity to our oceans, our rainwater, our soil. Practices like natural gas mining (also known as *fracking*) and disasters like the British Petroleum oil spill in the Gulf of Mexico have made our environment radically toxic. Add to that the shift in our dietary habits over that same century. This century saw the rise of processed foods, sugar substitutes, genetically modified foods. Steroids artificially fattened animals for maximum profitability. Insecticides became a staple of industrial farming, which also robbed the soil of the nutrients which vegetables and fruits require. Tobacco was modified with chemicals for a variety of diabolical reasons.

Our paleolithic systems were never designed to process such an array of toxins, so the liver and kidneys can't be relied upon to do the job. Hence, the need to cleanse. And not only should a cleanse eliminate collected toxins, it would therefore make way for the body to intake new nutrients in their place.

The basic way a detox works is to eliminate specific foods and food groups. This allows the system to stop processing those toxins and heal from the corrosive effects of toxins on the body. The solid foods are replaced, usually with drinks comprised of various natural ingredients, each recipe designed with a certain approach to the body. Some of these ingredients include lemon, cayenne pepper, maple syrup, green tea, or fresh vegetable and fruit juices. Cleanses may last from a single day to an entire month.

Caveats of Cleansing

As we've pointed out, there is little in the way of clinical trails tracing the effectiveness of cleansing. Unless you're suffering from gastroparesis or Crohn's disease, skipping foods in unlikely to generate any healing, according to doctors. The fiber in vegetables and fruits slows digestion and helps the body absorb nutrients and remove toxins through the stool. The digestive tract utilizes fiber's probiotics to nourish the intestines with bacteria, needed for a strong immune system.

And, as we've noted, weight loss from cleanses (as from long-term fasting) is usually temporary. It's mostly water weight and stored stool, which is naturally replaced. The rest of that weight is basically stored carbohydrates, and a dietary change would be needed to prevent that from recurring. Most dietary regiments include some carbohydrates, and exercise is necessary to prevent carb storage.

Athletes should avoid cleansing, as they actually use the stored carbohydrates their bodies carry. Athletic bodies don't use the keto dietary method of using fat as fuel, as their bodies often don't have that much stored fat.

In fact, experts recommend that nobody who is fasting should exercise at the same time. Nor should athletes cleanse while recovering from sports injuries, for the same reason. The body needs those nutrients.

Pros and Cons of Detoxing

Cleansing requires some commitment; of time, of money, of your personal health. You're well-advised to know the pros and cons of your new exploit. Just to remind you; consult with your doctor before changing your diet or exercise protocol.

The pros of cleansing include an increase of minerals and vitamins from fresh juice supplements, and new insight into food sensitivities by process of elimination and reintroduction

The cons of cleansing include lack of energy and disruption of blood glucose levels and disruption of the metabolic rate. Frequent bowel movements and gastrointestinal distress are also common. These diets are also protein deficient. And, as we've discussed, cleansing makes exercise unwise, and this can cause atrophy, sloth, ultimate weight gain, and other related conditions.

No matter which type of cleanse or detox you prefer, these tips will maximize the efficiency of your campaign and ensure a healthier transition to a healthier lifestyle.

1. Limit your alcoholic intake. The liver processes about ninety percent of alcohol, and when the liver enzymes do metabolize alcohol it becomes acetaldehyde, which is a chemical known to cause cancer. The liver then coverts that toxin to the harmless acetate, later eliminated from the body. Excessive alcoholic intake damages the liver, making it unable to process acetaldehyde to acetate, leading to various cancers (including liver cancer). Fatty buildup, scarring, and inflammation are other was alcohol can damage the liver.

Health authorities recommend no more than two drinks a day (for men) and one drink a day (for women) and two for men. This isn't a recommendation to start drinking if you don't drink now, however.

2. Get more sleep. The body gets a lot done when it is at rest, including various detoxification processes. It's good for the brain and for the psyche as well. During a fast, getting adequate sleep is especially important.

The brain reorganizes and recharges during sleep, but it also removes toxic byproducts. One of these is the protein beta-amyloid, a major factor Alzheimer's disease development.

Lack of sleep may also contribute to:

- Anxiety

- Stress

- Heart disease

- High blood pressure

- Obesity

- Type 2 diabetes

Experts recommend seven to nine hours of sleep per night.

A number of things may interrupt or prevent sleep, including erratic scheduling, light from electronic devices, caffeine, stress, and anxiety.

3. Drink more water. Water has several health benefits which are especially crucial during a cleanse. The benefits of drinking more water include:

- Thirst quenching

- Body temperature regulation

- Joint lubrication

- Digestive aid

- Nutrient absorption

- Natural detoxification

- Waste product removal

Experts recommend and 91 oz (2.7 liters) for women and 125 oz (3.7 liters) for men, though this may vary depending on activity level, diet, and environment.

4. Limit sugar intake. Excessive sugar intake is closely linked to obesity, cancer, heart disease, and diabetes. These are the diseases often preventing the body's ability to detoxify by damaging the organs responsible for detoxification, like the kidneys and liver.

5. Increase antioxidant intake. Oxidation is the breakdown of matter by loss of molecular electrons. If you've ever seen metal rusting, you've witnessed the oxidation process. And this happens inside the human body as well. Molecules lose electrons and become free radicals. While some free radicals are beneficial, as in the digestive process, an excess of free radicals can do damage the body in various ways, including tearing at the inner walls of veins and arteries. Pollutants, alcohol, the chemicals found in tobacco smoke, and poor diet can create excessive free radicals. Free radicals are associated with deadly diseases and conditions including heart disease, dementia, asthma, liver disease, and various cancers.

6. Antioxidants introduce new electrons to correct the free radicals and make them fully functioning molecules again.

Popular antioxidants include:

- Vitamins A, C, E

- Selenium

- Lycopene

- Lutein

- Zeaxanthin

  These are commonly found in:

- Fruits

- Berries

- Vegetables

- Cocoa

- Spices

- Nuts

- Coffee

- Green tea

7. Listen to Your Gut. No, we don't mean your gut instinct, but your actual gut. This part of your body is crucial to your overall health, as it is central to digestion and vital to detoxification.

And central to good gut health are good bacteria called prebiotics. These produce short-chain fatty acids, nutrients which are very beneficial to overall health.

But antibiotics, poor dental hygiene, and quality of diet can create an imbalance between good and bad bacteria. This may weaken the detoxification and immune systems and may increase the risk of inflammation and disease.

Foods that are rich in prebiotics include:

- Artichokes

- Tomatoes

- Bananas

- Onions

- Asparagus

- Garlic

- Oats

8. Limit salt intake: Too much salt causes the body to retain fluids. This can be complicated by conditions of the liver or kidneys, or in the case of insufficient water consumption. Given insufficient water and too much salt, the body creates and secretes an antidiuretic hormone which prevents urination. This can cause bloating and general discomfort. Increased water intake actually helps flush out water weight caused by too much salt by instigating urination, washing out the salt as well.

The effects of too much sodium can be counterbalanced by eating potassium-rich foods such as:

- Bananas

- Spinach

- Kidney beans

- Squash

- Potatoes

9. Reduce inflammation. Inflammation does have its proper place, such as wound recovery. But excessive inflammation of internal tissues can contribute to a number of life-threatening conditions, including cancers, high blood pressure, heart disease, stroke, and type 2 diabetes.

Exercise can be tricky during a cleanse (and is to be avoided during a fast) but it can help control inflammation. Experts suggest between150–300 minutes (per regular dietary week) of moderate exercise (like brisk walking) or 75–150 minutes (per regular dietary week) of vigorous physical activity (like running).

10. Use more spices: Consider eating and cooking with sulfur-rich foods like broccoli, eggs, onions and garlic. These promote glutathione production in the body and help the body excrete heavy metals such as cadmium. Glutathione is a master antioxidant. Chlorella is an algae which helps eliminate toxins such as heavy metals. Cilantro also enhances toxic excretion, particular heavy metals, insecticides, and phthalates.

11. Use natural cleansers: Baking soda and vinegar are just as effective as commercial cleansers and lack a lot of the harmful chemicals.

Let's take a closer look at these chemicals and the risks they pose.

1. Phthalates are found in dish soap, air fresheners, and toilet paper, among other products. It's part of the products fragrance and so won't be listed as an ingredient. Phthalates are endocrine disruptors. In men, higher phthalate levels correspond to reduce sperm count.

2. Perchloroethylene or *perc* is found in spot removers, dry-cleaning solutions, and upholstery and carpet cleaners. It's classified by the EPA as a possible carcinogen. Side effects from exposure are loss of coordination and dizziness, among others.

3. Triclosan is most commonly found in so-called *antibacterial* hand soaps and liquid dishwashing detergents. Triclosan is a possible carcinogen and its runoff has proven dangerous to algae.

4. Quarternary Ammonium Compounds, or *quats*, are found in antibacterial household cleaners and fabric softer liquids and dryer sheets. Quats are skin irritants and may have links to asthma and other respiratory disorders.

5. 2-Butoxyethanol is found in multipurpose cleaners, as well as kitchen and window cleaners. It's been linked to sore throats, pulmonary edema (caused by excess fluid in the lungs), narcosis, severe kidney and liver damage.

6. Ammonia is found in metal and porcelain polishing agents, and glass cleaners. It may have an immediate detrimental effect on those who suffer from lung issues, asthma, bronchitis, or other breathing problems. It can also interact dangerously with bleach, creating a poisonous gas much like chloroform.

7. Chlorine is found in toilet bowl cleaners, laundry whiteners, mildew removers, toilet bowl cleaners, and household tap water. Chlorine is a thyroid disrupter.

8. Sodium Hydroxide is often found in drain openers and oven cleaners. It can be extremely corrosive to skin and eyes, nose and throat.

But here are some healthier cleaning alternatives for the home!

- Choose fragrance-free or all-natural organic products

- Skip air fresheners, open a window

- Take dry-clean clothes, sheets and drapes to a wet cleaner, find one online

- Buy cleansers using liquid carbon dioxide (CO_2)

- Avoid antibacterial cleaners

- Use alcohol-based hand sanitizers without triclosan

- Use vinegar as a natural fabric softener

- Use antifungal, antibacterial tea-tree oil (mixed with vinegar and lavender for scent) as an all-purpose cleaner

- Clean windows and mirrors with diluted vinegar and newspaper

- Use Bon Ami powder as an alternative to commercial cleansers

- Use vodka to polish metal or mirrors

- Use toothpaste as a silver polish

- Use baking soda and vinegar to clear clogged drains

Natural soaps and body care products have the same benefits. Industrial makeups, deodorants, shampoos, moisturizers, and shampoos often contain questionable chemicals such as:

1. Parabens: Chemicals such as propylparabens, methylparabens, ethylparabens, and butylparabens, which preserve shelf-life. Parabens are commonly found in makeup, body wash, night cream, face wash, shampoo. They mimic estrogen and create hormonal imbalance. Parabens are also closely associated with breast cancer and fertility/reproductive issues.

2. Phthalates increase flexibility in cosmetics. They're commonly found in deodorants, lotions, and hair spray. Phthalates are endocrine disrupters and may cause birth defects.

3. Fragrance is a collection of dangerous chemicals and is most often found in hand creams, moisturizers, and hair products. It can cause allergies, reproductive issues, infertility, and hormone disruption.

4. Sodium Laureth Sulfate (SLES) and/or Sodium Lauryl Sulfate (SLS) are found in body wash, shampoo, and bubble bath. They can trigger allergies and cause skin irritation.

5. BHT are synthetic antioxidants which extend shelf life. They're most commonly found in lipstick, diaper creams, moisturizers. BHT are likely carcinogens, hormone disrupters, and may cause severe live damage.

6. Retinyl palmitate and Retinol (aka, Vitamin A) found in anti-aging skincare creams and moisturizers. It may speed skin tumor growth and damage DNA.

7. Lead is a neurotoxin and heavy metal found in lipstick, lip gloss, and Vaseline. Lead is closely tied to learning and behavioral problems.

8. Formaldehyde is commonly used in most cosmetics. It's a known carcinogen and is closely linked to neurotoxicity, asthma, and developmental toxicity.

A new natural retinol alternative, bakuchiol, has come out and has incredible anti-aging benefits. It gives you similar results to retinol without the irritation. This is the skincare line I've been using while pregnant and my skin has never looked better—never thought I'd say that while pregnant!

Here are some healthy alternatives to the dangerous cosmetics and soaps. Take note that these are specific brands and we as publishers have no association with them, privately or publicly. This is not a commercial endorsement, and we recommend you research all these products thoroughly as part of your own due diligence:

- Pure Deodorant

- Citrus Mimosa Body Butter

- Volume & Shape Mist

- Adaptive Moisture Lotion

- Citrus Rosemary Body Oil

- Hydrating Body Lotion

- Citrus Mimosa Hand Cream

- Sea Salt Spray

- Daily Shampoo

- Citrus Mimosa Body Wash

- Kid's Body Wash

- Baby All-Over Wash

- Sheer Lipstick

- Nourishing Day Cream

- Calming Diaper Rash Cream

- Dew Skin Tinted Moisturizer

- Antioxidant Soft Cream (Day Cream)

- Tripeptide Radiance Serum

- Overnight Resurfacing Peel

- Tetrapeptide Supreme Cream

- Ultra Renewal Eye Cream

- Sheer Lipstick

- Sheer Lip Gloss

- Color Intense Lipstick

That's another big boatload of information, we're well aware. But don't be daunted. Remember that this book is a much a reference book as anything else, designed to be re-read and reviewed as needed. However, it should hardly be surprising, with fasting and cleansing and other related practices becoming more popular, that cleansing/detox kits would be made available, virtual one-stop-shops for at-home treatment. Without any endorsement, let's look at some of the leading and easy ways to pursue cleansing your body of toxins.

CHAPTER NINE: Popular Cleanses

It's easy enough to use water for a cleanse, but there are also cleansing kits made available from different producers for different purposes. So let's take a look at some of the popular cleanses which are prepacked to give you the maximum nutritional value and impact. Remember that we're not associated with any of these producers. We're here for you, not for them. But one or more might just be perfect for your needs. We're here to give you choices, to give you information. Use it well! Always consult with your doctor before changing your dietary or exercise protocols!

Juice Cleanses

Juice cleanses are popular, varied, and controversial. Some are steadfast supporters and a lot of detractors. Holistic nutritionists support the idea that juices cleanses help the body to take a break from the heavy foods and potentially allergenic foods in favor of easily digested and assimilated nutrients of pure vegetables and fruits. The juices detoxify and hydrate at the same time, a clear plus.

Raw Generation has the standard juice cleanses, the company also offers a signature Protein Cleanse. Available in three-, five-, and seven-day options, the cleanse proports to cleanse the body without sacrificing the adequate consumption of protein or the energy which goes along with it. The options sell for between $100 and $250 or so and contain six juices and 40 grams of plant protein.

Pressed Juicery has been a respected name in juice cleansing for years. They offer an extensive menu of over 20 juice blends and cleanse packages in three bundles. Their beginner cleanse, most popular cleanse, and experienced bundles all sell for about $30 dollars.

The company Suja offers a signature 3-Day Juice Cleanse for about $100, which features healthy breakfast recipes and a seven-juice cleanse.

Juice Generation is the purveyor of Citrus Super C, a delicious and well-missed beverage. They currently offer thee Cooler Cleanses, in one-, three-, and five-day packages costing from roughly $60 to roughly $300. These cleanses focus on the juices, unlike Suja. Their Blend It Yourself offering, the ingredients are delivered to you to mix at home, reducing plastic consumption and lowering your carbon footprint.

Juiced offers an affordable and convenient juice cleanse which is designed to jumpstart and energize healthier lifestyle habits. Introducing blended, raw veggies and fruits into the user's daily routine for as long as a full week, their Jumpstart Cleanse costs less than $30 a day. This cleanse proports to improve response to stress, break the sugar-craving cycle, boost focus and mental clarity, and more. This regiment offers seven juice drinks a day, plus unlimited raw fruits and vegetables.

Project Juice' has organic juice cleanses which include three different five-day options, plus the user has the option to create a custom regiment. The company offers a beginners-level Classic Reset Cleanse and an experienced-level Advanced Reset Cleanse. Each costs about $75 per day and includes six juice drinks a day. The company's premium package is their Immunity Reboot Cleanse includes two very potent wellness shots every day at roughly $85 per day.

Lemonkind has a 3-Day Reset Core Juice Cleanse which features 24 juices (eight per day for three days). The cleanse is designed to break bad habits, detox the body, jumpstart a healthier diet. The regiment calls for a hearty juice drink every two hours, which makes it more satisfying and easier to follow.

Squeezed is an excellent choice for those unwilling to commit. The company offers various options to ease the user's transition into the cleanse. They have programs that go from one day to seven, at roughly $30 per day. Raw vegetables and fruits are permitted during the week.

Three Cleanses to Avoid

Not everybody agrees about the all-juice cleanse. People have tried it and recorded their experiences online and they are often anything but glowing. A diet of warm lemon water and several bottles of juice may provide less than 1000 calories, leaving a lot of people feeling hungry, irritable, and weak. This can also lead to headaches and a distinct lack of sociability. Many experts believe that juices the fruits rob them of the fiber and nutrients the whole fruits offer.

The tea cleanse also has its detractors. Stomach cramps and sleep deprivation are often reported with these cleanse types. Tea is also a laxative, so it may evacuate residual feces and water, but it won't change the fat-to-muscle ratio.

Drinking tea can have a lot of positive effects, but being a full-body cleanser simply isn't one of them.

There's a cleanse known as The Master Cleanse, but it makes some outrageous claims. According to the purveyors of this plan, the human body can survive off nothing more than six to 12 glasses of a concoction made of maple syrup, lemon juice, cayenne pepper, and water, for up to ten days. The claim is that up to 20 pounds can be lost in those ten days. The Master Cleanse seeks to help users overcome a psychological need to eat. And while there are connections between psychology and eating disorders, there are physiological needs to eat which have to be addressed. Ten days is longer than almost any expert will recommend going without eating.

Dedicated Cleansing Kits

A product called zuPOO proports to be able to flush out between five and 20 pounds of fecal matter from the bowel. This is important for the body, as we've seen, one of the many reasons for a colon cleanse. It's important to remember that fasts and cleanses in general achieve this same thing. Whether zuPOO is more effective than more DIY cleanses will be for the user to decide. It certainly should deliver a smoother digestion once the bowels are cleared, in any case.

The company offers a powerful blend of minerals, vitamins, herbs, and barks which it claims flush waste matter out of the system. This evacuation is said to begin with one to two days of administration, and the product is recommended for use in a 15-day cycle to fully flush out the bowels. (Keep in mind this includes good bacteria as well as bad.) The formula includes six natural ingredients with special functionality:

Cascara Sagrada, a gentle, natural laxative, is proven effective against constipation, a potent boost to the immune system, and a good way to promote probiotic bacteria.

Bentonite clay draws waste out of the body and passes it. The clay includes magnesium, calcium, sodium, silica, iron, copper, and potassium, all beneficial minerals.

Aloe ferox is well-known for its colon-cleansing powers. A 2004 study found that 30% of participants using the aloe demonstrated improvement or clinical remission. Only one percent of participants who took a placebo presented the same results.

Milk thistle is known to be a powerful fortifier of the liver, supporting liver function and tissue health.

Cayenne pepper, which we've already looked at briefly, has been shown to have a very positive effect on the human digestive system. It encourages saliva production, important for good digestion and fighting bad breath. Cayenne pepper is also known to stimulate enzyme production, essential for proper digestive system functionality. Cayenne pepper is also proven to stimulate gastric juices which aid the human body's metabolism of food and toxins.

Slippery Elm Extract has demonstrated a 20% increase in frequency of bowel movement frequency. Users have also reported less abdominal pain, bloating, and straining, and improvements in the consistency of stool. It can improve digestion and aid in weight loss.

It's taken in capsules, one or two in the evening before bed. Gas may build up in the first day or two. Flushing should begin after 12 hours or so.

Fiber is important. Eat enough brown rice, organic fresh vegetables and fruits, including:
- Beets
- Radishes
- Artichokes
- Cabbage
- Broccoli
- Spirulina
- Chlorella
- Seaweed

Protect and cleanse the liver with herbs such as:
- Burlock
- Dandelion root
- Milk thistle
- Green tea
- Vitamin C
- Glutathione

Experts recommend:
- Drinking two quarts of water per day or more
- Deep breathing for oxygenation of the system
- Emphasizing positive emotions to transform stress
- Hydrotherapy, in the form of a hot five-minute shower followed by 30 seconds of cold water (do this three times in a row and go to bed for at least 30 minutes)
- Saunas to encourage sweating to eliminate waste
- Dry-brush skin or use foot spas/baths which remove toxins through the pores of the skin.

And that's about it for cleanses. And once your body is cleansed, it's time to move on to picking the right diet. Because cleansing and fasting may help you lose weight, but it won't keep the weight off and it likely will not get off all the weight you want to lose. These are ways of kickstarting your new lifestyle, but a good diet is the way to make it a reality. So let's move on to the subject of perhaps more self-help books than any other.
Dieting.

SECTION 4: DIETING

CHAPTER TEN: Ketogenic Diet

Think back to the ugly statistics about obesity and ill-health. You already know the importance of a good diet by now, and you likely had some idea before picking up this book. But a good diet is both effective for weight loss and for weight management, and some are particularly good for an intermittent fasting lifestyle.

Keep in mind that fasting itself is a kind of diet, a crash diet of only water, minimal caloric intake, etc. But a diet is a regiment, and one of the most popular regiments these days in the ketogenic diet.

We looked at the ketogenic diet briefly. To remind you, the body generally uses carbohydrates as a preferred source of fuel, allowing fat to collect. Denying the body carbohydrates leaves the body to use its resources of energy from carbs and turns to using fats for fuel. Once the body goes through ketosis and reprograms itself to use fat as the preferred source of fuel, creating brain-feeding ketones, fat stores are used and no longer collect so readily. The ketogenic diet lowers levels of insulin too, and that is beneficial for boosting blood sugar management and insulin sensitivity.

The ketogenic diet has a high fat content, moderate protein content, and low carbohydrate content. It only takes a few weeks for the shift to occur.

Ketogenic staple foods include:

- Meat

- Butter

- Cheese

- Fish

- Eggs

- Heavy cream

- Nuts

- Oils

- Seeds

- Avocados

- Low-carb vegetables

It's probably no surprise that a lot of those foods seem familiar, especially from the cleanses and post-fasting foods. This is what makes the ketogenic such a good diet for before or after fasting. The ketogenic diet eliminates nearly all (and also familiar) sources of carbohydrates, including:

- Rice

- Grains

- Potatoes

- Beans

- Milk

- Sugars

- Fruits

- Cereals

- High-carb veggies

Does it work? The ketogenic diet has been shown to lower insulin levels, increase fat burning, and producing brain-nourishing ketones. It may create fat loss, muscle gain, and improve disease markers. Some studies suggest that, given the same calorie intake, a ketogenic diet can be more effective for weight loss than a low-fat diet. One study produced a similar results: volunteers on the ketogenic diet lost over two times more weight than volunteers on a low-fat, low-calorie diet. HDL (high density, or good) cholesterol, and triglyceride levels also increased. Calories in both groups were reduced equally.

A 2007 study compared a low-carb regiment to the dietary guidelines of Diabetes UK. dietary guidelines. The low-fat group lost 4.6 pounds (2.1 kg). The low-carb group lost 15.2 pounds (6.9 kg). Over 3 months, the low-carb diet generated three times more weight loss over three months.

Specialists aren't certain as to whether these results are from a metabolic advantage to the ketogenic diets or simply higher protein intake. There's also some question about long-term results from the ketogenic diet.

The ketogenic diet works through a series of processes to promote weight loss:

- Higher protein intake, which has many weight-loss benefits

- Gluconeogenesis, converting fat and protein into carbohydrates for fuel, burning calories

- Appetite suppressant, supported by changes in leptin and ghrelin and other hunger hormones

- Improved insulin sensitivity, improving metabolism and fuel utilization

- Decreased fat storage by reducing lipogenesis, the process of converting sugar into fat

- Increased fat burning

Ketogenic Diet and Metabolic Diseases

We took a brief look at metabolic syndrome, common risk factors for type 2 diabetes like obesity, and heart disease. Others include:

- High blood pressure

- High waist-to-hip ratio (excess belly fat)

- High levels of LDL (bad) cholesterol

- Low levels of HDL (good) cholesterol

- High blood sugar levels

Many of these risk factors may be improved or eliminated with some lifestyle and nutritional changes. Insulin plays a big role in metabolic diseases and diabetes in particular. Ketogenic diets are known to lower insulin levels, particularly for sufferers of prediabetes or type 2 diabetes. One study revealed that after two weeks of being on a ketogenic diet, insulin sensitivity was improved by 75% while blood sugar dropped considerably, from a high of 7.5 mmol/l to a low of 6.2 mmol/l. Another study revealed a 16% blood sugar reduction. Seven out of 21 volunteers stopped using diabetic medication after the study. Other studies in animals and humans found the ketogenic diet reducing total triglycerides and cholesterol levels. It's important to note that some studies found negative effects of the ketogenic diet in children. Also, research indicates that saturated fat intake as happens in the ketogenic diet may increase levels of LDL (low-density, or bad) cholesterol, a big risk factor for heart disease. Other studies demonstrate a connection between cancer and some fats.

Impact of the Ketogenic Diet on Metabolic Disease

Key factors of the ketogenic diet effect certain markers of metabolic disease, including:
- Fewer carbs: High carbs mean higher insulin and blood sugar, decreasing insulin resistance

- Decreased insulin resistance: This causes high trigiyceride levels, inflammation, and fat storage

- Ketone bodies: These protect against cancer, epilepsy, Alzheimer's, and other diseases

- Reduced inflammation: The ketogenic diet reduces inflammation, linked to metabolic syndrome

- Fat loss: Abdominal fat, a staple of metabolic disease, is vulnerable to the ketogenic diet

- Restoration of insulin function: Healthy insulin levels fight inflammation

Is the Ketogenic Diet Right for You?

Diets vary, as do people. No diet is perfect for everyone. The right diet depends on a variety of factors, including lifestyle, heredity, tastes, and so on. The ketogenic diet is also not suitable for sufferers of:
- Liver failure

- Pancreatitis

- Carnitine deficiency

- Fat metabolism disorders

- Pyruvate kinase deficiency

- Porphyrias

Dieters should also be wary of the so-called *keto flu*, a collection of flu-like symptoms including:
- Low energy

- Digestive discomfort

- Nausea

- Poor exercise performance

- Poor mental function

- Increased hunger

- Sleep issues

- Dehydration

There may also be risks to liver and kidneys after extended periods on the ketogenic diet, though the research is lacking in this department.

A ketogenic diet isn't always easy to stick to. Carb cycling or a low-carbohydrate diet may be preferable. Athletes may find the use of fat inconvenient, as they rely more on carbs, and vegans and vegetarians may balk at the reliance on meats and dairy.

As we've seen changing the body's energy source from carbohydrates to fat can increase ketones in the blood. This so-called *dietary ketosis* is different from *ketoacidosis,* a very dangerous condition.

Too many ketones may cause ketoacidosis (DKA). DKA is prevalent in type 1 diabetes, where excessive blood glucose can occur from lack of insulin. It's also possible in type 2 diabetes when ketone levels get too high. Being on a low-carb diet like the ketogenic diet while ill may increase the risk of DKA. DKA is considered a medical emergency. Symptoms require immediate medical attention, as the sufferer may fall into a diabetic coma.

DKA warning signs include:

- Dry mouth

- Consistently high blood sugar

- Nausea

- Frequent urination

- Breathing difficulties

- Fruit-like odor in the breath

We've already taken a look at the keto-friendly foods, but let's be a bit more specific, as we're about to move on to an entire keto-friendly menu!

A ketogenic diet should center around these foods:

- Eggs: Organic, pasteurized whole eggs are best

- Poultry: Turkey or chicken only

- Shellfish: Oysters, shrimp and scallops

- Fatty fish: Herring, mackerel, wild salmon

- Meat: Venison, bison, pork, venison, grass-fed beef, organ meats

- Full-fat dairy: Butter, yogurt, and cream.

- Full-fat cheese: Mozzarella, cheddar, brie, cream cheese, goat cheese

- Nuts and seeds: Almonds, macadamia nuts, walnuts, peanuts pumpkin seeds and flaxseeds

- Nut butter: Natural almond, peanut, and cashew butters

- Healthy fats: Olive oil, coconut oil, avocado oil, sesame oil, coconut butter

- Avocado: Whole avocados

- Non-starchy vegetables: Broccoli, greens, mushrooms, tomatoes, peppers

- Condiments: Pepper, salt, lemon juice, fresh herbs, spices. vinegar

Keto-friendly beverage choices include:

- Water: The best source of hydration

- Sparkling water: A good replacement for soda

- Unsweetened coffee: Flavored with heavy cream instead of sugar

- Unsweetened green tea: Especially green tea

The following foods should be restricted:

- Breads and baked goods: Breads, cookies, crackers, rolls, and doughnuts

- Sweet, sugary foods: Ice cream, sugar, maple syrup. candy, maple syrup, coconut

- Sweetened drinks: Juices, soda, sports drinks, flavored teas

- Pasta: All forms of noodles

- Grain products: Rice, wheat, cereals, oats, tortillas

- Starchy vegetables: Butternut squash, potatoes, corn, sweet potatoes, pumpkin, peas

- Beans and legumes: Chickpeas, black beans, kidney beams, lentils

- Fruit: Grapes, citrus, pineapple, bananas

- Sauces: sweet salad dressing, barbecue sauce, dipping sauces

- Some alcoholic beverages: Sugary mixed drinks, beer

- Unhealthy fats: margarine, vegetable oils like corn and canola, shortening

- Processed foods: Packaged foods, fast foods, and processed meats

- Diet foods: Preservatives, artificial colors, sweeteners like aspartame and sugar alcohols

A One-Week Sample Keto Menu

Note: The recipes which follow are all based on reasonable portions. While proportions of one ingredient over another depend on taste, we're basing these meals on a few standard measurements which should be applied across the board. Salad recipes are based on two cups of greens. Limit salad dressings to two tablespoons. Cream cheese or nut butters should be limited to one tablespoon. Cheese portions should be limited to two slices or one ounce. Vegetable and fruit portions between one and five pieces, depending on the size. Meat portions are generally six to eight ounces. All diets recommend six to eight glasses of water each day.

This menu was put together by dietary experts. It offers fewer than 50 grams of carbohydrates per day.

Monday
- Breakfast: Two fried eggs (pastured butter only) with sauteed greens

- Lunch: Grass-fed burger patty (no bun) topped with mushrooms cheese, and avocado on a bed of greens

- Dinner: Pork chops, sauteed green beans (coconut oil)

Tuesday
- Breakfast: Mushroom and cheese omelet

- Lunch: Tuna salad (with celery), a slice of beefsteak tomato, served on a bed of greens.

- Dinner: Roast chicken topped with cream sauce and served with sauteed broccoli (pasteurized butter)

Wednesday
- Breakfast: Stuffed bell pepper (cheese and eggs)
- Lunch: Arugula salad topped with turkey, blue cheese, hard-boiled eggs, and avocado
- Dinner: Grilled wild-caught salmon served with sauteed spinach (coconut oil)

Thursday
- Breakfast: Yogurt (full-fat) with Keto granola and/or blueberries
- Lunch: Steak bowl (cauliflower rice, herbs, cheese, salsa, avocado)
- Dinner: Bison steak with broccoli in a cheese sauce

Friday
- Breakfast: Baked avocado and eggs (whole)
- Lunch: Caesar salad with grilled chicken
- Dinner: Roasted or grilled pork chops with apple sauce and roasted vegetables

Saturday
- Breakfast: Cauliflower toast with avocado, cheese, and ground pepper
- Lunch: Wild-caught salmon burgers drizzled with pesto
- Dinner: Zucchini noodles and meatballs with parmesan cheese

Sunday
- Breakfast: Coconut milk chia pudding topped with walnuts and coconut
- Lunch: Cobb salad (greens, avocado, hard-boiled eggs, turkey, cheese)
- Dinner: Coconut chicken curry with cauliflower rice.

That's a week of satisfying and keto-friendly meals. But everybody likes to snack every now and then. So here are some healthy ketogenic snacks:
- Cheddar cheese and almonds
- An avocado half stuffed with homemade chicken salad
- Low-carb vegetables with guacamole
- Unsweetened trail mix
- Cocoanut chips
- Hard-boiled eggs
- Sliced salami and olives (green or black)
- Kale chips
- Peppers and celery with cream cheese dip
- Berries topped with heavy whipping cream
- Beef jerky
- Greens with avocado and high-fat dressing

- Macadamia nuts

- Avocado cocoa mousse

- Keto smoothie made with coconut milk, cocoa and avocado

The Ketogenic diet certainly has gotten a lot of attention, and that is only fitting. You'll note how elements of this diet recur in other popular diets. And there are other popular diets, after all. Let's take a closer look at them now.

CHAPTER ELEVEN: Other Popular Diets

The Paleo Diet

The paleo diet (also called the paleolithic or the *stone age* diet) is based on foods which are similar to those available during the paleolithic era, which lasted between 2.5 million to (as recently as) 10,000 years ago. This includes fish, lean meats, vegetables, fruits, seeds and nuts. Since farming became popular about 10,000 years ago, at the end of the paleolithic era, dairy products, grains, and legumes are also included (unlike the ketogenic diet).

The reasoning behind the paleo diet is that the body's genetic makeup does not fit its modern, processed diet. It holds that our bodies are basically unchanged from the paleolithic era, though our environment has changed drastically, as we've already discussed. This is called the *discordance hypothesis*.

People who choose the paleo diet often have similar goals, and a full body detox is often one of them. You may want to lose weight or to maintain an optimal and healthy body weight. Others may want assistance in meal-planning.

Like the ketogenic diet, the paleo diet comes with some variation, which makes it more flexible. In general, a new paleo dieter will be looking forward to eating the following foods:

- Fruits

- Vegetables

- Fruits

- Lean meats (grass-fed or wild game)

- Nuts and seeds

- Fish (salmon, albacore tuna, mackerel, any that are rich in omega-3 fatty acids

- Olive oil or walnut oil

The paleo diet basically avoids these foods:
- Grains: Wheat, barley, and oats

- Legumes: Lentils, beans, peas, peanuts

- Salt

- Dairy products

- Potatoes

- Refined sugar

- Processed foods

A Typical Paleo Diet Daily Menu

Just a reminder: These following recipes also follow reasonable-portion measurements. Salad recipes are based on two cups of greens. Limit salad dressings to two tablespoons. Cream cheese or nut butters should be limited to one tablespoon. Cheese portions should be limited to two slices or one ounce. Vegetable and fruit portions between one and five pieces, depending on the size. Meat portions are generally six to eight ounces. All diets recommend six to eight glasses of water each day.

With that in mind, here's a look at the first of several different sample menus, this one delineating what you might eat during a typical day following a paleo diet:

- Breakfast: Broiled salmon served with cantaloupe.

- Lunch: Broiled pork loin served with a salad (romaine, cucumber, carrot, walnut, tomatoes, tossed with lemon juice dressing).

- Dinner: Beef sirloin tri-tip (roast), steamed spinach or broccoli, salad (mixed greens, avocado, tomatoes, onions, topped with almonds and tossed with lemon juice dressing), and strawberries for dessert.

- Snacks: Celery stalks, carrot sticks, an orange.

A One Week's Sample Paleo Menu

Monday
- Breakfast: Kale, avocado, apple, banana, and almond milk smoothie
- Lunch: Mixed salad with fried seabass and pumpkin seeds, tossed in an olive oil dressing
- Dinner: Roast chicken with stuffing (carrots, onions, rosemary)

Tuesday
- Breakfast: Scrambled eggs with grilled tomatoes, spinach, and pumpkin seeds
- Lunch: Mixed salad with roast chicken, tossed in an olive oil dressing
- Dinner: Baked salmon with broccoli and asparagus (fried in coconut oil)

Wednesday
- Breakfast: Chopped bananas with almonds and blueberries
- Lunch: Mixed salad with salmon and tossed with an olive oil dressing
- Dinner: Stir-fry beef with onions and mixed peppers (fried in coconut oil)

Thursday
- Breakfast: Coconut oil-fried broccoli with a poached egg and toasted almonds
- Lunch: Mixed salad with boiled eggs, tuna, olive oil, and sesame seeds
- Dinner: Harissa-baked chicken legs or wings, served with steamed broccoli

Friday
- Breakfast: Spinach, mixed berries, and coconut milk smoothie
- Lunch: Broccoli, tomato, and butternut squash omelet, served with a mixed salad
- Dinner: Salmon stir-fry with broccoli, red pepper, baby corn

Saturday
- Breakfast: Eggs, bacon, and tomatoes pan-fried in virgin olive oil

- Lunch: Chicken and vegetable soup, served with turmeric

- Dinner: Lamb chops (grilled or roasted) with spiced red cabbage and spinach

Sunday
- Breakfast: Mushroom, tomato, and spring onion omelet

- Lunch: Mixed salad with avocado, chicken, olive oil, seeds

- Dinner: Beef stew and mixed vegetables.

Between meals, drinking water and getting plenty of exercise is recommended. The diet also emphasizes drinking water and being physically active every day. Several clinical trials compared the paleo diet to the Mediterranean Diet and the Diabetes Diet. They showed that the paleo diet may provide special benefits, including:
- Greater weight loss

- Improved blood pressure levels

- Greater glucose tolerance

- Better appetite management

- Lower triglycerides

The Mediterranean Diet

The Mediterranean diet is popular among doctors and nutritionists for the prevention of disease and maintain better health for longer. The Mediterranean diet is inspired by the foods of the countries surrounding the Mediterranean Sea, including Italy, Greece, and France. The diet emphasizes these foods:
- Fish

- Healthful fats

- Legumes

- Nuts

- Olive oil

- Vegetables

- Fruits

- Vegetables

- Whole grains

- Red wine

- Purple grapes

- Dark chocolate

The diet de-emphasizes these foods:
- Dairy

- Eggs

- Meat

- Refined grains (white flour)

- Refined oils (including soybean and canola oils)

- Sugary foods (pastries, sodas)

- Processed meats (hot dogs, deli meats)

- Packaged or processed foods

Like the ketogenic diet, the Mediterranean diet has a higher percentage of calories from fat than other diet regiments. Those are monounsaturated fats (like olive oil) so it may not be right for people watching their fat intake.

A One Week's Sample Mediterranean Menu

Note: With every day, a breakfast option of Greek yogurt with walnuts and blueberries is allowed.

Monday
- Breakfast: one fried egg on whole-wheat toast with grilled tomatoes and sliced avocado

- Lunch: Mixed salad greens with cherry tomatoes and olives on top and a dressing of olive oil and vinegar whole-grain pita bread 2 ounces (oz) of hummus

- Dinner: Whole-grain crust pizza with tomato sauce, various grilled low-carb vegetables, low-fat cheese, small pieces of ham, or chicken.

Tuesday
- Breakfast:1 cup of Greek yogurt with half a cup of fruits, such as blueberries, raspberries, or chopped nectarines. For additional calories, add 1–2 oz of almonds or walnuts.

- Lunch: Whole-grain bread sandwich with grilled vegetables (zucchini, eggplant, union, bell pepper) and spread with hummus or avocado.

- Dinner: Baked salmon or cod with black pepper and garlic, one roasted potato drizzled in olive oil and sprinkled with chives

Wednesday
- Breakfast: Whole-grain oats with dates, cinnamon, and honey topped with low-sugar fruits (blackberries or raspberries) shredded almonds (these are optional)

- Lunch: Boiled white beans with garlic, laurel, and cumin. Raw arugula tossed in an olive oil dressing and topped with cucumber, tomato, and feta cheese

- Dinner: Whole-grain pasta with olive oil, tomato sauce, grilled vegetables, Parmesan cheese

Thursday
- Breakfast: Two scrambled eggs (with onions, bell peppers, tomatoes topped with queso fresco

- Lunch: Roasted anchovies on whole-grain toast with lemon juice, served with a warm salad of steamed tomatoes and kale
- Dinner: Steamed spinach with herbs and lemon juice, a boiled artichoke with salt, garlic powder, and olive oil.

Friday
- Breakfast: Greek yogurt with honey and cinnamon, shredded almonds and chopped apple
- Lunch: Quinoa with sun-dried tomatoes, bell peppers, roasted garbanzo beans (with thyme and oregano), olives, topped with avocado or feta cheese crumbles
- Dinner: Steamed kale with cucumber, tomato, lemon juice, olives, and Parmesan cheese, grilled sardines served with a slice of lemon

Saturday
- Breakfast: Whole-grain toast (two slices) with soft cheese (queso fresco, ricotta, or goat) add chopped blueberries or figs
- Lunch: Mixed greens with cucumber and tomato, roasted chicken, olive oil, lemon juice
- Dinner: Vegetables roasted in olive oil (carrot, artichoke, eggplant, zucchini, tomato, sweet potato), served with one cup of whole-grain couscous

Sunday
- Breakfast: whole-grain oats with dates, cinnamon, maple syrup, low-sugar fruits
- Lunch: stewed yellow squash, zucchini, potato, onion, topped with a tomato/herb sauce
- Dinner: Spinach or arugula with olives, olive oil, tomato, a portion of white fish

Suitable snacks include:
- A small portion of nuts
- Whole fruits (oranges, grapes, plums)
- Dried fruits (figs and apricots)
- A small portion of yogurt
- A small portion of hummus with carrots, celery, or other low-calorie vegetables
- Whole-grain toast with avocado

The Atkins Diet

The Atkins diet, like the ketogenic diet, promotes low-carb intake for weight loss, though it may also improve or prevent various health conditions, such as heart disease and high blood pressure.

The Atkins diet was first created in 1972, but it's evolved a lot since then. Today, fifty years later, there are two distinct Atkins diets. Atkins 20 is the original diet, described below and based on a net carb intake of only 20 grams. The new Atkins 40 is not as and allows 40 grams of net carbs, double that of the first regiment.

Both versions of the diet consist of proteins, healthy fats, and vegetables (comparable to the ketogenic diet). In fact, some people consider the Atkins diet as a precursor to the ketogenic diet.

The Atkins diet features a Food Guide Pyramid, prioritizing food from bottom (to be eaten more) to top (to be eaten less). The pyramid includes whole grains such as oats, rice, and barley.

The pyramid does not include so-called *white foods*, including:

- White rice

- White sugar

- White potatoes

- White bread

- Pasta made with white flour

The Atkins diet is constructed and applied in phases. Net carbs vary in each phase.

Phase 1: Induction. This is where the regiment is the strictest. Dieters must forgo, entirely:

- Bread

- Fruit

- Starchy vegetables

- Grains

- Alcohol

- Dairy products (other than butter and cheese)

Phase 1 allows 20 grams of net carbs per day. The FDA recommends 300 grams daily. The idea is to increase the body's fat-burning ability. It's effective and motivational.

Phase 2 is notable for ongoing weight loss even as a few whole food carbs are reintroduced to the diet. These include:

- Legumes

- Berries

- Tomato juice

- Nuts

- Yogurt

Phase 2 allows 25 to 50 net carbohydrates per day. Phase 2 goes on until the dieter is within roughly 10 pounds of their target weight.

Phase 3 focuses on pre-maintenance and continues to add a increasing variety of carbohydrates, including more fruits, whole grains, and starchy vegetables.

Phase 3 allows between 50 to 80 net carbohydrates per day. This phase continues for roughly a month after reaching target weight.

Phase 4 is lifetime maintenance employing a low-carbohydrate (80-100 net carbohydrates daily) diet for the rest of the dieter's life.

If all this sounds familiar, it's because the Atkins diet relies on the same process of ketosis which the ketogenic diet uses.

A Journal of the American Medical Association study found that women on the Atkins diet lost 10 pounds on average and showed lower blood pressure and improved triglyceride levels.

But the Atkins diet suffers from the same drawback as the ketogenic diet; high fat intake is a danger to liver, kidneys, heart, and other organs and various systems throughout the body. Potassium and vitamin C are notably missing from the Atkins diet as well.

A One Week's Sample Atkins Menu

Like the current ketogenic diet (and really, Atkins is a ketogenic diet at heart), the Atkins diet is made up of 60–70% fat, 20–30% protein, and five to ten percent carbs. Net carb intake is limited to between 20 and 40 grams daily, mostly from mineral- and vitamin-rich vegetables. This sample diet averages about 20.5g daily net carbs.

Monday
- Breakfast: Scrambled eggs with cheddar cheese and sautéed onions
- Lunch: Deli ham over mixed greens with avocado, 5 large black olives, sliced cucumbers, and blue cheese dressing
- Dinner: Baked Catfish served with broccoli and butter
- Snacks: Atkins Peanut Butter Fudge Crisp Bar, 3/4 sliced zucchini and provolone cheese

Tuesday
- Breakfast: Atkins Frozen Sausage Scramble
- Lunch: Tuna salad with mixed greens, 3 cherry tomatoes
- Dinner: Lean pork chop served with cauliflower and cheddar cheese
- Snacks: Sliced red bell pepper with ranch dressing, celery with cream cheese

Wednesday
- Breakfast: Swiss cheese and spinach omelet
- Lunch: Grilled chicken over baby spinach, tomato, and avocado salad
- Dinner: Sauteed beef and vegetables over a bed of romaine
- Snacks: Atkins strawberry shake, ham with cream cheese, and a dill pickle spear

Thursday
- Breakfast: Spinach and cheese omelet with avocado and salsa on top
- Lunch: Atkins frozen crustless chicken pot pie
- Dinner: Hamburger topped with pepper jack cheese, small tomato, avocado, and romaine lettuce
- Snacks: Atkins French vanilla shake, Zucchini and Monterey jack cheese

Friday
- Breakfast: Two eggs, shredded cheddar cheese, salsa cruda
- Lunch: Atkins frozen chili con carne served with mixed greens and Italian dressing
- Dinner: Half of a cobb salad with ranch dressing
- Snacks: Atkins cafe caramel shake, sliced red bell pepper with ranch dressing

Saturday
- Breakfast: Red bell pepper stuffed with eggs scrambled with spinach and onion

- Lunch: Tuna salad (celery, dill pickle spear, mayonnaise)

- Dinner: Italian sausage, sliced onion and red bell pepper, served with baby spinach, sliced mushrooms, and blue cheese dressing

- Snacks: Atkins strawberry shake, one portobello mushroom cap stuffed with salsa cruda, and pepper jack cheese

Sunday
- Breakfast: Pumpkin pancakes

- Lunch: Grilled chicken breast served over romaine hearts with radishes and creamy Italian dressing

- Dinner: Baked Salmon served with charmoula and broccoli

- Snacks: Whole snap peas and cheddar cheese, celery and cream cheese

The Diabetes Diet

The diabetes diet is a plan for eating healthy that helps control blood sugar. Like a lot of the diets we've looked at so far (and all the best diets there are), the diabetes diet suggests eating only the healthiest food in moderate portions at regular mealtimes. The diet is rich in nutrients and low in calories and fat, relying heavily on whole grains, vegetables, and fruit. It's excellent diet for anyone on diabetes, naturally, but comes highly recommended for fasting, weight loss and weight management, and overall longevity. The diet may reduce risk of certain cancers and cardiovascular diseases. Consuming low-fat dairy products may reduce risk of low bone mass (osteoporosis loss of bone tissue).

Other benefits of the diabetes diet include:
- Control of blood sugar levels

- Control risk factors of heart disease and stroke

- Control high blood pressure

- Control high blood fats

- Prevent hyperglycemia, which can lead to kidney, nerve, and heart damage

The diet is great for these benefits, basically to control blood glucose levels, and weight loss.
The diabetes diet consists of three meals per day and always at regular times, which aids in insulin use. These meals focus on good fats, fish, fiber, and healthy carbohydrates.

Healthy carbohydrates? Sure! Carbs have their place, and not all carbs are the same. Sugars are simple carbohydrates, starches are complex carbohydrates which break down into blood glucose. So focus on healthy carbohydrates, such as:
- Vegetables

- Fruits

- Whole grains

- Legumes (peas and beans)

- Low-fat dairy (cheese and milk)

Fiber-rich foods include plant food and other things which the body doesn't absorb or digest and it helps moderate levels of blood sugar. High-fiber foods for this diet include:

- Fruits

- Vegetables

- Nuts

- Whole grains

- Legumes (peas and beans)

Heart-healthy fish are suggested for twice-weekly consumption. These include the fish we've looked at before (salmon, tuna, mackerel, sardines). Their wealth of omega-3 fatty acids may prevent various types of heart disease. Avoid frying the fish.

Just as there are healthy carbs, there are good fats, which we've already looked at in this book. These are the polyunsaturated and monounsaturated fats which lower cholesterol levels. Foods with these good fats include:

- Avocados

- Nuts

- Olive, peanut, and canola oils

Things to Avoid on the Diabetes Diet

Foods to avoid on the diabetes diet include any with saturated or trans fats. Saturated fats come from animal protein and high-fat dairy products. These include beef, butter, sausage, bacon, hot dogs, also palm kernel and cocoanut oils. Trans fats are found in baked goods, processed snacks, stick margarines, and shortening.

Avoid sources of cholesterol. They include organ meats, egg yolks, high-fat animal protein, and high-fat dairy products. The diabetes diet calls for 200 milligrams (mg) of cholesterol per day or less.

Avoid sodium. This diet calls for fewer than 2,300 mg daily. Sufferers of high blood pressure should consume even less.

Diabetes Diet Meal Plans

The American Diabetes Association has a simple and interesting way to balance meals on the diabetes diet. They call it the plate plan. It works by dividing your plate into quadrants for different foods: Half the plate is for non-starchy vegetables (carrots, spinach, tomatoes). One quarter of the plate with protein (lean pork, chicken, tuna) and the remaining quarter with a whole grain (rice) or starchy vegetable (green peas). Nuts and avocados may be added in small amounts. A serving of fruit or dairy may be added, and a glass of water or unsweetened coffee or tea.

A Sample Diabetes Diet Menu

This weekly menu provides 1,200 to 1,600 calories per day. It may be tailored for those who require more calories per day.

- Breakfast: Whole-wheat bread with jelly, shredded wheat cereal with one-percent percent low-fat milk, one piece of fruit, one cup of coffee

- Lunch: Roast beef sandwich (wheat bread, lettuce, tomato, low-fat American cheese, and mayonnaise) one apple, water

- Dinner: Salmon, small baked potato, carrots, green beans, one dinner roll, unsweetened iced tea (add milk to taste)

- Snack: Popcorn with margarine

The Hormone Diet

We've taken a look at how integral good hormonal balance is to overall good health, and how impactful hormonal imbalance can be. But hormones are complex; they're varied and diverse in form and function. For example, hormones can affect weight and can be affected by it. So whether a dieter is concerned about correcting hormonal imbalance or losing weight, both are likely to be affected by a change in diet.

It's well-known, for example, that hormonal fluctuations likely affect weight gain (particularly belly fat), sluggishness, lagging libido, stress, sugar cravings, and other health problems.

Some experts favor a variant on the Mediterranean diet, which proports to be good for weight loss and energy levels.

This approach, known as the glyci-med diet, starts with the Mediterranean diet but adds foods which are low on the glycemic index (these foods raise blood sugar slowly, whereas foods high on this index raise blood sugar quickly).

The hormone diet has proven beneficial for those suffering from diabetes, hypertension, and heart disease.

Like the Mediterranean diet, the best diet for hormone health includes:

- Lean protein (eggs, chicken breasts, wild-caught fish)

- Vegetables and most fruits (most nuts, flaxseeds, chia seeds, flaxseeds)

- Olive oil (unsaturated oils like canola)

- Whole grains (buckwheat, quinoa, brown rice)

Meanwhile this minimizes or eliminates:

- Alcohol

- Caffeine

- Processed meats

- Fried foods

- Peanuts

- Full-fat dairy

- Saturated fat

- Artificial sweeteners

- Hi-GI carbohydrates

This diet does not indulge fasting. Dieters eat every three to four hours. The healthy meals will be consumed at a rate of 80%, leaving two meals out of ten as *cheat meals* to make the diet more sustainable. Some people observe the diet six days out of the week and give themselves a *cheat day*.

You'll eat often -- every 3-4 hours -- making healthy food choices at least 80% of the time. But you do get one to two "cheat meals" a week.

Like some of the other diets, the hormone diet is progressive. After a few weeks at the beginner level described above, dieters will advance to a medium-level regiment. It takes more effort, but it brings it better results. Note that it's best done progressively and it's not advised to jump into an advanced level without doing the beginning level first. This holds true for all the diets and regiments in this book.

For this next level, dieters abandon all alcohol, caffeine, diary, sugar, gluten, dairy, and most oils for at least two weeks. Instead, dieters add supplements, such as calcium, magnesium, vitamin D3, and omega-3 fatty acids.

As with all these diets (except the Atkins), the hormone diet relies on organic or whole foods, cooked fresh and not processed.

Since this diet is not a fast, getting regular exercise isn't a problem. This diet recommends about half-an-hour, six days a week. Full-body strength, interval training, cardio, and yoga are all recommended.

The diet is especially convenient for vegetarians and vegans, those who live gluten-free. Some of these organic and gluten-free ingredients will be more expensive than other foods, dieters should be warned. And as this is a hormone diet, hormone tests may be advisable to track progress and check for unexpected results. Those tests may not be covered by the dieter's insurance and could turn out to be rather costly.

This diet, like others, favors:

Cruciferous vegetables, which help livers metabolize the hormone estrogen and prevent estrogen-dominant cancers (Brussels sprouts, cauliflower, cabbage, kale, and bok choy)

Salmon and albacore tuna, which have the cholesterol needed to make male sex hormones such as testosterone and healthy omega-3 fatty acids, which help hormonal communication (Albacore tuna, flaxseed, walnuts, olive oil, chia seeds, avocados). Salmon also stabilizes the body's hunger hormones, controlling appetite

Avocados are rich in beta-sitosterol, to balance cortisol levels and positively affect cholesterol levels. Plant sterols influence progesterone and estrogen, hormones responsible for ovulation and menstrual cycle regulation.

Organic vegetables and fruits avoid the hormone-killing pesticides and chemicals like glyphosate, known endocrine-disrupters which reduce fertility, among other detrimental side-effects.

High-fiber carbohydrates (vegetables, fruits, whole grains) are known to clear out excess hormones, as well as facilitate chemical bonding and subsequent removal of active but unbound estrogens. Sweet potatoes, carrots, squashes, and other root vegetables are popular choice.

As we've discussed, probiotics are the so-called good bacteria in the gut. Prebiotics, on the other hand, are fibrous foods which those bacteria eat and thrive upon. To give you an idea of how important they are, the gut is the human body's largest endocrine organ. It creates and secretes over 20 hormones, each of which play a role in metabolism, appetite, and satiety (fullness). Prebiotic foods such as raw oats and garlic, dandelion, asparagus, apples, almonds, chicory, bananas, and Jerusalem artichokes. Kimchi and yogurt are rich in prebiotics as well.

On the other hand, there are foods which may only complicate a dangerous hormonal imbalance. They include fried foods, processed foods, sugar and sugar substitutes. These may ultimately impact the balance of the hormones ghrelin and leptin. Alcohol is a hormonal disrupter on a number of levels, from estrogen metabolism to blood sugar management.

So now we have a better idea of foods and how to use them, as that is truly what a diet is all about. But no diet protocol can cover every need your body will have. Not even the most clever dieter can get by just on the ketogenic diet or any other. Because as a diet progresses toward its target, especially in the early part of the diet, supplements may be crucial to success, even to survival. They're important during fasts, during diets and for overall wellness management. So lets take a look at the supplements you may be in desperate need of, some you may know well and some which will be entirely new to you.

Vegetarian and Vegan Diets

When well-planned, a vegetarian diet can be a very healthy way to meet daily nutritional needs. They continue to be popular for their various health benefits, including a reduction of risk of some cancers, diabetes, and heart disease.

They also parallel a lot of the other practices in this book, including fasting. And there are different kinds of vegetarian diets too, catering to different needs and different tastes. Lacto-vegetarian diets cut out fish, meats, eggs, poultry, but not dairy products such as cheese, milk, butter, and yogurt.

The ovo-vegetarian diet excludes meat, seafood, poultry, and dairy products, but it allow eggs. The lacto-ovo diet excludes fish, meat, and poultry, but it allows eggs and dairy products. Pescatarian diets exclude poultry meat, eggs, and dairy, but it does allow fish.

Vegan diets exclude poultry, eggs, meat fish, and dairy products, and all foods which contain any of these products.

The flexitarian diet is a plant-based diet, but it includes occasional, small portions of meat, dairy, eggs, poultry and fish.

A good vegetarian diet gets the most out of a spectrum of plant-based, healthy foods. Include fruits and vegetables, nuts and legumes, whole grains. Sugar-sweetened fruit juices and refined grains should be avoided.

This vegetarian diet offers daily portions based on 2,000-calorie diet Food group. As with all our recipes, observe the consistent measurements: vegetables and fruits at 1.5 – 2 cups (2 – 3 in these cases, as there is no meat in the diet), dressings to two tablespoons, pieces or slices of fruit and vegetables sides to between 1 and 5, salads at two cups of leafy greens. But here is where this diet differs, at his has significant grain and dairy portions which diets like the ketogenic diet do not have. Six and a half ounces of whole grains are recommended, dairy at three cups a day, protein foods at 3-4 ounces a day. The vegetarian diet also requires oils, from nuts or olives, at about 25-30 grams a day.

This diet, and the related vegan diet, also require a bit more supplementation, as they reduce or eliminate the natural sources of:

- Calcium and vitamin D: for strong bones and teeth, found in dark green vegetables, soy

- Vitamin B-12: necessary to producing red blood cells and preventing anemia

- Protein: maintains healthy bones, organs, muscles, and skin

- Omega-3 fatty acids: important for hearth health

- Iron and zinc: crucial for red blood cells

- Iodine: a vital component of thyroid hormones

Monday
- Breakfast: Overnight baked eggs bruschetta (baked in a casserole dish)

- Lunch: Arborio rice and white bean soup (arborio rice)

- Snacks: Cheese and fruit kabobs with yogurt

- Dinner: Grilled vegetarian pizza

Tuesday
- Breakfast: Shakshuka (poached eggs with onion, cumin, and tomatoes)
- Lunch: Roasted sweet potato salad with a honey-maple vinaigrette dressing
- Snack: Portobello bruschetta drizzled with rosemary aioli (caramelized onions and broiled peppers)
- Dinner: Vegetarian enchiladas (eggplant, corn, summer squash)

Wednesday
- Breakfast: Protein parfaits (yogurt, nuts, and fruit and nuts)
- Lunch: Mediterranean bulgur bowl (bulgur wheat, veggies, cheeses)
- Snack: Deviled eggs (with horseradish)
- Dinner: Lentil tacos

Thursday
- Breakfast: German Apple Pancake
- Lunch: Roasted sweet potato with chickpea pitas
- Snack: Stuffed mini peppers (with cheese and chives)
- Dinner: Pepper ricotta primavera (garlic, herbs, and pepper, ricotta cheese)

Friday
- Breakfast: Oatmeal waffles
- Lunch: Mozzarella-stuffed mushrooms and garlic toast
- Snack: Roasted beetroot with garlic hummus
- Dinner: Veggie pad Thai

Saturday
- Breakfast: Mushrooms Florentine (portobello)
- Lunch: Quinoa-stuffed squash (quinoa, garbanzo beans, pumpkin seeds)
- Snack: Chewy Honey Granola Bars
- Snack: Chewy Honey Granola Bars
- Dinner: Black bean tortilla pie

Sunday
- Breakfast: Black Bean & White Cheddar Frittata (with salsa, chipotle pepper)
- Lunch: Spinach quesadilla
- Snack: Homemade guacamole
- Dinner: Grilled bean burgers (garlic, cumin, chili powder)

Now here's a seven-day menu for those on a vegan diet. Note: For this diet plan, snacks should be limited to moderate portions of whole fruit or vegetables. Recipes should follow comparable recipes, or they'll be easy to find in many variations online.

Monday
- Breakfast: Mixed fruit smoothie

- Lunch: Hummus wrap

- Dinner: Spaghetti with shishito pepper and charred tomatoes and shishito peppers

Tuesday
- Breakfast: Peanut butter banana oatmeal

- Lunch: Portobello soup

- Dinner: Pizza burrito

Wednesday
- Breakfast: Avocado toast

- Lunch: Low-fat mashed chickpea sandwich (with vegetables)

- Dinner: Black bean enchilada burgers

Thursday
- Breakfast: Cacao smoothie

- Lunch: Black bean burrito

- Dinner: Low-fat taco bowl

Friday
- Breakfast: Berry Cobbler Overnight Oats

- Lunch: Balsamic spinach wrap (balsamic, salt, maple syrup, smoked paprika) over avocado and spinach

- Dinner: Pizza with veggies, chickpea sausage crumbles and creamy drizzle

Saturday
- Breakfast: Avocado pizza toast

- Lunch: Mediterranean wrap

- Dinner: Enchilada burrito

Sunday
- Breakfast: Banana split overnight oats

- Lunch: Flatbread with white bean puree with asparagus

- Dinner: Leftover easy black bean enchilada burger

CHAPTER TWELVE: Natural Supplements

Our look into autophagy, fasting, weight loss, the molecular details of fats and cholesterol, and diets optimal health must now bring us to the realm of vital nutrients, vitamins, and minerals, and where to find them for your diet.

Holistic, organic, or natural healthcare may sound like far-out concepts, but chances are you or someone you know is already relying on it. According to the World Health Organization (WHO), 65 to 80 % of the global populace uses naturopathic, holistic medicine as their primary type of healthcare. In the United States alone, 38% of adults and even 12% of children have received one type of alternative medicine or another.

Keep in mind here that volumes have been written about these essential vitamins, minerals, herbs, and proteins. Each has a number of purposes, benefits, and side effects. As always, we strongly recommend you work closely with your specialist or physician before introducing anything new to your diet regiment. If there are any significant risks, we will include them here. But we will have to focus on the benefits as they relate to the subject of this book; fat burning, fasting, autophagy, hormonal balances. So while a lot of these nutrients may have benefits of other sorts, we're going to limit our study to the most relevant applications of each; weight loss, fat burning, fasting, and cellular regeneration.

Proteins, Enzymes, Vitamins, Minerals, Nutrients

Amino Acids: Amino acids are known as *the building blocks of all proteins*. They are intermediates in metabolism and must be ingested every day.

Beta-carotine: Beta-carotene is one of a group of natural chemicals known as carotenes or carotenoids. Beta-carotine boosts immunity and combats high blood pressure, its most applicable functions to our purposes here. It also aids immune-enhancing activity, proper cell communication, reproductive health, and is powerful antioxidant.

Vitamin B Complex: Vitamin B is compromised eight compounds: thiamine, niacin, riboflavin, folate, biotin, vitamin B6, folate, vitamin B12, and pantothenic acid and biotin: The vitamin B complex.

Thiamine: Thiamine (Vitamin B1) aids in the metabolism of carbohydrates and amino acids.

Riboflavin: Riboflavin (Vitamin B2) converts proteins, fats, and carbohydrates into energy.

Niacin: Niacin (Vitamin B3) helps synthesize fat and cholesterol, aids in the metabolism of carbohydrates, proteins and fat.

Pantothenic Acid and Biotin: Pantothenic Acid and Biotin (Vitamin B5 and vitamin B7) work together to convert carbohydrates, proteins and fats into energy.

Vitamin B-12: The body requires vitamin B12 for using certain amino acids and fatty acids which are essential to make DNA in your cells.

Vitamin B-6: Vitamin B-6 helps metabolize certain enzymes and make proteins. Vitamin B-5 helps to preserve normal immune and gastrointestinal function. Patients who are recovering from heart attacks are not advised to take vitamin B complex.

Conjugated Linoleic Acid: Conjugated Linoleic Acid (CLA) helps burn body fat, combat cardiovascular disease, fight high blood pressure, lower triglycerides and high cholesterol, boost insulin resistance and reduce inflammation.

Coenzyme Q10 (CoQ10): CoQ10 is an enzyme naturally found in every mitochondrial cell. About 95% of the body's energy is produced by these cells, converting fats and sugars into energy. Most of the body's CoQ10 is found in the internal organs, where they're needed most. CoQ10 is used to treat high blood pressure, obesity, diabetes, high cholesterol, heart disease, and immunity disfunction. CoQ10 is an energizer and an antioxidant and energizer, preventing free radicals and scavenging for those already free.

Curcumin: Curcumin is an anti-inflammatory agent which as ant-carcinogenic, antioxidant, anti-inflammatory, and antimicrobial properties are exceeded by it's applications against gastrointestinal disorders, cardiovascular disease, gastrointestinal disorders, and liver disease. Curcumin is also a free radical scavenger and reduces free radical production. Curcumin has shown promise for cholesterol, treating diabetes and supporting heart health.

Vitamin C: Vitamin C promotes wound-healing and is to develop and maintain connective tissues like muscle and fat. It has anti-cholesterol and anti-diabetic qualities as well as being a powerful antioxidant and a booster to overall metabolism and detoxification.

Vitamin D: Vitamin D is used treat conditions of the heart and blood vessels, including high cholesterol and high blood pressure. It's beneficial for weight loss too, and is also used for a host of other conditions and diseases far too long to go into here.

Vitamin E: Vitamin E is popular for preventing and treating heart and blood vessel diseases including hardening of the arteries, heart attack, high blook pressure, diabetes, and other maladies. Vitamin E is sometimes used for improving physical endurance, increasing energy, reducing muscle damage after exercise. It is also an antioxidant.

Glutathione: Glutathione is recycled in the body, except when the toxic load becomes too great. Glutathione collects and cools off the free radicals and recycles other antioxidants.

All toxins cling onto glutathione, which carries them to the stool and the bile and out of the body. Higher glutathione levels reduce recover time, decrease muscle damage, and increase strength and endurance to shift metabolism away from fat production and toward muscle development.

Magnesium: Magnesium is essential to good health, the fourth most-abundant mineral in the human body. Approximately 50% of total body magnesium is found in bone. The other half is found predominantly inside cells of body tissues and organs. It maintains normal muscle function, heartbeat, regulate sugar levels and normal blood pressure. It may be connected to energy and protein metabolism.

Melatonin: Melatonin is a sleep aid, ideal for helping distracted fasters sleep through some hungry nights. It may also help with weight loss on its own. It's also used to treat high blood pressure and diabetes. Melatonin is possibly unsafe for use during pregnancy. Children should not use Melatonin.

Quercetin: Quercetin is a powerful antioxidant which may protect against heart disease, high blood pressure, respiratory infections.

Resveratrol: Resveratrol is an anti-inflammatory, antioxidant, anti-inflammatory substance found in red wine and dark chocolate, green teas, and some nuts. Resveratrol lowers cholesterol and protects against LDL oxidation. Resveratrol may also reduce inflammation, reverse obesity and diabetes and obesity. Resveratrol turns on a cell's natural survival pathways, Which prevents damage to individual cells. It may also aid in nutrient intake, weight loss, and remove accumulated toxins.

Zinc: Zinc, a metal, is known as an essential trace element, and is useful in treating type 2 diabetes.

Herbs

Alfalfa: Alfalfa is an excellent natural diuretic and laxative. It detoxifies the urinary tract and fights urinary tract infections. It's a very good neutralizer of intestinal acids and eases digestive problems including gastritis and indigestion. Alfalfa contains high levels of enzymes ideal for digestion. It may lower bad forms of cholesterol and stabilize blood sugar levels. Alfalfa Leaf is a powerful natural source of many essential vitamins including the entire complex of B-vitamins, A, E, D, E and K which is important for blood clotting.

Artichoke Leaf: Artichoke leaf treats chronic gastrointestinal and some gallbladder and liver conditions entailing high blood fat values. It's an antioxidant and choleretic.

Cascara Sagrada: Cascara Sagrada may improve the colon walls' muscle tone in addition to its powers as laxative.

Corn Silk: Corn silk is used to treat diabetes, congestive heart failure, and high blood pressure.

Ginger: Ginger relieves gas pains, indigestion, stomach cramping, and diarrhea, It stimulates blood circulation, removing toxins and cleansing the kidney and bowels.

Pollen Extracts: Pollen extracts are known for their smooth muscle relaxation and anti-Inflammatory action.

Reishi: Red Reishi may enhance your immune system and improve your blood circulation. It's also used to high blood pressure, anxiety, high blood pressure, among other things.

And there's a virtual cookbook for necessary proteins, vitamins, nutrients, what they do and how to get them. Keep this chapter bookmarked for easy reference, as you may want to go back to it time and again.

And when you're ready, you can move on to the other big step on your journey toward wellness. You've been through fasting, stimulating autophagy, defined our goals as to fat and cholesterol, chosen a diet, chosen the right supplements. Now it's time tor the next big step on your journey to total wellness.

Exercise.

SECTION 5: EXERCISE

CHAPTER THIRTEEN: Exercising During Fasts

We've looked at various sorts of fasting, the benefits and the risks. Some of our analyses have touched upon exercise, when it was well-advised and when it was not. We never recommend lethargy, but over-exertion when the body's resources are depleted can have dangerous and even deadly effects (on the heart, for example, as we've seen). There are risks, and there are benefits, and there are specific regiments which are better for some types of fasting than others. So let's take a closer look at this crucial part of a cleansing regiment and of a healthy lifestyle.

Exercising for Intermittent Fasting

Exercising is especially important when intermittent fasting. Because the dieter is still taking considerable amounts of calories (sometimes only half of their usual intake). That means their exercising regiment shouldn't be reduced by any more than half as well. In fact, exercise at this time will invigorate autophagy and reset the body for a more vigorous, energetic lifestyle. It also redirects the body's energies toward muscle growth, and muscle loss is a risk of fasting of any kind.

It's more than just the advantages of exercising during fasting, but the detriment to the body if one does not exercise during intermittent fasting.

Lethargy during fasting not only resets your body to a lethargic pace, but body reads this as a signal that the body is weak, too weak to manage a healthy fast (even if it is).

It tells your body you're too weak to handle a fast. In our paleolithic past, fasts were followed by a hunt, so this is what the body expects. Change your body's expectations and soon it will expect and deliver nothing but lethargy. Just as your body can reprogram itself during ketosis, it can reprogram its body during fasting. Lethargy tells the body not to develop body mass. That will have effects on hormonal production and begin a cycle of slowed metabolism, weight gain, and greater lethargy.

This can convince the dieter (just as the dieter has convinced their body) that fasting is unhealthy and to be abandoned. This, of course, only furthers more destructive habits of overeating, lethargy, imbalanced blood sugar levels, all the things which inspired the decision to fast in the first place. The dieter has also taken one of their most potent weapons for longevity off the table, psychologically speaking at least.

Weight lifting is, by and large, a good exercise for fasting, as it focuses on muscle development. They're great for intermittent fasting, as there are always enough biological resources to divert attention toward muscle growth.

During intermittent fasting, general daily exercise is almost certainly adequate, perhaps even optimal. The body is already going through some extreme changes with the fasting, it doesn't need extreme physical exertion as well. Anything up to twenty-four hours in considered intermittent, and whatever the preferred mode of exercise is, it should suffice. Walking is always a good moderate form of exercise, though it's not very intense. Jogging is a bit higher impact, though anybody should check with their doctor before starting a jogging regiment. It can be hard on the joints and the heart. And since fasting can deplete essential minerals like calcium, care should be taken before running for extended periods.

Moderate calisthenics such as sit-ups, push-ups and pull-ups are also idea for exercise during intermittent fasting.

But some intermittent fasting requires abstinence (from caloric intake) for more than 24 hours, so they require a bit more of a deliberate application for maximum effectiveness and minimal risk. The longer the fast, the more care needs to be taken.

1. Walking: For longer periods of fasting, walking is all the more important as a form of exercise. It works muscle groups for growth, it burns calories, it instigates autophagy, increases metabolism. The movement

is good for digestion. It's good for the circulatory and respiratory systems, and helps clear toxins out of the body through perspiration and, later, urination and bowel movements.

Walking is also an excellent distraction. It gives a dieter time to think about other things besides fasting (and how hungry they are). Walking is famous for its opportunities to reflect, to think about other important things in life; social relationships, career challenges, plans for the future. Walking has a famously meditative quality, a calming effect that we'll look at in greater detail shortly.

Morning walks in particular are recommended during fasting. In fact, the fasted morning walk is an old bodybuilder trick for cutting body fat. The idea is to consume no calories before the walk and let the body use only reserves. After fasting through the night, the body will be ready to start using its resources. A fasted jog or even a cycle session forces body fat our of reserve and into circulation, to be expelled. Insulin is also generally low in the morning, aiding if fat burning.

2. Weights: As we've said briefly, lifting weights is a great way to preserve muscle during longer fasts. Strategies for weight lifting differ depending on whether the dieter is fasting intermittently or long-term. And, as we've said, the longer the fast, the more care has to be taken with exercise. So if you're fasting for 16 hours at a time, just go on lifting weights as you might normally do. Think about upping your reps, if you feel comfortable doing it.

But here are some tips if you're doing fasting for longer periods and you're concerned about muscle loss:

- Lift at higher intensities to lower the amount of reps in a single cycle

- Don't lift to failure (lifting until the final rep can't be completed)

- Don't max-out your repetitions during a longer-term fast

- Don't max-out on effort either. On a one-to-ten scale, keep it somewhere between six and eight

- Favor full-body exercises over isolated reps.

The whole body is undergoing autophagy, the cells and muscles of every part of the body are affected. So it only makes sense to spread that energy equally over every part of the body. And remember that fasting resets the body, and you don't want to instruct your body to focus on one part at the expense of the others. Your weightlifting regiment should match that.

Cardio: While fasting, so-called *easy cardio* is ideal, especially for extended fasts. And the longer the fasting goes, the easier the dieter should go with the exercise. Cardio is shorthand for endurance training, which is idea for fasting (which requires its own kind of endurance). During a long-term fast, keep your cardio intensity in the so-called *aerobic zone*, the heart rate at which the body is burning calories primarily from body fat. It's a moderate-to-high heart rate, but one which is sustainable and not overly intense. There's a handy equation to find your ideal aerobic heart rate: Your age subtracted from 180. If you're 50 years old, your ideal aerobic rate of beats per minute is 130. If you're 20 years old, your ideal beats per minute (BPM) is 160. Don't exceed these BPMs if you're fasting.

You won't feel overly taxed, which is good. That means your body is using fat as fuel, the easy way, instead of increased sugar cravings or using glycogen stores.

When fasts get longer, stay away from intense endurance training. Sprinting and jogging are likewise not recommended.

But it's not just what you eat, but when you eat it. All of the diets we recommended suggest regular eating times. And when you're exercising, that should be timed in correlation to eating windows.

Even during short-term fasting, you'll want to time your workouts a bit more deliberately. One study demonstrated that males on eating-window regiments who lifted to failure eight to twelve reps over four sets consumed 650 less calories than those who were not observing fasting eating windows. They retained and even improved muscle mass. However, the non-fasting group showed greater size gains.

A study in women found resistance training let to muscle gains even on a time-restricted eating schedule, as long as intake of protein and calories were maintained.

Most specialists suggest not breaking a fast immediately after a workout to augment the release of growth hormone, which burns fat and maintains tissues.

Exercise During Long-term Fasting

The longer you fast, the more careful you have to working out, right? So let's take a closer look at the potentially dangerous practice.

First, let's go back to the other caveat about fasting and working out. The longer you've been fasting, the less you want to exert yourself. It's also worth pointing out here (once again) that if muscle-building is your goal, fasting may not be your best approach. If you hope to slim down and then bulk up, fasting will help slim you down and working out will help you bulk up, those are two consecutive goals, each with a proper strategy, not one goal with an improper strategy.

If your goal is to maintain muscle mass during a fast (a good idea) then your reps and cycles and weight intensity should only be in accordance with the duration and intensity of the fast. If you're fasting a bit longer, lift a bit less. But do lift, as it prevents lethargy and atrophy. Consider a regiment of one to two days a week of full-body workouts while intermittent fasting.

Time workouts for the middle of an eating window so you can go home and have a good meal and replenish your nutrients.

Fasted cardio, which we touched on briefly before, is a favorite of athletes who are fasting. Their morning hours for fasted cardio are usually between seven and ten in the morning.

You may never have wondered what actually happens to fat when you exercise. As we've seen, stored glycogen is the first choice for the body's energy. After about a half-hour to an hour, the body begins burning fat.

Experts recommend at least 30 minutes of cardio two to three times a week. For weight loss and proper management, physical activity of up to an hour a day is often recommended, given normal dietary and medicinal intake.

(Remember to act responsibly with these or any exercises and consult your doctor.)

An Important Note

This is crucial for using this book from this point forward. We're about to start introducing exercises into this book, to use the knowledge you're accumulating and put it to real, physical use. Here, as they say, is when we start putting boots on the ground (or hands on the matt, as it were). And up until now, the likelihood is that you've been reading this book as a solitary endeavor (the way most books are written). But while you can read the upcoming exercise or yoga instructions and memorize them, that will be in conflict to the very goals of those applications. And nobody I've ever known could read and meditate at the same time. The two things are practically antithetical. And you certainly can't read to yourself during hypnosis.

So we have two recommendations for implementing the applications which are to follow. The idea is that you'll need somebody reading these yoga courses while you perform them, you'll need a voice to guide you while you meditate and during hypnosis.

One choice is to record your voice. It's as easy as downloading a smartphone voice recording app. Read the directions for the exercises and practices into the app and play them back for yourself. This frees you up to clear your mind and perform the often-complex maneuvers which these practices sometimes require. The benefits of this approach are: Convenience, since nobody else needs to be inconvenienced by your workouts; privacy, which fasters, dieters, and self-care practitioners crave and deserve; and self-control, since you can record the directions at the pace which suits you.

The drawbacks to this approach are that you lack the input of somebody who can see what you're doing wrong. That objective viewpoint is something you will be harder pressed to do for yourself, even with an adequate mirror.

These things do often require a certain amount of expertise to avoid injury and maximize the benefits. That's why so many people see yogis, exercise trainers, meditation coaches. Each of these schools have their own subtleties and challenges and many of us just don't know enough to work our way through it, DIY.

It's also a bit isolating, which it is sometimes meant to be. Other times, group support is helpful and even necessary.

Another approach is to include a second person in your workouts and meditations (and especially hypnosis). They don't have to be experts, as we'll provide the expertise. They just have to be willing and able. This approach has a lot of benefits and a few drawbacks too.

A second person provides support, encouragement, and perhaps expertise. But a second person can also improvise and contribute a perspective which no prerecorded voice can do. It's flexible, and flexibility is key to the systems we're manipulating and the way in which we manipulate them.

There is also the presence of a second person, which can't be underestimated. Feelings of isolation may lead to a sense of weakness, helplessness, and that may discourage further application.

It is also reciprocal in its own way. After your partner guides you on an exercise or a yoga session, you can turn around and guide them. That will only increase your understanding, even mastery of these techniques. This will give you the objective perspective you necessarily lack when engaged in your own exercises and applications. Having a partner means you can be a partner.

Drawback include convenience. A lot of people like you and me just don't have a second person on hand at all times of the day or night. A lot of these exercises require a certain amount of juggling to work into your schedule. Working them into two different schedules can be more than twice as difficult.

Also, you shouldn't be relying on anyone else for your progress. This is about you and you alone, at least at first. After you've made some progress you can help others, but the onus is on you to take those first steps, and you just may have to take them alone. If you do, you can still make the most of it.

In point of fact, your pursuit of these things may naturally take you from an isolated practice to one filled with support. Individual exercises will likely draw you to classes, to other like-minded people whom you can work with to achieve your mutual ends.

Either way, it would take a stone-cold genius to read and memorize these instructions and then instruct themselves while practicing to optimal effect. If that's you, congratulations! If not, start to think now about how you're going to help yourself through the more complex exercises and applications you're about to face.

But don't be discouraged by this. Don't be tempted to believe that you've gone as far as you can go and just give up. See it as an opportunity to reach out to others, to increase your social circle, to help others and to learn to accept help when its offered. These are milestones toward greater wellness on their own, even being willing to admit that help is needed is a significant step forward for you and any one you know. For now, there's still a bit more reading to do. Finish the book, familiarize yourself with what will be expected of you. Educate yourself. You may want to get a support friend or an exercise partner after you've finished reading. You may want that person to read this book to, so you're on the same page (if you'll pardon that expression). Of, if you can't wait, then download a voice recording app (to your laptop or desktop or tablet if you don't have a smartphone), roll up your sleeves, and prepare to get down to it.

Exercise Apps

Before you follow our exercise instructions, be aware that we're far from the only source of such things. In fact, we suggest use of apps and other books, videos, anything that will help you along on your journey to full-body wellness. Here are the best ones we could find online, and what they have to offer. Keep in mind that, as with all our lists of apps, detox kits, or any other product, we have no connection to any of them. We are not endorsing any specific brand or product, simply giving you the best information we can find to help you make the best decisions you can.

Keep in mind that, unlike previous apps, these apps are not all free. Some of them are quite pricey, actually.

Apple Fitness Plus is truly the head of the pack when it comes to monitoring your exercising via computer electronics. The subscription fitness service works for the watch and other devices such as the iPhone. The subscription is $9.99 per month.

PEAR Personal Fitness Coach is free and available for Android or iOS and it's free, but the subscription is $5.99 per month. Its specialties include:

- Hands-free, eyes-free audio coaching

- Guided workouts at a variety of levels.

- Wide variety of workout packages

- Performance tracking

- Sharing with other apps

Fitbit Coach is available for Android and iOS for a subscription of $39.99 per year or $7.99 per month. It allows the user to:

Log daily activities

Recommend exercise activities

Enjoy dynamic workouts which intuitively increase in difficulty according to input

Workout Trainer, free for Android and iOS: Free, plus different subscription rates starting at $6.99 per month). It offers:

- Training routines and exercises for newbies and veterans.

- A simple questionnaire

- Recommended workout plans and exercises personalized to the user's fitness goals.

- Reminders and notifications

- Streak tracking

- Stat tracking

- One-on-one trainers hired for various fitness specialties.

Peloton is available for Android and iOS for $12.99/£12.99 monthly. This app helps you conveniently (and safely) take advantage of what Peloton offers without the expensive (and allegedly dangerous) treadmill. The app is:

- Free to download

- Offers a 30-dayfree trial

- Guided workouts in just about everything from cardio to yoga to stretching.

- Group workouts

- Tag joining

  Fit Radio, for Andriod and IOs, has a number of unique features:

- It generates new playlists for every workout, designed to inspire.

- It serves different workouts from ellipticals to bike rides to low-density to high-density interval training

- Seven-day free trial ($9.99 after that)

Shred is available for Android and iOS for $12.99 monthly. As the name suggests, it's a favorite of fans of intense workouts. This is a good supplemental app to a traditional gym workout. Some benefits of the app are:

- Workout types options (bodyweight, gym, cardio)

- Shred community

- Interactive visuals

- Activity logging

- 7-day free trial

Seven, free for Android and iOS, offers:

- Seven-minute-a-day training

- Connection to friends to track progress

- 3D guides

- Subscription Seven Club ($9.99 monthly or $79.99 annually)

JEFIT is free to download for Android and iOS and specializes in bodybuilding and strength training. Special features include:

- Thousands of routines

- Routines sorted by target body part

- Detailed instructions

- Workout planner

- Progress tracker

- Exercise log

Belly Fat Exercises

1. Burpees: This is a great exercise for the core, and also for the chest, lats, shoulders, quads, triceps. In involves explosive plyometric movement and will get your heart pumping!
Note: When you do these exercises, the beginning stance is generally with your feel shoulder-distance apart. In other words, each foot is precisely under its corresponding shoulder.
So, with the burpee, you'll stand (feet being shoulder-distance apart) and push your hips back. Lower your body in a slow, low squat. Put your hands flat on the floor just outside of where your feet are. Then quickly push your feet back and straighten out, letting your chest touch (but not rest) on the floor. Push your hands flat and lift your body into a plank. Now reverse it and pull your feet back to where your hands are and stand up, all just as fast as you did the first half. The explosive nature of the cycle is crucial to its effectiveness. The move includes elements of the push-up and the power-squat.

Some people accentuate this exercise by holding a medicine ball. It's held in the hands at first before being lowered and left on the floor through the planking portion of the exercise, then picked up and raised at the end of the rotation.

2. Mountain Climbers: Like burpees, this moving plank exercise works a variety of muscle groups but focuses on the core.

Get into the same high-plank position you used for Berpees, wrists directly under the shoulders. Keeping the core tight, draw the belly button inward toward the spine. Drive the right knee inward toward the chest, then return the foot back to straighten the leg, bringing it back to the plank position. Then drive the left knee inward toward the chest, then return the leg to plank. Alternate right and left sides as many rounds as you wish.

3. Overhead medicine ball slams are great for the core, for endurance, for the heart rate. The heaviest ball you can manage, the better.

Stand with your feet hip-width apart (instead of shoulder width) and hold the medicine ball tightly with both hands. Stretch both arms up over your head, stretching your body. Slam the ball down and forward and down, bending your knees slightly as you hinge forward. Squat a bit to pick up the ball and stand again. Raising the ball again starts the cycle again.

4. Russian twists are great for the core and also improve definition and strength.

Start by sitting on the ground in a sit-up position, a medicine ball in both hands held at the chest. Raise your feet up off the floor, lean back to a 45-degree angle. Twist your torso right and left while holding the medicine ball in both hands, keeping your feet above the floor.

5. Running on an incline is a great way to burn fat. Running itself is good cardio, but an incline may increase that burn by as much as 50%. You might try start off with a walk or jog for five or ten minutes, then start jogging or even running. There's a lot of benefit to slowing to a walk for five to then, then jogging from five to ten, then alternating again. As you get stronger, consider extending the running portions of this rotation to twenty or thirty minutes or more, keeping the walking stretches to ten or even decreasing them to no more than five.

6. Rowing machines are a great way to work up the heart rate, burn calories and melt fat while you build muscles in the back, shoulders, arms, legs and core.

Here's an effective 4-minute cycle: Start with 20 seconds' rowing and ten seconds' rest. Remain in the rowing position when at rest, and note the miles or meters traveled. Repeat the cycle eight times, each time trying to improve your distance. After the eight rest, go for a quick 500 meters and see how long that takes. Try to beat this number the next time.

7. HIIT is based on the idea that short bursts of intense cardio are best for burning fat, as opposed to sustained periods of lower-intensity cardio.

After a 10-minute warm-up, do 30 seconds of as many repetitions as you can manage of any one thing: Push-ups, squats, single-arm rows, or kettlebell swings. Rest for 30 seconds and choose a different exercise for another 30-second round. Do this for ten rounds, ten different exercises. Make sure you choose the exercises to work different muscle groups.

8. Strength Training is a good way to lose weight too. While most weight lifting isn't designed to burn fat exclusively (that may be the goal but the effect is merely secondary). While moderately heavy weights are usually used for cardio or weight management, and very heavy lifting is designed for putting on muscle mass, there is an area in between which is perfect for burning fat.

If you're not lifting any weights, get some and start lifting; just a few hand weights at home will do the trick. If you're already lifting, increase the weight and duration of your workouts. This creates the afterburn effect, wherein fat is being burned even after the workout is over.

9. Walking has appeared before on our list of exercises for a variety of things, and that should come as no surprise. Walking is good for the body and the mind. It's good for metabolism, for autophagy, for virtually every system in the body.

Experts recommend between 45 and 60 minutes of brisk walking daily to improve metabolism. It also may prevent overtraining. Overtraining may lead to an excessive production of cortisol, the stress hormone which contributes to belly fat. Experts suggest that one hour's worth of rapid walking per day may generate one lost pound of fat per week.

From diet to exercise, our journey can only take us to one logical place, and that's Yoga. Yoga and fasting interconnect in a number of intriguing and educational ways. The mind and body have been getting closer and closer, from autophagy to fasting and then the rest, it's all been a long and complex intermingling of mind and body, with the mind continuously guiding the body toward more effective autophagy and greater overall wellness.

And, looking ahead, our next step will take us naturally to the one after that. At this point, it's important to note how one thing builds upon the one before it, and prepares one for what is next to come. This is why the stages aren't to be skipped, at least not in the first reading. Everything is mindful and deliberate to deliver you to the future you envision for yourself, which we'll get to in greater detail later.

For now, it's onward and upward (literally) into the world of yoga as it relates to fasting and the dietary practices you've been implementing. So unroll your matt, stretch out, and open your mind and your heart … and your hips. It's yoga time.

SECTION 6: YOGA FOR FASTING

CHAPTER FOURTEEN: Yoga for Fasting

Fasting Meets Yoga

Yoga and fasting actually have a lot in common. Each entail a great deal of discipline and physical stamina. Both are good for physical fitness and psychological wellness. Yoga requires the kind of meditative mindset which is critical to a successful fast, as we have seen.

And both are centered around the idea of detachment, or rising above the daily scurry of life to achieve a higher physical and mental state.

Both yoga and fasting ask us to resist temptation, to eschew instant gratification. If yoga is your principle focus, your main challenge may be to overcome lethargy and stay on the map. If fasting is your course, your challenges may be focused around your efforts to overcome hunger. Yoga is great for either, and there are certain yoga regiments for a fasting-friendly approach.

As we know, fasting allows our digestive functions to rest and to reinvigorate. Most of us run our systems around the clock and never think twice about it, much less give it a deliberate rest. But this book is all about being deliberate, being mindful.

There's another connection between fasting and yoga which makes them go perfectly together. Fasting rids the body of a lot of extra mass, either water weight or accumulated fecal matter, or fat reserves around the belly. Fasting for any duration rids the body of these obstructive weights. True, it takes more than fasting or yoga to keep the weight off, the loss of the weight makes the body more flexible, more capable of the elasticity yoga requires. And yoga, in return, stretches the muscles and keeps them growing, essential during a fast.

Fasting also has meditative qualities, as we've discussed. It calls upon users to recalibrate their relationships with food, and with our needs and desires to eat. It gives a faster more time to walk and to think about other things, if for no other reason than to distract the mind from the belly.

A lot of fasting is religious, some of it political. It's main purpose in these cases is to focus the mind by focusing the body. But the benefits of fasting are much broader, paving the way toward deeper states of awareness. All the world's major religions feature some form of fasting. Jews fast during Yom Kippur, Christians deny themselves certain things during the Lenten period before Easter Sunday, Muslims have Ramadan. In the lineage of Tantra Yoga, one of the niyamas has a direct relation to food consumption. Inspya Yoga's teacher training requires a ten-day detox.

Politically, Bobby Sands drew worldwide attention to the plight of the Irish Republican Army in the early 1980s. In 2021, Russian anti-Putin protestor Alexi Navalny staged a hunger strike after being arrested in Moscow.

But it's the spiritual realization of fasting which is particularly potent when it comes to yoga. Even when not in a spiritual or religious context, fasting brings mental clarity. We know this because of the autophagy which happens in the brain, improving performance (as it does for every organ). And that clearing of the mind is the hand and yoga is the key to unlock that spiritual realization.

As it is with fasting and diet and exercise, all things work together for the improvement of the whole in a well-balanced system.

So yoga can give the faster strength even as the faster brings improved flexibility. Focus and strength improve in both areas of life.

Both yoga and fasting give a person a feeling of accomplishment as well, verifiable and even immediate rewards for the efforts. The body feels better during and after yoga, as it does during and after a period of fasting (either short- or long-term).

Yoga is also right in line with intermittent fasting. In yoga, the suggested break between meals is a full eight hours. (This is to allow the excretory system to function properly.) That's breakfast, dinner, and no lunch. This is already one of the favored types of intermittent fasts we read about earlier. Just another way fasting and yoga seem to go hand-in-hand. In fast, fasting is a very common practice among yogis.

Yoga embraces various long-term fasting techniques, including water and juice fasts, as well as dry fasts for up to several days. A healthy person can manage a wet fast for up to five days. As long as or more than seven days is not recommended for anyone.

Here are a few tips to keep your yoga regiment going smoothly while you're fasting.

While motion is key to yoga, and some physical activity is important to fasting, there will be times when you may feel too weak or unmotivated for a lot of energetic movement which is sometimes required of yoga. In that case, and these may strike during a fast, there is always *seva* (selfless service or karma yoga), *pranayama* (breathing exercises), meditation and concentration. You might even spend some time simply reading and learning about yoga, which is definitely a part of the practice (and perfect if you just don't have the energy). If you find you consistently lack the energy for even a mild yoga session, you may be following a regiment lacking in proteins, healthy carbs, or healthy fats.

Make sure the timing is right for you. You may be choosing the wrong time of day or the wrong day of the week. Remember that timing and regularity are important in working out while fasting, and the same applies here. If you're consistently lacking in energy in the evenings, you may want to get up early and do your yoga sessions before the work day begins. If you're skipping lunch during your eight-hour fasting window between meals (a yogi practice as we've seen) you may spend your lunch hour doing yoga. If your work days are simply too busy with other things, you may consider doubling up on your yoga sessions on the weekends. If you're too tired from your work week and your diet is adequate, you may be working too hard. Meditation may be a good alternative to yoga, one we'll look at shortly.

If you're committing to a yoga regiment, start slow. If you're new to it, find some guidance if you can. There are lots of classes for people at different levels and it should be easy to find the right class for your level, location, and schedule. But don't get locked into a slower regiment. The whole idea of fasting, dieting, yoga, meditating, any of the practices we discuss, is to keep going with them, to let your practices evolve as you evolve. The more you need, the more you should take. The less you can handle, the more you should leave on the table.

Beginners may start with a couple of rounds of sun salutation and five or so other poses of choice, and investigating more static and gentler practices like Yin Yoga (where in each pose is held for between three and ten minutes). Yin Yoga is ideal for releasing connective bands and tissues around the muscles. This provides a better opportunity for the body to relax, promoting circulation and clearly blockages.

These practices help reduce *tamas* (darkness, chaos) and *rajas* (passion, confusion) and promote *sattva* (purity). So fasting may include keeping one's surroundings and one's body clean, abstaining from lying or gossip, controlling negative emotions such as anger and a cranky mood.

Some *Pranayama* (breathing exercises) which can be easily perform while fasting include Diaphragmatic Breathing (yogic breathing), which calms the mind and brings focus in times of distraction. Another is *Bhramari Pranayama* (bee breath) for a deepen of concentration and preparation for meditation.

Here are other good poses for yogic fasting:

- *Bhujangasana* (Cobra pose)

- *Setu Bandhasana* (Bridge pose)

- *Balasana* (Child's pose)

- *Ardha matsyendrasana* (Seated spinal twist)

- *Paschimottanasana* (Seated forward fold)

- *Shavasana* (Corpse pose for relaxation)

Admittedly, this is hardly an encyclopedia of yoga terms and positions. Entire books have been written on that subject, and you're well-advised to get one, preferably an illustrated book (there are lots of them).

But we hope you've achieved a working knowledge of what yoga is, why you might be doing it, and how to get the most out of it while fasting. We've also tried to show how yoga will help you get the most out of fasting.

Before we put all that to use on your body and mind, let's take a quick look at popular yoga apps.

Yoga Apps

Yoga Studio is a top-ranked yoga app which has a number of impressive benefits, including:
- High-quality content

- Ease of use

- Excellent value

- Numerous custom classes

- Focus on balance, flexibility, strength, and relaxation

- Ideal for back pain

- Custom flow creation

- Schedule and track classes

- Library of over 280 poses

- Choose or create music tracks

- Subscriptions by the week

Down Dog is also popular, mostly for these features:
- Useful as you progress

- Routines and lessons for all levels

- Different practice durations (from ten minutes to 110)

- Generates new sequences

Daily Yoga specializes in community motivation and support. It's most popular features include:
- Weekly activities for motivation

- 200 guided yoga classes, 500 asanas, 50 work out plans (with subscription)

- Multi-week programs

- Constant additions of new videos and programs

Glo is a popular app for yogis and those who are too busy for regular studio classes. It offers:
- Five-, Ten-, or 20-minute classes

- User friendly app

- Challenging and beginner friendly classes

Simply Yoga is great for kids (and adults) who are at the beginner level. It offers:
- Sequences of 20, 40, or even 60 minutes

- Easy-to follow instructions

- 21-day or 30-day challenges

That should be enough info to get you started on finding the best yoga app. Now let's put this knowledge into some serious practice with a specially designed program for yoga during fasting.

CHAPTER FIFTEEN: A Program for Yoga During Fasting

We're already seen the benefits of periodic fasting. And practicing yoga only amplifies the power of the resets of autophagy which comes about during fasting. So here is a program to cleanse the mind and the body in more powerful ways.

As always, the usual caveat apply: Consult a doctor, follow prescribed guidelines, do not strain yourself to the point of injury.

This program is flexible. If you're planning a one day fast, just practice the first day's exercises. Feel your way through the week and stop if you feel you need to. Both yoga and fasting require gradual assimilation, and that's even more important when you're doing both at once. Re-evaluate after your third day, if you get that far, and see if you shouldn't take a break in your fast and repeat those three days the following week, to take it further then if you feel up to it. Good change is gradual change.

This program is a three-, four-, or five-day program wherein you remove a food from your diet and add a yoga practice in its place. The duration is flexible upon the user's requirements and abilities.

This program offers two yoga classes from which to choose, one more rigorous and one more gentle. The rigorous classes gradually decrease in intensity as energy reserves decrease. But one body may be more energetic one day and less so the next, so the options make the most of this natural tendency. And if you repeat the program, you can switch every class from the one you did the cycle before, giving you an almost-endless combination of classes in any given week. Remember to do one class per day only, don't try to do two or three options in a single day.

The program also includes a meditation option for each day, as meditation is an important part of what yoga and fasting are all about. And just as being active helps to properly reset the body after autophagy, meditation resets the mind on the right track in the same way. We will look at such meditative practices as they relate to fasting in the next chapter, but they belong here as part of the week-long program.

This program is ideal for those interested in the mental and physical benefits of fasting, beginning and advanced yoga practitioners, and anyone interested in complimenting their health regiment with yoga.

Note that the program entails one yoga position after the next, but we also understand that you might not know all the positions by name. So we'll lean toward describing the action and naming the positions when we can.

Day 1
Gentle Option: Toxic Twist

This detox class is first exercise for a reason; it's great for setting the body's reset button. It's hard work and really gets your juices flowing to kickstart a new detoxification regiment.

Twisting the body cleanses the liver and the kidneys. And there are plenty of twists in this class in different variations and with different variations. Drink plenty of water during and particularly after the toxic twist or its more rigorous option.

Start with a downward-facing dog position, which is feet and hands on the floor, legs straight, head down. Exhale. Lower your body flat on the floor, touching down before curling your spine to lift your head up, hands on the floor at the sides of your chest. This is the tall cobra position. Arch your back and raise your head, inhaling, then lower back down while you raise your up off the floor. Keep your knees and hands on the floor, arms straight, head down, breathing deeply. Then return to downward-facing dog pose again.

Raise the left leg up behind you as far as you can, keeping the leg straight and the toes extended. Then bring your left leg back and all the way in, touching your left knee to your chest, hands still on the ground. Left foot on the floor, lift up your body, raising your hands above your head. Lower your hands to your heart and look down.

Put your right hand on the floor and twist to reach up with your left hand as you exhale. Hold and stretch, then return your left hand to the floor as you exhale. Return your right hand to the floor and straighten your right leg back. Return to the downward-facing dog position.

Exhale and straight your body as you lower your belly and chest to the floor, exhaling. Curl your back up in tall cobra position, hands flat on the floor as you pull yourself up, spine arching, head back, inhaling. Hold that position.

As you exhale, keeping your hands and knees on the floor, push yourself back, facing down. Your weight is on your calves in this position, you knees wide apart. Turn your palms upward to twist your arms and shift your hips a little to one side, then the other.

Now we'll do the same to the right side.

Raise the right leg up behind you as far as you can, keeping the leg straight and the toes extended. Then bring your right leg back and all the way in, touching your right knee to your chest, hands still on the ground. right foot on the floor, lift up your body, raising your hands above your head. Lower your hands to your heart and look down.

Put your left hand on the floor and twist to reach up with your right hand as you exhale. Hold and stretch, then return your right hand to the floor as you exhale. Return your left hand to the floor and straighten your right leg back. Return to the downward-facing dog position.

Exhale and straight your body as you lower your belly and chest to the floor. Curl your back up in tall cobra position, hands flat on the floor as you pull yourself up, spine arching, head back, inhaling. Hold that position.

As you exhale, keeping your hands and knees on the floor, push yourself back, spine parallel to the floor, head facing down. Your weight is on your calves in this position, you knees wide apart. Turn your palms upward to twist your arms and shift your hips a little to one side, then the other.

Repeat as desired.

Rigorous Option: Soft Heart with A Twist; Chaturanga Free Practice

Trusting our legs and core to be strong, yoga allows the heart to be oft. The movement to ease the heart space is the backbend. Twists and side bends expand space in the ribcage and in the heart. This practice is wrist-friendly.

Start with arms up, knees slightly bent. Lower the body to rest on the knees. Bring the right knee forward and up, foot on the floor and raise the left arm up straight. Then lean to the right, stretching your left arm as you breathe deeply. Hold that position.

Then twist and lower your right arm to touch your right elbow to the outside of your left knee. Your left hand is pointing up toward the ceiling, palm flat. Now raise your right arm and place your right hand flat against your left, palm-to-palm. Allow your right hip to move toward your left knee. Press your left elbow into your right knee. Turn your face rightward toward the ceiling and look up. Expand the capacity of your lungs, the capacity of your heart. Exhale. Straighten your spine and reach up, arms straight. Lower your hands, palms to the floor as the left knee rises. Inhale as you half-lift your body, right leg straight, toes and fingertips on the floor.

Bring your feet together, legs slightly bent at the knees. Exhale as you lean fully forward and drop your head, hands touching the floor by your feet. Reach up and stand, legs slightly bent as before. Legs still bent, lower your arms and then reach back behind you (the airplane position).

Bring your arms forward and then up in front of you until they're reaching straight up to the ceiling and, in the same motion, raise your right leg. Find your balance at the outside of your left foot. Allow your right hip to descend, twist to the right with your left arm in front and your right arm stretched out behind you. Reach down with your left hand and press it against the outside of your upraised right knee, your right arm still outstretched behind you. Pull your right knee in with your left hand. You may choose to let your left arm float, that will work the core even more.

Release and return to a standing position, facing forward. Return to the original position, arms upraised and knees slightly bent.

Now do the same for the other side.

Start with arms up, knees slightly bent. Lower the body to rest on the knees. Bring the left knee forward and up, foot on the floor and raise the right arm up straight. Then lean to the left, stretching your right arm as you breathe deeply. Hold that position.

Then twist and lower your left arm to touch your left elbow to the outside of your right knee. Your right hand is pointing up toward the ceiling, palm flat. Now raise your left arm and place your left hand flat against your right, palm-to-palm. Allow your left hip to move toward your right knee. Press your right elbow into your left knee. Turn your face leftward toward the ceiling and look up. Expand the capacity of your lungs, the capacity of your heart. Exhale. Straighten your spine and reach up, arms straight. Lower your hands, palms to the floor as the right knee rises. Inhale as you half-lift your body, left leg straight, toes and fingertips on the floor.

Bring your feet together, legs slightly bent at the knees. Exhale as you lean fully forward and drop your head, hands touching the floor by your feet. Reach up and stand, legs slightly bent as before. Legs still bent, lower your arms and then reach back behind you (the airplane position).

Bring your arms forward and then up in front of you until they're reaching straight up to the ceiling and, in the same motion, raise your left leg. Find your balance at the outside of your right foot. Allow your left hip to descend, twist to the left with your right arm in front and your left arm stretched out behind you. Reach down with your right hand and press it against the outside of your upraised left knee, your left arm still outstretched behind you. Pull your left knee in with your right hand. As with the other side, you may choose to let your right arm float, that will work the core even more.

Release and return to a standing position, facing forward. Return to the original position, arms upraised and knees slightly bent.

Repeat as desired.

Meditative Option: Meditate & Cultivate Calm

This 15-minute-long meditation is perfect for beginners and advanced meditators and anyone in between. The practice focuses on enjoying the meditative process without getting hung up on meditating correctly. Remaining connected to the breath will make you will feel calmer, lighter, and clearer.

Sit comfortably with your legs crossed, knees out and ankles in. A good tip to have your knees in line with your hips, or even lower. That's central to the lotus position, to keep the knees low. Use a pillow or yoga block for greater comfort if you like. Place your hands on your knees with palms up, take a deep breath, Feel your tailbone lower, as if it were connected to the earth. Then feel your heart rise up, through your head and up as if it were connected to the heavens.

Take a deep breath brough your nose and right into your heart center. Relax your shoulders and exhale. Repeat as desired.

Day 2

Gentle Option: Reset Refuge; Bliss Out and Be Blessed

Experience the bliss of this smooth and soft and practice. This class combine hip openers and gentle flow, self-massage, twists, *mudra* and *pranayama* and enhance the body, soul, and mind.

Stand on your knees, facing forward. Pull the right knee back to a 45-degree angle behind you, pelvis lowered, right leg in front and bent at the knee, foot on the floor. Lean back and inhale while extending your arms to your sides, then bending the elbows to raise the hands upright at the sides of your head. Keep your elbows at a point behind your shoulders.

Set your left hand on the left knee and twist, bringing your right arm across to the left side of your body. Bend the right arm and press the right elbow against the outside of the left knee. Make a fist with your right hand and cover it with your left hand, left elbow up. With the right elbow against the left knee, twist to the left with greater force. Turn your torso up and toward the left. Take a deep breath right in to the belly and then slowly and gracefully release. Don't rush that.

Walk (or inch) your left foot toward the right, then lower yourself down by straightening the right leg and pressing the left knee to the floor. The left calf is also against the floor, horizontally in front of you. Beware of any pain in the left knee.

With both hands on the floor, lean forward over your left calf, head down and forward. Hold and breathe deeply. Place your elbows and lower arms flat on the floor in front of your left calf and foot.

Let this be a soft pose. Release unnecessary tension in your body and dive into your breath. Direct the breath to the place of sensation, the left hip or inner thigh, which is what you're stretching most. Hold that pose. Often and surrender, release and receive.

Slowly lean back, pulling your left leg back and replacing your left knee to the floor, Push up until you're standing on your knees, spine upright.

Now let's do the same to the other side.

This time, pull the left knee back to a 45-degree angle behind you, pelvis lowered, left leg in front and bent at the knee, foot on the floor. Lean back and inhale while extending your arms to your sides, then bending the elbows to raise the hands upright at the sides of your head. Keep your elbows at a point behind your shoulders.

Set your right hand on the right knee and twist, bringing your left arm across to the right side of your body. Bend the left arm and press the left elbow against the outside of the right knee. Make a fist with your left hand and cover it with your right hand, right elbow up. With the left elbow against the right knee, twist to the right with greater force. Turn your torso up and toward the right. Take a deep breath right in to the belly and then slowly and gracefully release. Don't rush that.

Walk (or inch) your right foot toward the left, then lower yourself down by straightening the left leg and pressing the right knee to the floor. Now your right calf is also against the floor, horizontally in front of you. Again, watch out for any pain in the right knee.

With both hands on the floor, lean forward over your right calf, head down and forward. Hold and breathe deeply. Place your elbows and lower arms flat on the floor in front of your right calf and foot.

Once again, let this be a soft pose. Release unnecessary tension. Direct the breath to the place of sensation, this time the right hip or inner thigh, which is what you're stretching most. Hold that pose. Often and surrender, release and receive.

Now slowly lean back, pulling your left leg back and replacing your left knee to the floor, Push up until you're standing on your knees, spine upright.

Repeat as desired.

Rigorous Option: Yoga Alchemy; The Axis

In this practice we'll look at locating the true center of the being, the essence nature, the divine self. We'll begin with potent core work, vigorous, decidedly physically, to draw attention from the external to the internal; away from turbulent emotion to implacable, incorruptible self.

Start in a downward-facing dog position, with feet and hands on the floor, legs and back straight, pelvis upraised. Raise your right leg up and back and bend at the knee, extending your toes toward the left side of your body. Stretch and hold, breathing deeply. Keep the shoulders square. Keep the left foot strong, the left leg straight and firm. Hold that position and breathe deeply.

Return your right leg to an extended position behind you, straight and strong, before pulling it back in all the way to your chest. Extend your right leg again, back and up and straight. Hold it before bringing it back in to your chest. Repeat this five times, slowly and pausing between positions.

When you bring your right knee in the last time, put your right foot on the floor, keep the left leg extended behind you. Lean back and raise both arms up and back, keeping them straight. Reach upward, stretching your muscles. Hold the position and breathe deeply. Avoid tension in your upper body.

With your hands up, hook your thumbs together and wave your hands and fingers to stretch under-utilized arm muscles. Gently draw your arms back a bit more as you open up your heart center. Release them and let your arms stretch out to the sides to open your chest. Hold and breathe deeply.

Raise your arms to the sky, then bring them together over the heart. Put your hands on the floor and pull both knees in.

Now let's do the same thing to the other side.

Assume the downward-facing dog position, feet and hands on the floor, legs and back straight, pelvis upraised. This time raise your left leg up and back and bend at the knee, extending your toes toward the right side of your body. Stretch and hold, breathing deeply. Keep the shoulders square. Keep the right foot strong, the right leg straight and firm. Hold that position and breathe deeply.

Return your left leg to an extended position behind you, straight and strong, before pulling it back in all the way to your chest. Extend your left leg again, back and up and straight. Hold it before bringing it back in to your chest. Repeat this five times, slowly and pausing between positions.

When you bring your left knee in the last time, put your left foot on the floor, keep the right leg extended behind you. Lean back and raise both arms up and back, keeping them straight. Reach upward, stretching your muscles. Hold the position and breathe deeply. Avoid tension in your upper body.

With your hands up, hook your thumbs together and wave your hands and fingers to stretch under-utilized arm muscles. Gently draw your arms back a bit more as you open up your heart center. Release them and let your arms stretch out to the sides to open your chest. Hold and breathe deeply.

Raise your arms to the sky, then bring them together over the heart. Put your hands on the floor and pull both knees in.

Repeat as desired.

Meditative Option: Meditate with Gratitude

Here one sits to reflect on what one is grateful for; the things which bring joy and calm in a frantic world. You can do this as an option to the other yoga practices, or do it before or afterward or even both.

This is a very simple exercise. Sitting in the lotus position, comfortable with back straight and hands on the knees with palms upturned, simply focus on your breathing as you would in any transcendental meditation session. Feel the breath come in, hold it in the lungs, feel it being expelled in an exhalation. Feel the sensation of the oxygen entering your lungs, your bloodstream, passing through your body.

But with this exercise, once you're relaxed and in tune with your body, focus on slowing down your breath. Do it gradually, and not to extremes. The idea is to slow the process, to be more mindful, to have more control of the mind over the body, and this is what meditation is all about, especially for our purposes here. You can take as much time as you want, go as slow as you want. But remember to come out of it slowly. Any jarring shift into hyperactivity could be dangerous. Good change is gradual, and a transitional period into and out of this exercise is highly recommended.

Day 3

Gentle Option: Gentle Renewal Flow

This class renews energy, stretches the body, and gently tones muscles. There's a flow from one posture into the next. It includes postures like Warrior 2 and Triangle Pose, then single-leg balancing, along with long holds of hip-opening postures like the Half Pigeon and the Frog/Garland Pose (*Malasana*).

Start with downward facing dog, with feet and hands on the floor, legs straight, hips up and head down. Exhale. Be a step behind your breath, surrender to it. Step your feet to your hands. Rise halfway, gently. Fold deeply, head down and hands on the floor. Inhale as you rise, stretching your arms out at your sides and then up over your head as you stand up straight. Hands together, exhale as you fold forward, bringing your arms in as you lower to the floor, head and hands down (while keeping your legs straight). Raise your left leg in the air as you inhale, lean back and into a lunge position, with your left leg back and straight and your right knee in front of you, right foot on the floor. Lower your right knee to the floor and arch your spine, raising your arms up and back into a crescent moon position.

Twist right and extend your arms to your sides, exhaling. Inhale as you raise your arms upright again and turn to face forward, Hold your left wrist with your right hand and lean to the right while you exhale. Inhale and return to crescent moon position, leaning back with your arms still outstretched above and behind you. Lean forward and return to downward-facing dog.

Now go through it again, this time for the other side.

This time raise your right leg in the hair as you inhale, lean back and into a lunge position, with your right leg back and straight and your left knee in front of you, left foot on the floor. Lower your left knee to the floor and arch your spine, raising your arms up and back into a crescent moon position.

Twist right and extend your arms to your sides, exhaling.

Repeat as desired.

Rigorous Option: Deep, Slow, Mindful Flow

This thorough, full-body class moves at a reasonable pace, but it's still fairly challenging and rigorous. The class seeks to cultivate a balance between ease and effort. It involves twisting and heart-opening balance. Breath is a priority, and the class is suitable for all levels.

Start in a plank position. With fingers and toes on the floor, legs and body straight, hands outside the shoulders. Pull the left leg in so that the outer thigh is against the stomach. Inch the left foot inward so it's to the right of the left hand, but keep the left knee further left of the arm. Your calf should not be in a straight up and down position, but angled so that the knee is projecting to the left. If you think of your leg as two hands on a clock, from your perspective the would read 11:25, not 12:30.

Lean forward just a bit to stretch the muscles and unlock the joints. Now move your left foot to center so that your calf is straight up and down.

Back into a plank position, lower yourself halfway down, inhale and push your head up and back, arching the spine. Take a few deep breaths in this position. Push your toes down and your head back, stretching your core.

Lift your hips and tuck in your head, back into a downward-facing dog position. Lift your heels and stay on your tiptoes as you lean your heels to the right and return them to the floor. Your feet are now horizontal to your body. Feel your beath from your left hand to your left hip joint. Hold that position and breathe deeply. Then shift your heels from the right to the left, keeping your toes firmly fixed on the floor. This time feel the pressure from your right hand to your right hip. Hold and breath before returning to downward-facing dog.

Walk step your feet back to your hands and slowly rise to a standing position.

Repeat as desired.

Meditative Option: Living the Dream; A Vision Meditation

This option has the practitioner looking into the future to envision an ideal condition or situation for their lives. This prepares the mediator for the life they want.

Sitting comfortably (or laying down) and obtaining a calming, regular breathing rhythm, close your eyes and imagine yourself stepping into an elevator. The doors close and you rise; you rise above the worries and complications of your current circumstance. You let go of the pressures and constraints of your present reality. Look up above the doors and see the lights advance, right to left as it takes you higher and further from your anxieties and stresses.

Now the elevator stops and the doors slide open. You are now looking at your idealized life. For you, this is heaven on Earth. What do you see? Is it tropical or mountainous or metropolitan? Where do you live? How is it decorated?

Who's there with you to share it? Where are you? How are you all dressed? There are no constraints, no limits, it's the very maximum of whatever your heart desires. How do you feel?

When you've spent time there, know you'll have to return to your present reality. And transition here is as important as anywhere. Wave goodbye to your family and friends for the time being, knowing you'll see them again soon. Take that elevator back to the ground floor, where you're once again grounded in reality. Your feet may be on the ground, but your head and your heart may remain in the clouds. And isn't that a wonderful thing?

Day 4

Gentle Option: Yin Yoga for Stress Relief

This class offers stress relief through a series of nourishing yin postures which are sequenced so as to unwind your whole being, returning it to a balanced state. The practice will ground you in breath awareness and will take you through a sequence of yin poses to quiets the mind. These postures are carefully chosen to help the joints, relieve lower back pain, and stimulate the parasympathetic nervous system to decrease stress and release anxiety.

This is just one of several stress relief posses which can be held for prolonged periods of time and are great for easing tension. It's the sphynx pose, or the seal pose (they're actually a bit different). Lay flat on the floor, facing downward, with toes extended, elbow and lower arms on the floor in front of you.

For the least amount of back-bend, stack your forearms in front of you with each hand over the opposite elbow. Lower your forehead to rest on your forearms.

For more bending of the spine, pull your elbows back and rest your forearms on the floor in front of you facing either inward with your palms pressed together in the center; or put your arms out straight ahead of you with your palms down. These are variations on the sphynx position. In this position, let your head drop down to stretch the spine and neck and release tension.

Comparable is the seal position, pressing palms flat on the floor in front, straightening the arms and arching the spine, raising the head.

These can all be done with cushions to alleviate soreness and accentuate bending angles more comfortably. Place a yoga cushion under the area of focus and achieve the position. Once there, hold the position and breathe deeply. This position can be held indefinitely, or the cushion can be moved to different spots in rotation.

Rigorous Option: Hatha Yoga; Strength & Freedom

An all-levels Hatha yoga class, this class will tone, warm, and open the body. It's a slow-moving class with long posture holds which strengthen and stretch.

Start with a standing forward bend, legs straight with body bend forward, hands touching the floor. Bow down as deep as your body will allow. Fold inward. Bring your feet together and raise into a chair pose, with knees bent and spine straight but forward-leaning, lifting your arms straight out and up over your head for balance. Reach up as far as you can. Take a deep breath and then, as you exhale, clasp your hands in front of you and bring them to your heart. Lean forward, hands still clasped and knees still bent (even a bit more for balance).

Now twist to the right so that you can place your left elbow outside of your right knee. If you can't do this, put your left hand on the outside of your right knee and place your freed right hand on the small of your back.

Either way, now pull your right shoulder back. Set your hips down a bit and hold this position, breathing deeply. Now go into a forward fold, the position you started with, and do the same for the other side.

Cycle through from the chair position to bringing your hands to your heart. Lean forward, hands still clasped in front of you, knees bent a little more for balance.

Now twist to the left so that you can place your right elbow outside of your left knee. Or put your right hand on the outside of your left knee and place your freed left hand on the small of your back.

Pull your left shoulder back. Set your hips down a bit and hold this position, breathing deeply. Now go into a forward fold, the position you started with, and do the same for the other side.

Repeat as desired.

Meditative Option: Transform Tension to Vitality

This meditation is designed to be done during fasting and during periods of regular diet and weight management. It helps achieve a more restored state to help move the *prana* (life force) through the entire being. This one can be done as an adjunct to another class or on its own.

Sit in a comfortable position, lotus of possible, lying down if necessary. Start with a very deep breath. Now feel your self, your energy, lowering down through your body and into the ground, deep into the Earth. Now feel it coming up again, from the earth and into our body, through your open chest and to the crown of your head. Now exhale, feeling your energy descend back into you and travel downward back to your core. The more you exhale, the further that energy descends. Then inhale again, slowly and naturally, and feel the energy rise. It rises in conjunction with the speed and depth of the breath. The more you inhale the higher it goes, the slower you exhale you lower it descends. This unites the self with the earth below and the sky above, observing the oneness of all thing. But note that you're not controlling the breath, you're simply observing it, understanding it and yourself in a whole new way.

Day 5

Gentle Option: Yin Yoga for Energy and Clarity

Great for a depleted body or spirit, this one is great for when any faster is deep into a fast. This class's yin poses work with the body's chemical intelligence and gently detoxifying the spinal column, kidneys, and enhancing internal organ blood flow.

Begin by lying flat on your back. Pull your right leg up, knee to the chest, placing both hands on the calves just below the knee. Pull gently and breathe deeply. Let your left arm drop down to the floor. Extend your left arm out to your side while your right hand guides your left knee across your body, twisting the lower body to your right. You may have to adjust the angle of your left arm for comfort. Your weight should be on the side of your pelvis with your lower back strong and straight.

Now stretch your right arm out as well, letting your upper body stretch. Now turn your head to the left. Hold and breathe deeply, feel the effects of the twist. Hold this pose as long as you like before returning your head to look directly upward and uncrossing your left leg, once more lying flat with your arms at your sides and your legs together.

Now do the same thing with the other side. Pull your left leg up, knee to the chest, placing both hands on the calves just below the knee. Pull gently and breathe deeply. Let your right arm drop down to the floor. Extend your right arm out to your side while your left hand guides your right knee across your body, twisting the lower body to your left. You may have to adjust the angle of your right arm for comfort.

Now stretch your left arm out as well, then turn your head to the right. Hold and breathe deeply, feel the effects of the twist. Hold this pose as long as you like before returning your head to look directly upward and uncrossing your left leg, once more lying flat with your arms at your sides and your legs together. Repeat as desired.

Rigorous Option: Earth Yoga

The grounded yoga practice uses gravity to connect the self to its bodily roots and then beyond to its earthly roots. This is a moderately challenging *vinyasa* flow practice which invites balance and stability and which appreciates and honors all the different connections the Earth provides.

Start with downward-facing dog. Walk or hop your feet up to your hands, then halfway lift before going back down in a full forward fold. Rise up straight, arms reaching up, looking up, inhaling. Then exhale as you lower your arms, hands clasped (standing at attention). Release hands and raise them up along the sides and above the head, spine and arms straight.

Follow that up with a forward fold.

Halfway lift, put your hands flat on the floor and walk or hop your feel back, spine and legs straight in a plank position. Press the head back and up, spine arched and arms straight, in a tall cobra position. Inhale then exhale into a downward facing dog.

Inhale and raise the right leg up and back behind you, straight, rotating the right hip to extend the leg as high and straight as possible. Then bend the right leg at the knee, angled toward the left. Hold and breathe deeply. Then straighten the leg, square the hips, and bring the right leg down under the chest, foot on the floor. Extend the left leg, point the left foot outward, and rise up to a standing position with your feet splayed. Extend your arms to your sides, turn your head to look down your right arm to your right hand and beyond. Take your left hand and run it down the left thigh and point the right hand upward. Hold and breathe deeply. Slowly return to a standing at attention position, then lower yourself back into downward dog to repeat for the other side.

Inhale and raise the left leg up and back behind you, straight, rotating the left hip to extend the leg as high and straight as possible. Then bend the left leg at the knee, angled toward the right. Hold and breathe deeply. Then straighten the leg, square the hips, and bring the left leg down under the chest, foot on the floor. Extend the right leg, point the left foot outward, and rise up to a standing position with your feet splayed. Extend your arms to your sides, turn your head to look down your left arm to beyond your left hand. Take your right hand and run it down your right thigh and point the left hand upward. Hold and breathe deeply. Slowly return to a standing at attention position, then lower yourself back into downward dog. Repeat as desired.

Meditative Option: Morning Manifestation Meditation

This short meditation is designed to help energetically and mentally align with your goals for the upcoming day. It should help clear the clutter from your mind and connect to your best intentions and the utmost of your abilities.

Get into a comfortable position, get control of your breathing, locate your energy center and calm it so that it rests peacefully in the core of your being. Now concentrate on what follows; memorize it or have somebody read to you. Read it yourself into a voice recording app on your phone, if that helps. Then let the words pass through you and settle in your brain. Don't fight it; just do it.

Sift through the clutter in your mind. Shelve your to-dos, what's unfinished for now. Sift through the mundane and repetitive thoughts and patterns you may be stuck in so that you can reconnect with your inner intuition, your inner knowing. What emotion is in your space, mind or body or soul, that you don't need, that you want to clear away? Let it go. Acknowledge why it is there, then let it go, especially if it will not serve you today. Allow it to dissolve.

It's easy to imagine your new yoga regiment has you well on your way toward total wellness. You've achieved greater discipline and you've seen and felt the rewards. You're stronger, more capable, more well-informed, more confident. Your body and mind have been more deliberately enjoined and focused to work with one another toward the greater good.

But the journey's not over yet. There are two crucial steps on the journey toward total wellness, greater health and awareness, and master of mind over body. We're reaching the superego promised when the mind/ego controls the body/id. It requires every bit of strength and knowledge this book hopes to offer, and will only encourage both to greater heights. You may already have guessed where we're going, an what we'll be doing next.

Meditation for fasting.

SECTION 7:
MEDITATION FOR FASTING

CHAPTER SIXTEEN: Meditation for Fasting

If you're fasting and dieting and exercising and even doing yoga, you're probably pretty serious about resetting your body and your mind. All of the principles in this book coalesce and intertwine, and they lead us to the world of meditation.

Meditation is an ancient and robust tradition of mental and physical wellness which is derived from the notion that one can separate from one's circumstance, to transcend it, to reach a place of perfect spiritual wholeness.

Like diet, fasting, exercise, and yoga, meditation is easy to lose track of in our cluttered world and amidst our frantic lifestyles. While we're barraged with bad foods, dangerous electronic lighting, long hours and unyielding stress, increased pollutants, desperate economic demands, every opportunity for respite, relaxation, and resetting are robbed from us.

So once again we have to be deliberate and mindful, of what we're doing and how we're living. The paradox is that, while meditation is famous for removing all thought, it is still a mindful practice; more than most, in fact. And while yoga (and fasting) is certainly very deliberate, its goal is to achieve a kind of effortlessness which one can take into other, more challenging facets of modern life.

For this reason, meditation is a solid exercise in discipline. And that discipline is helpful when applied to fasting, exercise, yoga, or any of the things we're discussing in this book. Again, we see how every facet of what we're looking at touches on every facet of everything else. It all connects like some great web of psychological and physiological wellbeing.

Meditation and Weight Loss

Since the body and mind are connected in various ways. And the mind is as powerful a tool as the body. The hand reaches for what the mind allows it to reach for, after all (likely something unconstructive which may please but not benefit and could even harm the body, mind, or soul). And meditation focuses the mind, which makes it a sharp weapon.

Meditation may set the mind free to greater understand the reason the hand reaches for what it wants, the reasons it wants what it wants, reasons the mind does not intervene. When the brain understands what it is doing, it can change the entire chain reaction of behaviors. Meditation allows this the way few things (if anything) can. Along the way, meditation may bring the practitioner closer to core beliefs and childhood disruptions which may be affecting adult behavior. Eating is often a response to stress, anxiety, self-esteem issues, body issues, insecurity, depression, and a host of other destructive conditions and behaviors. Understanding this is the first step toward controlling it. Meditation may be the first step toward greater understanding.

How Meditation Works

For the uninitiated, meditation is grounded in a very simple practice. The idea is to find a relaxed physical condition, either sitting or lying down, standing still or even walking (a more advanced and yet the most pedestrian form of meditation, if you'll pardon the pun). Setting walking aside, imagine sitting still in a quiet place, with your body physically comfortable.

The meditator then chooses one thing to focus on, something very simple. Very often, a beginning meditator begins by focusing on their own breath. This is something which is always accessible to anyone at any time and in any condition. It also connects the meditator to their own body to achieve a kind of closed energy cycle and a stronger connection of body and mind.

The practitioner simply focuses on that single thing, the breath. They focus on the slow inhaling, holding the breath in the lungs, then releasing. The focus isn't on accomplishing the act, which is automatic, but on it is deliberate about breathing; deliberate about intaking the air, holding it for a short but regular count, and deliberate about releasing it. It's about being mindful of how the lungs feel taking in the air, how the blood feels holding it, how the body feels releasing it. It's about focusing on every facet of that often-overlooked but vital practice.

Not everybody chooses their own breath to focus on. Some may choose their own heartbeat, or do a kind of body scan which starts at the feet and guides the focus through every part of the body. Others choose a distant focal point, such as a tree top in the distance, a stain on the wall. Some focus on a monotone they utter, others on a mantra, a repeated phrase. Some focus on envisioning an ideal future for themselves, a perfect mate or house or a family photograph. Some focus on their idea of what God (or a comparable force) might look like.

Some prefer walking as a way of focusing, though there is rarely a single focal point to focus on. This kind of meditation diverts attention to the simple act of walking. Though one isn't so mindful about it as they might be about breathing. Breathing, one concentrates on the inhalation, the exhalation. Though this only lasts a short time, before the mind becomes free of thought as may roam to productive places. When walking, you're not likely to be focusing on the minutia of right foot, left foot. Instead, the focus is drawn by the surroundings, a combination of autonomous movement, breathing, energy management.

Walking is the most popular form of meditation, as people do it so often and it takes little training. People don't think of it as meditating, which is why they do it so often.

Another (but not at all healthy or recommended) type of meditation is the cigarette break. As dangerous and disgusting as this habit is, it does draw the practitioner's attention to breathing, feeling the breath (though chemically charged), savoring the exhalation. Luckily, fewer and fewer people are choosing this type of meditation. It certainly isn't recommended here.

And making that better choice brings us to being deliberate about what we do and how. One may think, for example, that fast food and snack foods are economical. But a USDA study showed recently that $2.50 a day is enough to buy all the natural fruits and vegetables to provide anyone with the recommended weekly caloric allowance.

It's all about being mindful and deliberate, which is what meditating is all about.

Being mindful during a dietary shift like fasting means making and sticking to a new eating plan and having the wisdom and discipline to stick to it. This might entail writing out the weekly menu and putting it on the refrigerator door. Support groups are also often helpful, especially for first-time meditators.

Meditation is Intermittent Fasting for the Mind

We've seen how intermittent fasting can assert mindfulness and deliberateness into our dietary lives, causing autophagy and stimulating the body to reprogram itself. Well, meditation does basically the same thing for the mind.

In fact, the body has two different nervous systems, the autonomic and the voluntary. Automatic behaviors include breathing. Voluntary behaviors include holding your breath. So breath is one of the few places where these two nervous systems meet. This makes it a perfect way achieve a greater connection between body and mind.

In fact, a lot of the potent meditative techniques involve a meeting of these two different aspect of the self, if you will (the automatic and the voluntary). Focal meditation uses the involuntary sense of sight, used in a voluntary way. Hearing is an automatic sense, so hearing your own voice can be said to be a meeting of voluntary and automatic nervous behaviors. Speech is also automatic. Normally, one doesn't have to concentrate on speaking. It's a pity more people don't concentrate on *what* they're saying, but they certainly don't give much thought as to how to say it. How they're saying it is immaterial. But when repeating a mantra, one is deliberate about the pace, the tone, the vibration of the tone in the mouth, the throat, the chest, even resonating throughout the entire body.

And once the body and the mind are more closely connected, the mind has more control over the body and the body less control over the mind. Why is this so? Because the automatic functions have little to do with the mind (but everything to do with the brain). Voluntary functions have everything to do with the brain and the mind. There's much we don't know about the so-called *mind*, so we're in danger of slipping down a rabbit hole here. What we know factually is that a person may be mindfully desirous of moving their hand, but a malfunction of or injury to the brail may prevent it. The brain and the mind are not the same, though they are closely related. And both have sway over the body and can also be swayed by it.

Think of the human being in Freudian terms. Sigmund Freud, the father of modern psychoanalysis, is famous for a number of different contributions to the field. It was Freud who coined the Oedipal and Electra complexes of complex sexual attraction of children to their opposite-gender parents.

Perhaps more famously, Freud has a theory that the human psyche was constructed of three different parts; the ego, the id, and the superego. Freud described the ego as the adult part of the psyche which deals with the outside world; practicality, social behavior. This is the practical adult part of the psyche. The id is the part of the psyche which deals with itself; immediate wants and desires without regard to consequence. This is the child part of the psyche. Freud speculated that every psyche has these two facets inherently. Some people have a stronger ego than others, for some the id is more dominant.

But Freud described a third aspect to the psyche, the superego. This is not inherent, but achieved. The superego is a moral perspective which can only be attained when the practical ego takes and retains control of the childish, selfish id. When the id is dominant, the ego spends all its time satisfying the id and cannot turn its attention to the higher truths and the clarity which is necessary for a strong moral perspective. When the ego controls the id, the superego becomes possible, then and only then.

Now let's think about everything we've looked at in this book so far, the total self. The mind represents the ego, the part of our self which deals with the outside world. It's deliberate, strategic, practical. The body is the id of the whole self, it wants immediate gratification and satisfaction, reaction automatically to stimulus entirely without reason. It reacts with sweat and goosebumps and nausea, hunger and thirst and any number of automatic responses for which it demands satisfaction. Complete wellness (for lack of a better term) is the superego, the moral high ground. It works going backward too; Complete wellness can only be achieved when the practical mind has control over the immaturely selfish body.

You can probably already see where this goes. Everything we've looked at here is about the mind gaining control over the body; fasting, diet, exercise, yoga, understanding hormones and other bodily systems, it's all been about how the mind can control the body.

And meditation is the epitome of the mind controlling the body.

Why is it so important? It brings us back to another phenomenon we've looked at often, and that's the interrelation of systems. One thing influences the other. The mind can control the body and strengthen it by discipline. The body's greater strength inspires the mind to a greater sense of possibility. The mind is rewarded for its efforts toward discipline, and this encourages more discipline, which affects greater strength, which in turn inspires greater discipline.

Let's look at the flipside. When the body gets what it wants all the time, it becomes weak and lethargic, overweight and prone to disease. Disease makes the body weaker. This physical dilapidation affects the mind, which falls into depression from anxiety, stress, and guilt. This generates self-medication (overeating, substance abuses) which further contribute to the maladies which are slowly destroying the body.

In short, these things come in cycles, and one affects the other. The body and mind are inextricably linked. It's only when were mindful of this that we can do something about both. We can see to our bodies through changes in diet and exercise, but meditation is the best way to fine-tune the other major part of the equation; the mind.

Another conundrum about meditation; it's about clearing the mind, but only to allow it to become occupied again. When one focuses on any stimulus, it is not thinking about the chatter of the outside world. It is finding clarity in the jumble of information. But once that clarity is achieved, it remains itself a means to an end. The mind, once cleared, moves on to start thinking about other things, mulling through that chatter and chaos, thinking things through. The clarity is a better way to approach a problem, not a way to avoid or deny it.

Nonjudgmental Awareness

There's an old saying: "All of men's problems arise from his inability to sit quietly for five minutes." This is truer than you may realize. Why? In the day and age people actually used this expression, the 1800s, there was little enough to do and plenty of time to sit quietly. These days, our lives are so hurried and demanding that five quiet minutes actually does seem like a luxury. And with the dominance of electronic entertainment in our culture, five minutes of quiet time is almost unheard of. If we're not letting the TV drone on at home, the internet at work, or our phones while we're on the bus, subway, or plane, we're never without entertainment or input of some kind of content. It's almost as if the powers that be don't want us to be alone with our thoughts. Perhaps they know the great strength there is to it, and how much of a manipulative hold they'd lose over such a huge buying audience.

Either way, finding five minutes to sit alone isn't as easy or as common as you might think.; unless you're mindful and deliberate about it. You might set a certain time aside every day, first thing in the morning or last thing before bed or tea time at four in the afternoon. You may do it opportunistically, when the moment arises. But it's important to do it.

Think of it as nonjudgmental awareness.

The key to it is that it's not really meditating in that it doesn't require a focus on a single focal point or bodily system or mantra. This is the kind of meditating one does on a walk. Instead of thinking precisely about one thing, one thinks basically of nothing. The same kind of clarity is still achieved, and it is automated in a certain sense. If you're sitting or walking or taking a shower, you're still engaged in a cluster of automatic behaviors, though when they're combined they're just a bit more deliberate.

If you're sitting looking out the window, don't think about trimming the trees or anything too deliberate. Just sit and stare. There are no answers on that tree, the answer is in the looking.

This is actually a common trick among various professionals, including those who have to puzzle over tricky concepts or principles. These can be lawyers circling around a tricky problem for their client, writers working out story questions, social workers and doctors and all manner of professionals. When one concentrates too much on a problem, a forest-for-the-tress problem sets in. Overthinking a problem can jam up the rational system. So stepping away from the problem to perform some perfunctory physical chore is a good way to distract the mind just enough. This is often called *thought showering* because taking a shower requires a group of fairly automatic but still voluntary actions which require just enough conscious though to distract the mind. This often frees up the mental jam and lets an answer become easy to find. Walking is a popular way to implement the same method of bringing body and mind together and letting one influence the other in a positive, deliberate fashion.

Another aspect to nonjudgmental awareness is actually about not judging what you see. It's more than just not being distracted by your tree branches, but your neighbor's yard. It's hard to be aware and not be judgmental. We're trained from childhood to have cognitive and critical thinking skills, and this requires a certain amount of information processing and problem solving. The problems are that (firstly) people are not problems, they *have* problems which can be solved; and (secondly) children are not equipped to understand the subtleties between understanding things and judging them. They're often never taught these differences, as often enough their parents don't know the differences either. It's another subject for another book, one of several on the subject from our own library perhaps. But for our purposes here, there is a difference between a person and their actions, opinions, mistakes. The clear mind will see this, and meditation will make that clear.

Transcendental Meditation

Here is the meditation we've all come to know, sitting quietly focusing on the breath, a focal point, a mantra. It's about stillness and quiet, focusing concertedly on one thing to the exclusion of everything else. It's great for clarity, for mental sharpness, for discipline in every way.

When thoughts do appear in the uncluttered mind, they are easier to understand, and so the answers are easier to see. This practice may be done for five minutes a day for clarity management, or for an hour or several hours at a time.

An hour a day is recommended for serious meditation. It's as good a way to spend an hour at night as, say, watching reruns of *South Park* or *Peep Show*. And the more you watch the news, the more the calming effects of meditation may be helpful and even required. So for that one hour, don't be fearful. We spend so much of our lives in fear. Our bodies and minds are guided by a fight-or-flight response, which is basically fear incarnate. Our society teaches us to be fearful of just about everything; strangers, social scorn, sexually transmitted disease, gun violence, terrorism.

But for an hour a day of meditation, give up the fear, transcend it. Focus on your selected point of interest; your breath, your mantra, your body, your stained wall. Let go of everything else, especially the fear.

There's also a matter of guilt. Because our lives are so demanding, because time is so short, it may be hard to justify taking an entire hour to do absolutely nothing. But we know meditating is so much more than nothing, it only appears to be that. The benefits are almost unending and are plain to see even in a short dissertation like this one. But it's easy to allow the pressures of life to infiltrate on that hour of meditation, even to prevent it. So it takes discipline and resolve to declare one's own right to this kind of selfcare. Don't be afraid, and don't be guilty, just do it.

Once you've let go of the guilts and the fears of the present, you can begin to let go of the fears of the past. Meditation of this quantity and quality will allow reflection and introspection to allow one to transcend emotional corruption and chaos and discover rational and reasonable clarity. Then you can rationally overcome those lingering pains and negative feelings which cause so much present-day misbehavior and self-sabotage.

Meditation is the best way to make those old, lingering pains clear and to exorcise them. It's a mental kind of autophagy, and it's even more beneficial to overall good health.

Along those lines, be nonjudgmental about the thoughts which your new clarity brings you to. Don't fight them or deny them or blot them out. If they face you, face them back. This is what meditation is basically for, after all. You have nothing to be fearful of nor guilty over.

It isn't always easy or convenient, but what is easy and convenient is also often harmful to us, body and mind, as we have seen. Be deliberate and mindful, use the discipline of the ego to control the immature id of your body. Achieve the superego's superior vision of better greater wellness.

All this meditation will bring you more closely in tune with psyche, your ego with your id. You'll learn to recognize how your mind and body may be disjointed and help you on the long road to reunion of the two. It won't happen overnight. Good change is gradual change.

But once you recognize your lesser self, once your mind has achieved control over your body (instead of the other way around), you'll be able to exercise that control with greater deliberation.

Before we move on to the specialized program we've arranged, let's take a quick look at some meditation apps, some of which will likely prove helpful to you in your quest for total wellness via intermittent fasting. Note: Some of these are free, others offer subscription add-ons. We suggest you double-check their prices, as these are subject to change.

Calm is considered the best of the best among experts. The app's guided meditations do more than lead you through anxiety and lack of focus, but they do a lot more than that! These benefits include:

- Different tools and modalities

- Well-being offerings such as sleep stories

- Celebrity voicings (including Matthew McConaughey)

Insight Timer offers features few others can match, including:

- Over 45K free meditations

- Filtering by need or goal, duration, or benefit

- Seven-day free trial/meditation introductory course

- Supportive community

Headspace Meditation & Sleep is popular for those trying to get to sleep, often a problem during a fast. It offers:

- Breathing exercises

- Wind-down practices

- sleep meditations

- dim, meditation-friendly lighting

Ten Percent Happier Meditation is based on the popular book. It's a good way to mainstream the meditation experience. It offers:

- Short, on-the-go sessions

- Mindful day tracking

Unplug is handy for those with little time to meditate. Even five minutes is enough to unplug with this popular app, which offers:

- User self-direction

- Ambient sounds and timers

- Ideal for refocus during stress

- 30-day challenge

Habit is perhaps the best for simple use. Modern users are often looking for more simplicity in their lives, not more complexity. So this app may be the best choice, offering:

- Quick, on-the-go meditation

- Extensive meditations library

- Clearly organized

- Special meditations to lessen stress and combat panic attacks

- Offline use (with premium subscription)

And now, as we did before, we'll apply all this new knowledge to some real-time physical applications. We've fasted, we've dieted, we've exercised, we've done some yoga. Now it's time to meditate. Of everything we've looked at, meditation may be the most user-friendly and the most beneficial. It certainly will tie all of your previous practices together.

CHAPTER SEVENTEEN: Meditation Programs for Fasting and the Immunity System

Meditation Program for Fasting

The purpose of this meditation is to guide your mind towards better health. Before we begin, find a comfortable position, either on the floor, in a chair, or on a bed. Let your back be straight and upright. Remain present and open minded. Close your eyes and take a long, slow breath in through the nose. Breathe in and out, long and slow, a few more times. The longer and the slower, the better.

Your mind is clear. Your awareness is here. You feel safe and relaxed while engaged in this meditation. When I talk about self, when you think about self, we focus on the awareness which is currently taking in these words, hearing them and feeling them resonate through the entire body.

If you're fasting, you are already healing your body and mind. You are extending your lifespan and improving the later years of your life. Imagine a life which becomes more enjoyable as we age. Obesity, heart issues, cancer, it's a long lit of ailments which fasting can prevent. Eating only when we are truly hungry creates the utmost self-respect. The idea of eating multiple small meals per day does not give the body time to begin the healing process. This process is vital to clean out the body's impurities. Abstinence of food gives us a new, sharpened mental discipline which converts itself into a force of freedom. By freedom, we mean freedom within your mental or physical health. Fasting and eating appropriately will provide extra vitality, and that is the essence of life. Now you can spend more time with family as a more energized, healthier individual who leads life to the fullest.

Relax your body and mind now, knowing that you are already well onward in your journey.

Feel what is through your senses. Understand that you are not your senses, you are only using them to observe yourself and your reality. Meditate. Listen to whatever sound there is in the room, even if that's only vague sounds leaking in from the outside.

Now take a deep breath in through the nose and let it out through the mouth. Do that again. You are fasting again, getting healthier with every passing minute. You mut keep the regime up, even though it will at times be difficult. The rewards are worth the effort. It's too important for you not to give up, however difficult it may be.

Visualize yourself living the best life possible, free of disease, high in energy and appreciation. Visualize yourself sharing it with those you know and love. Fasting will bring that reality to you, so let it guide you toward that ideal future and let that ideal future guide you through your fasting regiment.

Return your awareness slowly to the room, to your body. Center on your heart and then slowly bring your awareness outward to the rest of your body. Shrug your shoulders as you feel that energy pass outward through them. Bend your spine slowly from side to side, muscles gently pushing at the vertebrae to release excess tension.

Meditation Program for the Immune System

The purpose of this meditation is to improve your immune system through self-reflection and meditation. These are easy and effective ideas which may help you improve our immune system.

Allow yourself to be comfortable, but not too comfortable. You should be sitting up, with back straight, leaning on some pillows. Roll your head a few times to loosen your neck so you can be relaxed and focused.

Connect to the breath by inhaling through the nose and exhaling through the mouth, slowly and deliberately. Do this repeatedly until your body and mind are in a tranquil, open state. Bring your awareness into the center of your mind. Greet it, come to know it. Slow it down and connect with your immune system. Focus on connecting to the white blood cells, which govern your immune system. Greet them. Note how you feel when you familiarize yourself with the immune system.

Even considering the immune system makes it stronger, by focusing the body's attention on it. And considering it is a form of meditation. You're already on your journey toward tranquility and away from stress, getting further along with every breath in through the nose, every moment holding it, and every moment during the exhalation.

Begin concentrating on your feet. Feel your toes, move them around and flex them. Sense the bones, the tendons. Then move up to the feet, arch and twist them, roll them on your ankles. Then focus on your calves, the muscles pulling and contracting and releasing at your whim. Get a sense of the skin stretched over that muscle, the hair on that skin if there is any. Then move your attention upward. Feel your thighs, the strong femur bone, the tendons stretching from the knees to the hips. Feel your groin, the center of the body. Be aware of it, the physical and mystical power of the genitals, the base of the vital organs as you feel your way through your own digestive tract. Sense the congestion if there is any.

Remember to be breathing deeply but steadily as you do this meditative survey. Keep scanning up to your stomach, your kidneys and liver, your spine. Be mindful of every part of your body, what its function is and what its condition is. Be even more mindful of your breathing as your scan takes you to the lungs, expanding and contracting, your heart beating steadily. Is the heartbeat steady? Keep it calm without having to wrestle control over it. Work with it, not against it. Be aware of your bones, ribs strong and protective.

Feel your shoulders, is the tension still there from before? Scan down the length of your arms, down the muscles to the elbows, down the forearm to the wrist and hand, where tiny bones intermingle with tendons, nerves, and muscles in a most delicate way. Think about those frail bones which do so much work, so much of the time. Feel your nerves and tendons and bones right to the tips of your fingernails.

Now come back, revisiting the arms on your way back to the shoulders, the neck, the spine in this delicate area. Scan your head, your jaw and teeth, your ears and face, your nose and eyes. Bring your focus right up to the top of your head, completing the full meditative scan.

Now do it again, but this time you'll have some familiarity with how each part of your body feels. Start at the head and work your way down, revisiting areas which you'd overlooked for so long. It's on this second scan that things become more noticeable; little pangs or pains, twitches or stiffness or weakness now become more apparent. It's like re-reading something for errors. The more often you read it, the more errors you notice … and can correct.

Once you have scanned your body twice, pull back and see it as if for the first time. What does it look like, what does it smell like? Is it in its prime, or in clear decline? Make sure your body is as aware of it as you may now be, and direct your body's resources to those areas both with your body (physical exercises and yoga positions) and your mind (meditation, discipline).

Envision that future version of yourself and your life, as you did before. What does that you look like? What diseases have been rid of that version of you? Let those visions replace doubt anxiety and doubt.

Imagine yourself transforming into that person, becoming them with every breath, with every new or newly repaired cell, with every better dietary choice you make, with every walk you take.

Early morning walks and late-night bike rides are pleasant ways to exercise the body we currently inhabit. We must be mindful not to overstress it, to let its healthy functions take place. Daily exercise is crucial to a healthy lifestyle. There are no short cuts, no magic pills. A healthy body is a mindset, and a mindset is a state of mind. A state of mind is an awareness, and this is an awareness of who we are and who we could be; living a strong, peaceful, contented life with everything we want in life.

Take another deep breath in through the nose to focus on awareness before releasing a big sigh of awareness. We're focusing on making better decisions in our lives, and our immune systems will function better as a result. The exercises don't have to be strenuous, and heathy food tastes delicious. It makes us feel energized toward life, so we can live longer and appreciate the quality of life. It allows us to focus our attention on our internal heat. Heat fosters relaxation. Picture a sauna, relaxing the body, detoxifying through sweating, allowing autophagy and rebirth throughout the body.

Take another deep breath and bring your awareness back to your shoulders. Roll your head again on your shoulders as you did at the beginning of the meditation to bring your awareness back to your body, to remain loose going into the rest of the day.

One might think we've gone as far into the mind as we can, and in a way our journey has indeed gone from the physical (fasting, dieting, exercising) to the mental (yoga, meditation). But there's one step further to go, one which transcends both body and mind and yet draws them together in a way that nothing else can. It is neither nutritional nor dietary, nor is it recognized as an aspect of mental health or even psychology or psychiatry. It is the last frontier of non-traditional treatment which has already demonstrated a history of efficacy in a variety of ways. There things it can't cure and things it can. Once you come to know it better, to master it, you'll know if it can save your life or merely improve it. Prepare yourself, as you're about to go to the final step in our journey toward the ultimate reunion of body and mind, total wellness.

Hypnotism.

SECTION 8: HYPNOTISM

CHAPTER EIGHTEEN: Hypno-fasting

Hypno-fasting may sound like a new approach, and it may be, depending on how you look at it. Hypnosis itself is fairly new to the human experience, and there's a lot we still don't know or understand about it. But the link between hypnosis and weight loss is longstanding and well-established. As soon as people recognized hypnosis as a remedy, weight loss was one of the first maladies they turned it to. And that only makes sense. Both are often misunderstood, and weight loss has been such a stubborn (and increasingly threatening) problem that it only makes sense that seemingly drastic measures such as hypnosis would soon be taken. This was when diet and weight loss were not so well understood as they are today. Even so, hypnosis had proven a potent remedy for any number of things, for reasons still now quite known. It's too functional and effective to simply discount. And with our opened minds and opened hearts, with our greater understanding of physiological actions and reactions, its time to turn our attention to this final frontier of overall wellness.

Hypnosis.

History

As much of a post-psychoanalytic novelty as it might seem, hypnosis actually dates all the way back to the ancient empires Greece and Egypt. The word *hypnos* refers to a Greek God of the same name, and it is the Greek word meaning *sleep*. Keep in mind here that, though considered ancient and, by some, primitive, each of these bygone empires accomplished feats of engineering with the minimal tools of the age which today's modern computer technology could not hope to replicate. So consider the geometric perfection of the Pyramids of Giza or the deliberate imperfection of the Parthenon atop the Acropolis in Athens. (For those who don't know, the seemingly perfect geometry of the building is an illusion, using forced perspective to give the illusion of geometric perfection. In truth the building is riddled with deliberately inaccurate angles which will look perfect from afar.)

So if these cultures (which also pioneered brain surgery) took hypnosis seriously, perhaps we should too. Both the Greek and Egyptian cultures had religious centers where people sought consultation. Hypnosis of a sort was used to induce and interpret dreams, to envision oracles. Ancient writings are replete with references of the sort. Indeed, most of John of Patmos' Book of Revelation is said to have been written in an hypnotic, trance-like state.

In 2600 BC Wong Tai, the father of Chinese medicine, recorded techniques involving incantations. In 1500, BC, the Hindu Vedas chronicled techniques involving certain hypnotic procedures. Druidic, shamanistic, yogic, voodoo, and other religious practices rely on a trance-like state induced by some form of hypnotism.

Franz Mesmer (1734 – 1815) is said to be the father of modern hypnosis. The word *mesmerize* is derived from his name. He was maligned in his time (and often enough, today) but he was a pioneer and a genius. He was the man who developed the now-accepted theory of animal magnetism, which states that diseases are resultant from blockages of magnetic forces inside the body.

Mesmer became popular defining the image of a hypnotist; goatee, black cape, magnetic eyes. He was rebellious and theatrical, and we wouldn't have hypnosis (as we know it) without him.

London University professor John Elliotson (1791 – 1868), who introducied the stethoscope to England, was forced to resign after championing the use of mesmerism (soon to be called *hypnosis*). He went on to give numerous private demonstrations, furthering the increasing interest and literature on the little-understood subject.

Mid-nineteenth-century Britain James Braid (1795 – 1860) was a Scottish eye doctor when he found a patient staring into a lamp, seemingly dazed. He was responsive to Braid's commands, sparking Braid's interest in the field. Getting a patient to fixate on a certain thing (as one does in transcendental meditation) was a critical aspect of hypnotism. A swinging watch, a swirling disk, even the hypnotist's fingertips or eyes, are popular focal points to use during hypnosis. Braid's work remains a cornerstone for contemporary studies on the subject.

British surgeon James Esdaile (1808 – 1859) saw the potency of hypnosis on pain relief and actually performed many hundreds of major surgical operations using only hypnotism as an anesthetic.

Frenchmen J.M. Charcot (1825 – 1893), Ambrose Liébeault (1823 – 1904), and Charles Richet (1850 – 1935) also did impressive work furthering the art and craft of hypnosis. Emile Coué (1857 – 1926) pioneered auto-suggestion. He coined the phrase made popular in The Beatles' song, *Getting' Better*: "Day by day in every way I am getting better and better." He believed in guiding people toward self-healing, which is where hypnosis begins to work its way into our current field of concern. He believed, in fact, that there was no such thing as hypnosis, only self-hypnosis.

In a sense Coué also anticipated the placebo effect – treatment of no intrinsic value the power of which lies in suggestion: patients are told that they are being given a drug that will cure them. Recent research on placebos is quite startling. In some cases statistics indicate that placebos can work better than many of modern medicine's most popular drugs. It seems that while drugs are not always necessary for recovery from illness belief in recovery is!

Even Sigmund Freud (1856 – 1939) showed an interested in the advancing field of hypnosis, but his work took into the area of psychoanalysis, for which he became famous. For Freud, remedy was not found by the patient alone, but through careful guidance by a trained professional.

In the modern era, Milton H. Erickson, MD (1901-1980), advanced hypnosis after suffering with polio-induced paralysis as a child. It gave him a window into human psychology. Erickson's work remains the most popularly cited in the study and application of hypnosis today and his techniques are considered the most effective.

Experts now are more ready to accept the connection of hypnosis and medicine.

What is Hypno-fasting?

Hypno-fasting combines intermittent fasting with various techniques of hypnotherapy/hypnosis toward the specific goal of losing weight through fasting.

Intermittent fasting is proven to have beneficial effects, that's true. But it can be difficult for some people. We're trained throughout our lives to rely on three meals a day, and those meals get bigger and bigger while offering fewer nutrients. Psychologically, physically, and socially, we've become addicted to the habitual act of eating, regardless of nutritional necessity. It's more than just temptation for satisfaction, it's a matter of a lifetime of training. It can be hard to reverse such deeply engrained patterns.

Hypnosis can help with that, because habits are practiced in the body, but they're born of the mind. Once you've been through the practices in this book, your mind will be stronger, its relationship to our body should be more dominant. If so, that'll help with hypnosis during your fasts. If not, hypnosis will help you achieve that mental mastery.

Hypnotism as useful on the young as the old, and it works regardless of health, wealth, race, creed, or social strata. Rich or poor, fat or thin, hypnosis has no differential of efficacy.

Hypnosis is not mind-control or magic. A person cannot really be made to do something they do not want to do (sorry, fans of *The Manchurian Candidate*). Hypnotic blackouts are also mythological, as is the idea of being stuck in hypnosis and never snapping back to reality. Really, minor states of hypnosis happen all the time without any theatrics or swinging watches on gold chains. It may happen to you every time your mind just wanders, every time you lose yourself in thought. It may happen several times a day, depending on who you are, where you are, and what your mind is normally like.

Hypnosis is, like other things we've studied, a way to direct focus in order to block out other distractions, the basic principle of meditation. And, as with meditation, it's a conscious state, not a zombie-like sleepwalking state of perfect suggestibility. Those who have been hypnotized describe is as the feeling one has just as they fall asleep; awake, but so relaxed that even movement seems unnecessary.

Experts agree that nobody is truly beyond hypnotism. Some are more open to it, more responsive, some will naturally be more closed and more resistant. One thing is for sure; if you don't want to be hypnotized, you won't be. The subject (for lack of a better word) plays an active part in the process, and that requires an open heart and an open mind.

And, like intermittent fasting, this kind of hypnosis, hypno-fasting, can be sustained for an indeterminant amount of time; regularly for the rest of your life, if you like. You're developing parallel skills of self-discipline and self-awareness. Both are excellent for tightening your focus, and that will help you in other endeavors. The more you do both, the better you'll get at them, and at related practices as we've gone over here. Your exercising regiment should be accented by the discipline you've learned and earned during a fast, and that energy will transfer to the self-awareness you achieve during yoga and meditation. Hypnosis will not eradicate the hunger a fast brings on, that will come and go. But it will help you accept it instead of fighting against it. It will help you embrace that hunger as a necessary part of your life and as a necessary part of your growth.

Hypnosis Apps

We'll be going through some actual hypno-fasting courses soon, when you'll be able to put this fascinating concept into practice. But first, let's take a look at one of the newest revolutions in hypnosis, the hypnosis app.

This should come as a surprise to nobody. They have apps for everything, after all. We've already taken a look at apps for yoga and for exercise and even for fasting. And hypnosis is an ideal way to partake of this kind of practice without disrupting anybody else's schedule.

Some people don't like apps, or don't have app-worthy phones. Others prefer the company of others. Either way, there are apps for that, and here are the best ones:

Hypnobox is regarded by many as the best self-hypnosis app. It's designed to achieve a state of deep relaxation. This leans on the notion that being in a highly relaxed state makes one more open to suggestions of new behaviors and thoughts. The app can be customized with a male or female voice, and you can tailor your sessions and import your own background music.

Relax and Sleep Well Hypnosis focuses on techniques for relaxation and offers sessions on stress, anxiety, self-esteem, and mindfulness.

Harmony Hypnosis Meditation offers music, mantras, visual images, even sound effects.

Perhaps the best one for losing weight is the aptly named Lose Weight Hypnosis app. The app's audio sessions utilize suggestions to influence behavior and mindset subconsciously. User reviews suggest the app is useful for weight loss and relaxation both.

Digipill is well-known for relieving stress. It's also a well-known health and fitness app which uses psychoacoustics and the hypnosis style known as *neurolinguistic programming*. Psychoacoustics uses sound to induce psychological response. It's a type of neurolinguistic programming, which postulates a strong connection between sensory experiences, behaviors, and emotions. The app offers different programs for weight loss, stress relief, weight loss, motivation, and smoking cessation.

Anxiety Free's app seeks to relieve anxiety via self-hypnosis and guides users through activities meant to relieve stress. One study suggests self-hypnosis may be effective for ongoing anxiety and for situational anxiety, which occurs from a specific past, present, or future event.

Now let's get to it, shall we? You're probably already experienced in at least one or two of the practices in this book, though not necessarily. Don't feel bad if you haven't lifted a single knee. Feel free to read through these hypnosis programs first. You may be recording them on a voice recorder app, after all. But reading the material through first will let it sink in on one level before saying it helps the material sink in even deeper. Listening to it will give you a third listen in your first session, and that can only improve its efficacy. Repetition is what this kind of hypno-fasting is all about.

CHAPTER NINETEEN: Hypnosis Programs

 Now we present six one-hour hypnosis programs, one each for the things we've been discussing: Fasting, weight loss, food addiction, emotional eating, body anxiety, and sleep.

Some necessary notes here: These programs are meant to be spoken. Using whatever devices you used before, either pre-recording or using a partner, there are some things to keep in mind.

Read the text slowly. It is not meant to be rushed through, but to be languid and deliberate and mindful. The words have meaning, even the sounds of the words have meaning. When reading them, let the words linger on the tongue, let the speaker by mindful of their importance, of their rhythm.

Create a soothing tone with the text. Speak in a low tone, soft, not sharp or shrill. Imbue the reading with the nurturing and supportive spirit of the sessions. Whether or not you are prerecording the scripts, you may want to include background music, of course of a soothing nature. Sound effects may be appropriate too, including the sounds of wind, rain, birds singing, a babbling brook, whatever seems or feels appropriate. These programs are meant to help you, so you should have a say in how they sound. It could make all the difference in how they affect you.

True, reading them into a voice recorder app may not give you much creative flexibility, but you can always read the script into a a laptop with Garage Band or a comparable recording program and you can easily download and add whatever music or sound effects that you like. You can record and add your own music if you like.

If you have a partner reading the scripts, you can find plenty of sources of ambient sounds and music that are perfect for this practice. However you do it, there's no reason not to begin. You have nothing but choices and a beautiful, ideal future waiting ahead.

We'll begin with hypno-fasting and proceed from there. We do suggest you not skip ahead. Like the rest of this book, these are carefully sequenced to build one upon the other. Trust us, we know what we're doing.

Hypno-fasting

Fasting may help to improve the natural functioning of your brain. It may make you realize (and this escapes a lot of people) that you are only a humble human being. As your body's stored toxins are released, you will feel refreshed and ready to take on all the challenges that life has to offer.

Some doctors believe that pure water fasting may do more than detoxify cells and rejuvenate organs. It may actually cure some diseases. They believe fasting is nature's natural restoration mechanism.

Whyever you have decided to fast, you are going to use your creative subconscious mind to help you to maintain your resolve and to make fasting a pleasant, rewarding, and even an easy experience.

Visualization is the domain of the brain, its native language. In a moment, I will ask you to envision certain things. And I will ask you to envision the scenes as I describe them to you; envision them to the best of your ability.

Perceive any smells or sounds that accompany these impressions. You will find that, in envisioning the scenes, you may go further, deeper into a gentle hypnotic rest.

And with each of your breaths and each of my words, you will be drifting deeper into a calm. Your body becomes more at rest, more at ease. Your troubles are all faded and forgotten, your mind is at peace. Your heart is beating evenly, untroubled. Your blood moves easily in your veins, smoothly, your skin and your muscles feel relaxed.

You take a deep breath and hold it, let it refresh and relax you. Now release the breath again, feeling your chest going down as the air goes out, taking with it any trace of discomfort, any shadow of doubt. You have no preconceptions, you have no desires, you have no thoughts at all. You are loose, you are relaxed, your mind and body are at one and both are perfectly at ease as you listen to the sound of my voice. Your mind is receptive, your heart is open. You are ready for where you are about to go and what you are about to do. Your subconscious mind is set to go, there is nothing holding it back. There is nothing holding you back.

Envision yourself in your home. But this is not the apartment or house you live in. It is the room in your brain where your thoughts are stored.

You are surrounded by shelves of books, papers, and objects; all shapes and sorts and sizes. The books and papers cover a wide variety of subjects. Some of the books are old and others are new.

All the items on the shelves represent things you think about often.

There sits some paperwork relating to your job, piles of bills, photos of your friends and family, souvenirs from your vacation, items to represent your hobbies and interests and various other things. You are starting to fast, or you are about to begin fasting. Food is on your mind. But in order to help you succeed in your fasting, thoughts of food must be shunted, put aside.

One wall of the room has numerous cupboards, and a refrigerator and freezer.

Walk over to it. The cupboards are filled with the thoughts of all your favorite foods. You gather a few large empty cardboard boxes and begin filling them with everything to do with food.

The cupboards are bare; your mind has been emptied of all thoughts of food. You are left with filled-up boxes that you drag outside, ready to be carted off.

Go back inside, admire your accomplishment. Survey all the clean empty shelves. You have done something significant here, and you feel lighter inside, clean just as the cupboards are clean. You cannot quite remember what was on them, it does not matter. There are always new thoughts in your mind that need a shelf. And the new things you will store there will be better, fresher, made for new life and better times. They will be the memories of the better choices you make now, the better things you are now better able to do.

Since the shelves are empty and you have cleared the clutter, you may now move ahead with you fasting amid fewer distractions. Your mind is clear and your thoughts are positive. You enjoy detoxifying your body. It is an added bonus, but also crucial, to detoxify your mind. Fasting may help improve your mental clarity, concentration, and focus. It is a transformative practice for a better, more spiritual life.

You may not see a spiritual star in your life, but that does not mean there isn't one there. It could mean that you hasn't found it yet. Or, like all stars, it could be travelling light years across space and time to reach you, and it may not have appeared in your life's sky as yet. That does not mean that it is not there.

But you have nothing to fear either way. You are your own source of strength, your own star. You do not need a higher power, you already have access to a higher power within you. You are a higher power. All you have to do is look within to see everything that is without. That power allows you to go anywhere, see anything, do anything, even fasting.

Fasting requires self-discipline. This gives you a feeling of being in greater control of your life. It increases your confidence in the choices you make. It fills you with a new and yet familiar strength. It is the strength of the best you, the alpha you. This is the person you were designed to be, the person you were meant to be. Enjoy the feeling of that strength, in your blood, in your muscles. You are strong and you are getting stronger. Feel that strength increasing with every breath, gathering up to face any challenge, withstand any storm.

You recognize that your system does not need (nor does it want) to be overloaded with food. You enjoy a new feeling of lightness in your body and mind. Your blood insulin, sugar, and cholesterol levels are in balance. Your metabolism and fat-burning systems are slowly strengthening. Every part of your body, every cell, is working toward your optimal health. The body is healing and caring for itself because you are allowing it to. You are our own champion, and you are standing up for yourself at long last.

And you are fighting a grievous enemy; illusion. Illusion is at the heart of so much of what we're combating together on your journey to total wellness. It is illusion which manipulates our self-images. It is illusion which makes us think we will be satisfied by processed, fried foods. It is illusion which prevents us from investigating paths to truer consciousness, like yoga and meditation. This entire book is a rally against the illusions which are preventing you from achieving, from loving and doing, from living and from being.

Now you have the truth, which vanquishes illusion. Now you have the power to cast aside old pains which you believe still have power over you. But those things are gone, and their influence over you is the influence of an illusion. Now you are armed with the tools you need, the truth, to remove illusion as a road block on your journey to total wellness. It has held you back for too long, blocked your way and kept you from getting ahead.

But no more.

Even now, the changes are underway. Even now autophagy is replenishing your cellular supply. This very instant, your body is detoxifying, clearing away the old to make way for the new. This is a moment of revelation for you, body and mind. All the cellular changes are happening inside your body. Your body is cleansing and repairing itself. You feel an inner sense of peace, calm, and tranquility. Any problems that you have previously experienced in your life fade away. They become insignificant and you become connected to the higher forces around you.

Recognize this as an entity which you are comprised of; flesh and spirit. When you give your physical self the rest it craves, this allows the spiritual side of you to grow and refine. As it grows, you become more aware of your place in the Universe. Your relationship to others and the importance of love and kindness changes.

You enjoy fasting and savor the inner sense of satisfaction which may never be provided by food. You may decide to fast intermittently to encourage healing and transformation and promote peace and harmony at the very deepest level of your body-mind system. Visualize yourself going through a day of fasting in a calm and peaceful way.

Envision that you are starting to feel a bit hungry. Envision a balloon and place it in your stomach, right where the hunger was. Once your balloon is in place, you can pump it up by taking a sip of water. If water is not allowed, swallow your saliva.

The water travels to your stomach and inflates that balloon, relieving your stomach of its hungry feeling. It fills you. It leaves no room for anything else. It occupies your empty places. You are full, you have no need for more food. Your body craves fasting, it denies food. It knows that food would interrupt the good work it is doing. Your body is grateful for what you are doing for it, for allowing it to repair itself.

And you are glad to be able to help. You and your body have a healthier relationship now, a stronger alliance. You are its champion.

Look around the room. Look at the shelves which you cleared. If any thoughts of food have returned to the shelves, you clear them off once again and place them into another empty box, ready for disposal.

The suggestions are embedded in your subconscious mind. They grow stronger every day. You can fast whenever you wish to with complete willpower. You will know that no negative thoughts of hunger or food will be able to stand in your way.

And this will happen; not just because I say so, but because you have decided it will. That is correct; you have decided, you and your subconscious mind.

Trust yourself. You know by instinct when it is time to fast and when it is time to break that fast. When it is time to continue eating again, you will know the time is right. You eat healthier than ever, and you feel better each time.

You know the importance of maintaining a healthy diet and you know when it is time to have a rest from eating and give your body and mind time to repair. And fasting is easier for you and you enjoy it. You take satisfaction from being able to demonstrate your power of mental determination to yourself and to the world.

I'm going to count the numbers from one to five. At the count of five, you will be wide awake, fully alert, refreshed and ready to allow the suggestions to work for you. And the suggestions will grow stronger by the day, stronger by the hour, stronger by the minute.

Prepare yourself as I count up to five. You will come all the way back to me at the count of five.

One, two, three … begin coming back. Four … your eyelids are starting to flutter. And … five. Your eyes are opening, your mind and body are returning to your full conscious awareness. You feel alert and refreshed and ready to commence your period of fast.

End session.

Relax and reflect. Breathe deeply, give yourself some time to transmission out of your state and back to a grounded, healthy perspective. How do you feel after your first session? What did you learn about your powers to envision? Did you build on the visionary skills and abilities you developed earlier, in your meditations? Did you find solace in what you envisioned? How did you feel at the end of the session?

How does it make you feel during your fasting? Did you pick up some useful tools to get you through the more challenging aspects of the fast? Could you feel that balloon in your belly, pushing away any room for food? Did you sense the control of your mind over your body? Do you sense it?

Remember as you go on with your fasting that you are always in control. If you use these hypnotic techniques or if the other techniques in this book are going to be enough will be up to you. But even more important than any constructive tools you take away is the overall feeling you have as a result of the experiment. Savor the calm, the sense of unity with yourself. You have seen yourself in a new light, and you should be imbued with a new confidence, a sense that you have insight which others do not have.

And you have gained some invaluable experience just by participating in the exercise. Your question about hypnotism have been answered, your doubts have been allayed. You are not clucking like a chicken, right? You are not walking around like a zombie, bumping into walls. you know how it feels, you know what to expect. And you are ready to move on to the next program. From fasting, we move to weight loss, and then onward!

Weight Loss

Feel relaxed and at ease, your body loose and light. Your heart is beating evenly, your lungs gently expanding and contracting. Your body's systems are fluid, languid, all is well. You are in a safe place, your surroundings protecting you, freeing you to transcend your physical place and go to a place of the mind, to take a journey of the mind.

Your mind and your body are easy to attune, one integrated with the other. But it is your mind which is the stronger, and your mind is the key to the realm we are about to enter. You are receptive to my words, to the images I will suggest. You can summon memories of smells and tastes from the past. You can see faces from the past, faces of the future. You are at one with body and mind, and you are at one with space and time. Feel yourself lift up out of your own body, to rise out of the room you're in a go up into the sky. Look around at the clouds, the clear blue stretching out and up in every direction.

Lower yourself down now, in complete control of your mind-self as your descend. You are lighter than air as you return to your room, your body, entering as if sitting down into a comfortable old chair. You lean back, body perfectly comfortable, serenity and tranquility flooding through you. You are open and ready, your mind is eager, my voice is your guide.

For a long time, you have been acting and feeling in ways that are not your own, ways that have taken you away from your own, natural self. You have relied more and more on eating to help you through the negative feelings which you have been experiencing, and have done so to such an extent that you deny yourself your own true feelings.

Nobody feels on top of the world all the time. There will be days that could be better for you. It is only by experiencing some of life's lows that you can enjoy and appreciate life's highs. Blotting out your feelings with overeating does not solve anything, it only makes things worse. That is why you have decided that you have had enough of overeating, and you want help with that old problems of yours.

Focus on a part of your life that you feel happy with. Enjoy remembering some of the good things that happened to you, something that made you feel confident. Reflect on an achievement, or on some praise you received. Note how you feel; confident, proud happy. and allow those good feelings to grow stronger, while you relax, and let go.

And when those good feelings come, take a very deep breath, hold it, and squeeze your hand into a fist. Your subconscious mind memorizes these good feelings. You are imprinting this feeling, this moment, into your memory, into your body's memory, into your muscle memory. It is as if you have driven that feeling into your hand, an invisible diamond in your palm. Let it be the storage place for that memory, for that feeling. When you wish to enjoy this feeling again, all you have to do is take a long deep breath and squeeze your hand into a fist. You will release that feeling from the diamond in your palm and your mind will access that memory.

Envision yourself in a situation where you would reach for your first sugary snack. Note where you are, what you are doing, who is with you, if anyone is there, use your imagination to remember it with as much detail as you can manage.

Note your feelings as you reach for the fridge. Think of the feeling of helplessness you have always had, and how those feelings have affected your life. Now envision yourself walking away and looking out the window. Take a deep breath in through your nose and squeeze the other hand into a tight fist while you remember those good, confident positive feelings. Savor their familiarity, how they make you feel that you can meet any challenge, that you are the very best and strongest you that there is.

You feel good. It is good to be confident, and to know that you are finally free from your old, addictive way of life. You are free of the burden of having to eat constantly. You are free to move ahead with your life, to experience the highs and the lows. Knowing this will help you appreciate it when things get better.

Envision an alternative activity. It does not matter what it is just as long as it is a break from the norm. What are you imagining? Skydiving? Swimming in a turquoise sea? Do you see your slim body, tawny and muscular, as you glide through the water?

You are changing. Your old ways of behaving and thinking are improving, you are in command, you are taking charge, you are in control. You are free as a bird, you are free from the addictive way of life, and yes, there will be moments when you feel pain, but these moments will get less, and you will appreciate the pleasurable things in life, the little things that make you smile and feel good.

You can glide like a dolphin through an azure sea. You can fly up out of your own body and hover with the clouds. Your mind and your body work together, to take you anywhere and to face anything, to do anything. You are open and receptive, your mind able to conjure anything and any place. You can feel it, smell it, sense it.

Envision that you are standing at the bottom of a small flight of stairs, leading up into an attic. There are ten steps leading gently up and you feel drawn towards climbing the stairs to explore the contents of this attic. With each step, climb toward the attic, become more deeply and comfortably relaxed.

Take the first step and feel yourself becoming even more deeply relaxed.

Two … three … ascending higher … four … you feel light, floaty, and you are more deeply relaxed than before.

Five … you reach a small landing and turn as the stairs take you in another direction.

Six … note a pleasant familiar aroma of wood. It is almost like being at a carpenter's workshop. Seven … you are surprised by the warmth as you ascend.

Eight … nine … and ten.

You are at the top of the stairs and you note a door in front of you. The door is locked, and there are two keys hanging by the side of the door. Take one of the keys and slip it into the lock of the attic door.

It fits and you unlock the attic door, opening it carefully and turning on the light. Note are beautiful dark oak beams running across the ceiling of the attic, and when you look down you see rickety old floorboards that creak ever so slightly beneath your feet.

Just to your left is a large old brown, trunk (like a treasure chest). It is bound by leather straps, fastened by buckles.

You are curious about what the trunk contains. Undo the straps. The trunk is padlocked. You try the spare key you took from the side of the door. The trunk unlocks and you lift the lid and take a peek inside.

It is crammed with memorabilia; positive memories from times gone by, your hopes and dreams for the future, valuable lessons that you learned as a youngster, inspirational thoughts and ideas and dreams, and images of your ideal self, the person you will be when you have achieved your goal of a slimmer and healthier body.

You rummage through the trunk, musing over your childhood dreams. You admire the concept of a slimmer you; the you who is able to enjoy the activities that you love and live the life that you desire.

I will be quiet for a moment as you look through these memories and dreams.

There are so many memories here, from times that you thought were completely forgotten; so many good and happy experiences and so much joy for a future that is yet to arrive.

Your subconscious mind realizes that you can achieve your true potential, having succeeded already in so many things.

Select a memory that is associated with positive, happy and confident feelings, perhaps a time when you were your ideal weight and shape or maybe some other time when you had achieved a goal that made you feel good.

I'll be quite for a moment as you re-experience that situation in every detail.

Note how you looked at that time; your hairstyle, your clothes, the surrounding environment. Note who you are with (if anyone) and what you are doing. Remember any remarks that you or anyone else may have made (a compliments perhaps) that increase these good feelings.

There may even be a certain aroma or something else that you associate with this memory. I do not know what this memory is, but what I do know is that it is very special to you.

Enjoy the confident and positive feelings while I am quiet for a moment. Before we move on, label your experience, like the title of a movie or a book. It is time to descend the stairs from the attic of the past. Would be lovely to bring some of those positive experiences back?

You could place them into that bag lying near the door of the attic. Or you could put them in a jar. Or you could just keep them in a deep corner of your mind, or somewhere close to your heart.

Once you have saved those happy memories, close the lid of the trunk. Lock it and buckle the straps. Bring your container holding those confident memories to bring back with you. Close and lock the door to the attic and descend the stairs, counting as we go down.

Ten … coming slowly down. Nine … you are leaving the aroma of the wood behind you. Eight … you are bringing those experiences back, you have them with you always. Seven … you are feeling even more relaxed, more comfortable, more confident. Six … five … you pause for a second or two on the landing before continuing down the stairway.

Four … three … two … one … you are leaving the attic behind. You know that you can return on your own when you want, whenever you wish; to rediscover other valuable experiences that can help you in the present and in the future.

You know what it is to be healthy and slim. You have happy dreams and memories of your ideal self. You can achieve your goal with the power of your subconscious mind.

You find it easy to say *no* to anything standing in the way of achieving your goal weight. In the past, certain drinks or foods were considered temptations. But you feel and respond in a different way now. Everything is different now and it will go on being different in the future.

Something inside you has changed. You have all the motivation and determination you need to succeed, and you do succeed. You have succeeded at a good many things in the past. You will succeed again. If you need to, you may remind yourself of your many achievements just by recalling the label of your happiest memory from your chest in the memory attic.

Relax. Enjoy your memory in detail, with all the sounds, colors, smells. Focus on the good feelings and thoughts. Focus on the feelings of accomplishment, achievement, the pride of attaining your goals. Savor the positive sensations related to that good and happy time of your life.

It will be exciting for you to see how rapidly these good feelings return to you; boosting your confidence, increasing your determination and motivation to succeed and to achieve your ideal weight and shape. It will be gratifying to be able to wear stylish clothes of a smaller size. You will enjoy feeling comfortable in your own skin and being content and happy and with your life and with yourself.

Whenever you want or need to, just recall your key word, the label you gave to your happy time. This lets you be confident and to feel good about yourself. You are now more motivated and determined to succeed. It will be especially exciting when, in five or six months, you look back on your trip to the attic. You will be sure that you are well on your way. You may even have achieved your goal already, having reached your desired weight and shape.

You will realize that you were always able to be the person you wanted to be; your healthier, slimmer self. You will be able to use your own life experiences and realize your dreams. You can make these dreams come true in the way you wanted them to come true, and you'll do it by using the power of your subconscious mind.

This makes it easy to maintain your true size and shape. You already have the key to success (your key word). Think that word in your mind and you will reinforce these good feelings.

You find that something you may have thought was impossible has become as simple as one-two-three. You also note that, from this moment forward, new opportunities open up to you. Your mind is open, receptive to changes at a much deeper level. These are changes which can benefit you in countless ways. You can become a great achievers; because whatever your mind can conceive, you can achieve. Reaching your true, ideal shape and weight is just the start of a life-changing adventure.

With every breath you take and every word that I say, any and all stresses, tensions, worries or doubts about your ability to lose weight are disappearing. You are free of them now, weightless. There is nothing to constrain you, nothing weighing you down. You feel stronger than ever, more attuned to the connection of body and mind. You are secure, confident, certain that you can face even the most intimidating challenges with ease and aplomb. Remember that your friends and family know this too, they look to you for a better example, to help them be better people. You may think that they judge you, and if they do they do it with mercy and positivity. They judge you to be a good and worthy person, imperfect as all people are. And that support inspires you to show them just how close to perfection a person may get. You know you probably won't actually ever achieve perfection, but striving for it will get you closer than anything else will. You know that, and you know how much effort will be called upon. And you know you can muster that effort, that strength and power, that and so much more.

You have made a decision to take the journey to your ideal shape and weight. It is easy for you to stay on the path, doing all the things you must do to achieve your goal.

You eat smaller, healthier portions of food. You leave food on your plate without realizing it, without even thinking about it.

If you have ever snacked between meals then you already know you do not want or need to snack anymore. You have uncovered the secrets of snacking, the disguised motivators which you never knew before. But you know them now. Now you are better-equipped to change your behavior. Because you know why it has to be changed, and you know that you are the only one who can change it. You enjoy changing it. You enjoy the feeling of control, the rewards of self-discipline. You are the champion of your own body, and you relish being called upon to do your duty. You are looking after your body by exercising when you can. You are providing it is safe and appropriate for you to do so.

And your subconscious mind is helping you do this, helping you around the clock. You trust in your powerful subconscious mind. You know that it will not let you down.

It is time for you to return to normal, conscious awareness. You will be eager and ready to begin the journey toward achieving a healthier, slimmer body and a stronger, more powerful mind.

Remember that, as you go about your daily life, your mind-life also goes on. Your mind-self and your life-self must be partners, working in unity for the greater good of your general wellness. These suggestions, and others in other sessions, should remain with you. Let them linger. Live your life the way you would in your mind-realm; with a sense of control, of strength.

These suggestions are firmly embedded in your subconscious mind and grow stronger every day. They grow stronger by the day, stronger by the hour, stronger by the minute. You find that every time you listen to my voice. It gets easier to relax and to enter hypnosis. The suggestions will have more benefit. They are now a permanent part of your new reality.

Remember your key word, the label that you gave to your happy memory. Repeat it to yourself if and when you encounter a situation that might have prevented you from reaching your goal in the past.

Your key word is the key to the trunk, the treasure chest in the attic containing all your happiest experiences and memories. You can unlock it whenever you like to recover those feelings with the power of your subconscious mind.

But you can also leave it behind, move ahead without feeling weighed down by anything from the past, good or bad. You may use these things, draw strength from them. But true strength is in what you do today, not what happened before. You will always be able to handle any challenges from this point onward, no matter where you go or what you do. You will go on strengthening your powers until nothing dare stand in your way.

If you need the past, it is there for you. If you need the future, it is waiting. The present is where the two meet, and that is only now. Even the present cannot contain you. The present is ever-changing, just as you are ever-changing. You are all things, past, present, and future. Connect them as you did your body and your mind, let them work together. Let the past guide the present and help create the future instead of burdening the present and destroying the future. You are the champion of your body and of your life, of your future. You must create it, protect it, nurture it the way you do your body and your mind. Do not let others sully it, do not let yourself sully it either. You are stronger than that, you are stronger than yourself.

In a moment, I'm going to count to five. At the count of five, you will be awake. Beautiful feelings will flow through you, confident and calm thoughts filling your mind.

These confident and calm thoughts and feelings will stay with you. They remain within you, becoming stronger as the days goes by.

One … two … you're coming back slowly. Three … take a comforting and comfortable breath. Four … your eyelids are fluttering now. Five … your eyes open, you are wide awake, mind and body returning to normal conscious awareness.

Now let's relax and reflect. How did it feel going down those stairs? Are you comfortable with your key word? Do you feel ready and empowered to lose the weight? You should see now that you have incredible powers, powers of the mind, which you may never have realized were in you before. Now you know what kind of strength you can access. You can walk through any door, descend even the darkest staircase without fear. The demons which have plagued you have no power over you now. And if they do, or seem to, that power will soon recede as your own power advances. Everything about your life may well have changed, even if you do not realize it.

That is good. There's much you are only coming to realize, only now beginning to discover; about yourself, your body, your life. Keep learning, keep growing, keep trying.

Emotional Eating

Close your eyes and envision lying in a hot bubble bath. Feel the warm water caressing you, easing your tensions and relaxing your body, soothing you all over. You feel comfortable, your limbs and body are heavy. You are savoring the luxury of having nothing to do, nothing but to relaxing and just letting go.

Sense the warmth and that heaviness spreading over your entire body from your toes and your feet slowly up into the legs. Feel that warmth as it flows into your belly, abdomen rising and falling. Your breathing is regular and calm as your chest relaxes and your shoulders become limp and loose and relaxed.

Relax your arms as the comfort and warmth flow down from your shoulders. Savor the feeling, enjoy it.

Your throat and neck also relax, so do your little facial muscles. Your eyes become heavy, almost closed. But you can still focus on a single bubble in that bath, one particular bubble in all the thousands, the one that reflects beautiful colors from the sunlight which streams in through the window.

That little bubble contains every color in the rainbow, deep and pristine and clear. The reds are bursting, the blue deep and rich, the yellow hot and the green soothing.

Envision that bubble growing, expanding, more delicate than it was before. Note that the heaviness is gone and you can envision leaving your body through the crown of your head and floating up over the tub.

Float down and toward the bubble, head first and as your head reaches the bubble. The bubble turns inside out and engulfs you, your entire body. Now you are surrounded by gossamer film of color. You are floating back up and into a clear blue sky. You're lifting higher, not doing or feeling or thinking, only being.

You go higher, and you feel more relaxed and more comfortable. You are protected and safe in your bubble.

I will be silent so you can absorb the beauty and peace of this heightened awareness. When you do hear my voice once more, it will seem to be coming from outside the bubble. Your subconscious mind will be open, receptive to what you hear.

As you drift down deeper into hypnosis, your mind becomes receptive and open and to everything I say and everything I suggest. Your subconscious mind will listen intently. It will absorb any suggestions that are beneficial of your overall wellbeing and good health.

These suggestions will go deep. They will make a lasting impression. They will be ingrained in your mind, indelible. As these suggestions sink into your unconscious mind, they become a part of your life. They will influence the way you feel, the way you think, even the way you eat.

For a long while, you have been using food to cope with negative feelings. Whether these feelings are the result of sadness, loneliness, boredom, depression, anxiousness, frustration or anger, it does not matter.

When you eat when you are not hungry, you know it will take much longer to lose those extra pounds. If you look to food for comfort, that comfort will be short-lived. It solves no long-term problems, not for you or for anyone.

Deep down, you are aware of this. If food actually provided a true source of comfort, you would feel great all the time.

Emotional eating worsens your issues by generating extra weight that you do not want or need. You are learning that eating when you are emotional is only a temporary distraction. You start looking for healthier distracts.

You have full and complete control of the united efforts of body and mind, working together toward your overall wellness. You know they can meet any challenge, even the united efforts of emotional frustration and the temptation to overeat. They are also working together, to keep you on a downward spiral of mental and psychological decline. Your weight will go up while your confidence goes down. But your allied efforts are stronger. You will not be tempted or beguiled by these interlopers into your life. What are the reasons for your emotional tumult? How should you best deal with them?

You may begin by writing down your thoughts and feelings in a diary or journal. You realize this will help you to get them out of your head. You may recognize and identify the triggers which used to make you seek comfort from food.

You might call a relative or close friend for support. By sharing your problems, you find that they seem far less significant. Talking on the phone is also a welcome distraction from food. And it isn't polite to eat and talk at the same time, so you forgo that trip to the cupboard.

Clear your fridge and cupboards of junk food like cakes and chocolates. You substitute them for healthy snacks like fresh vegetables and fruit and low-fat food. You are done with emotional eating and you explore other activities which give you that good feeling.

You have many choices in life. You may join a club and meet other people. You may watch a feel-good movie. You might spend extra time cleaning your home, realizing that the exercise will help you lose weight while the smell of cleaning products will stifle your appetite.

You accept yourself as the unique person you are. You love your body. You like what goes into it. You treat it well by eating only small amounts of healthy food and exercising as much as you can. You treat yourself with respect and you expect others to treat you with respect in the same way. You have earned it and you deserve it.

Your emotions may wear the face of someone else, somebody who hurt you in the past. Picture that person's face, envision it. Perhaps your own face is the one you see, your disappointments turning against your own bad judgments and past mistakes. Either way, you are stronger now, strong enough to forgive. Forgive that other person. Even more difficult, forgive yourself. Forgive yourself for whatever you may have done and for whatever you may be feeling.

You also accept that your emotions are an essential part of your whole personality and you find constructive ways of expressing yourself. They are the voice of what is best about you; sensitivity, empathy, humanity. Your emotions are insights into your higher self. Accept them, embrace them, but do not let them control you. You do not let your emotions control you. Like your body, which you love and accept, you likewise love and accept your emotions. But you have gained control over your body so your body and mind can work together and not be at odds. So too must your mind and your emotions work together, and it must the subconscious and the conscious mind which makes that happen. It is your mind which makes that happen.

You exercise more, slowly at first if necessary. Your brain releases those feel-good hormones to make you feel calm, happy, more able to cope with the various challenges and issues that might crop up. You get stronger every day, in mind and body, strong enough to handle your emotions as you never could before. You do not need food to help you cope with feelings other than genuine hunger. The next time you feel emotional, when you might reach for the cupboard out of habit, you stop and reflect on the things I have been saying today.

You are not hungry, so there is no need for you to eat. Before you were eating just to have something to do, or to work out your emotions. There are plenty of other things to do with your time. There are other ways to work out your emotions. You put everything into creating a happier, richer, more fulfilling life. You can do everything you ever wanted to do plus so much more.

You no longer link emotions with eating. You eat merely when you are hungry. Your life is becoming so much more fulfilling now that you have no need to eat just for the sake of it.

You are not eating when you are emotional. You find that you have more energy, more vitality. You exercise more. You enjoy using your body. And the more you use it, the healthier your body becomes.

You need less food. You want less food. You have no taste for the junk food you used to eat. You have no interest in fatty, greasy foods that will damage your alley, your body. You have distaste for the sugary, processed foods you used to rely on. Your body craves better foods, nutritional foods. You mind knows your brain needs the too, and you are happy to do what you can for your body, your mind, your best self. Because not only do you deserve it, but you demand it. You've become too strong to be manipulated by things like memories or emotions. The unity of your body and mind is too strong a bond to be violated. It is too strong an alliance to be thwarted.

Look at yourself in the mirror and you'll see for yourself. Look at your body, leaner for having lost all those excess pounds. You are firmer, slimmer, toned. You are glowing with vitality and health. Note what you are wearing and how everything looks so good on your trim body.

Look at your face, with a brighter glow from the healthier foods, the better nights' sleep, the calm and repose from the yoga and meditation, the shine of inner peace. This is the real you, slowly rising from the ashes of the old you. This is the best you, the person you were meant to be. Little by little, the true self emerges from the illusions and frustrations of the old.

Your mind and body meet with your own approval. You are gratified and glad that you cut the link between eating and all those negative, emotional thoughts. You are proud to be a person who is strong enough to do such impressive things. You are accumulating accomplishments every day; with every pound lost, with every good night's rest, with every day's fasting. You have learned what you need and you are taking step to get them. That is something most others can never accomplish. You will never allow anybody to distort your opinion of yourself again. You are great and you are only getting better, every day and in every way.

You have an image of your ideal life, your ideal self, your ideal future. You have envisioned them, they are waiting for you. You know the effort it will take to cross the Rubicon and get to the other side, where paradise awaits; your personal paradise. And you know now that nobody can stop you, nothing can obstruct you. Nothing can or will weigh you down, not any more. It may have happened in the past, but things have changed. You have changed. And nothing will ever be the way it was before.

Every day you are moving closer to this new image. Every day you are more determined and you are more motivated to achieve your goal. Instead of eating in an attempt to fill some emotional void, you find more constructive ways of dealing with your feelings. You soon see a slimmer, happier you.

These suggestions are embedded in your subconscious mind. They grow stronger day by day. They are deeply embedded in your subconscious mind, where they will take effect at the earliest opportunity.

In a moment, I'm going to count from one to five and at the count of five, you'll be wide awake. One … two … three, returning to consciousness now. Four … your eyes are fluttering, opening. And … five.

Now let's relax and reflect. Has your hunger subsided? Do you feel strong enough to fight the pangs of hunger when they arrive? Do you fee properly empowered? Have you discovered a new relationship to food? Do you have a greater understanding of your strength? Do you have a better comprehension of your own emotional distress, and how you may be misguiding your own emotional expression? Food has real value, life-saving value. But it is not meant to be abused. It has no powers over the mind other than to befuddle and confuse. It is crucial to maintain control of the mind over the body, and this means control of reason over emotion. We said earlier that reason is a function of the mind, but emotion more a function of the body. So now you are well-poised to take greater control of your emotions by asserting the power of reason. You are better prepared to deal with your emotions in a constructive way, not a destructive way. Now you can face them head-on and re-establish a healthier relationship with your food … and yourself.

Self-Image

Close your eyes and take a deep breath. Feel your body and mind strengthen their bond with one another, creating your best mind-self. You are confident that you know what you are doing here. There is nothing dubious, nothing odd, nothing surprising now about these journeys into the world of the mind and beyond, all the way to the stars if you so choose. You are experienced, you are strong. You have come a long way in your journey and learned much. Your instincts are sharper, your insight is deeper. The eyes of your heart can see what the eyes of your head have turned from for so many years.

But even time is your domain, to use at your will. You are a traveler in time, into your own past and your own future. You are your body's champion. You are a conqueror. And now you lean back and relax, preparing to set forth again. Let my words guide you further down our life path, into the realm of the self. You travel inward even as you transcend. You will leave your body even as you have gotten closer to it. You have been forging a new relationship with your body, becoming its alley. It needs you to function at its best, to make the best decisions for feeding it or not, what and when. You now have the strength to make better choices, your mind well-able to take control, to lead where your body will readily follow.

You are ready to be kinder to yourself, to see yourself in a new and flattering light, a forgiving light. You are receptive, ready to take on any challenge, even the challenge of your own body. But you have done this before, and you know that you are more than able to prevail; for mind, body, and soul.

Take a deep breath and hold it, then release it in a cleansing exhalation. Breathe in and hold it, let it out again. Savor the relaxed feeling, the sense of ease that fills you. Nothing can stand in your way and nothing can hold you back.

Picture yourself outside in your favorite place in nature. It might be a tropical beach, it might be a lovely garden, or perhaps you could picture yourself laying back on a boat sailing on a beautiful river. It does not matter where you are, as long as it feels good to you.

Nod your head when you are thinking of that special place.

It is a beautiful day. The sky is a beautiful blue, very clear. It is a warm summer's day. A dazzling sun hangs in the sky. It is so bright and colorful that you want to close your eyes and feel the warmth of the sun on your body. Envision this.

You can direct the sun around your body. As you realize this, you direct the light from the sun over your face. You can feel the warmth of the light from the sun on your face, just relaxing those muscles around the eyes and the nose and the mouth.

Your facial muscles flatten as they relax, and you let go. It is a beautiful day. You move the light from the sun into your throat area, feeling the warmth of the light from the sun in your throat, relaxing all those muscles, letting go. And the sunlight moves into the shoulders and across the shoulders, making them feel loose and limp and comfortable.

You feel relaxed, comfortable and at peace with the world. Direct the light from the sun down the right arm, from the shoulders to the tips of the fingers, the right arm begins to relax and let go, relax and let go. It is a beautiful feeling to be here right. The warmth of the light from the sun penetrates nerves and bones and muscles of that right arm.

It is a beautiful day. Move the sun over to the left arm and guide the light from the sun down and up the left arm, from the top of the shoulders to your fingertips. Your left arm is relaxing, becoming heavy, and you feel even more comfortable and relaxed. Move the light across and into your chest area and relax the chest and all the muscles there. Relax your stomach, let that relaxation spread to your hips and your thighs and over to your right leg.

Relax your right leg. Let it feel comfortable and relaxed. Move the light from the sun down the right leg, up and down, from the top of the hips to the tips of the toes, and the right leg relaxes, and let go.

It is a beautiful day. Move the light into your left leg. Move it up and down your left leg, from the top of your hips to the tips of your toes. Your left leg relaxes, releases tension, it lets go. Your whole body is totally relaxed, from the top of your head to the tips of your toes.

As your body relaxes, so does your mind. As your mind relaxes, note that the sun is going down. The sun is going down, slowly descending. The sky is alight with colors, crimson and purple with yellow and blue streaks. It is a beautiful evening. Your mind lets go, releases all the stress of the day. You … just … let … go.

The sun goes further down, over the horizon, until the sky is black, like black velvet. And twinkling up there in the sky is a single twinkling star. Keep your mind focused on that star. Nothing else matters but this beautiful single, bright star in the sky.

It is a beautiful night. You feel safe, comfortable, relaxed. You feel at peace with the Universe. Envision yourself moving toward that star in the sky, moving up, and up and up.

Your body is weightless as you lift to the star, ascending to greater heights. As the star grows, you realize you are getting close to it … closer … closer. It gets bigger … brighter.

Then, all at once, you *are* that star in the night sky. That is right. *You* are that silver solitary star in the night sky. You become the star and the star is you. You are one, back from where you came. And it is a beautiful star. You are a beautiful star.

Let your mind go, set it free to wander. As you drift into this restful, calm feeling, I am going to talk about your self-image, which is somewhat different, slightly distorted from the way other people see you. I know you have difficulty in accepting other people's opinions of how you look when they tell you that you really do look good.

You see yourself as being fat and unattractive. No matter how many times you are told otherwise, you find it hard (if not impossible_ to believe. So you wind up walking through life with your eyes closed to the opportunities around you, oblivious to the rewards which could be yours for the taking.

But the world sees a better you. The world sees the attractive you which even you deny. The world sees the lean, attractive you, or the hearty, playful you. The world sees the person it wants to get to know. The world has never seen the person that you imagine yourself to be. That person does not exist, only in your mind. But your mind is now stronger, and combined with the strength in your body, you cannot be stopped. With your mind and body united, working together, you can see what the rest of the world sees. That's the real you, the better you. The person you imagine does not exist, but the person the world sees does exist. That's you. And you, mind and body strong, are no match for some imagined shadow of your true self, a distorted, funhouse-mirror reflection of reality.

You are missing out on so much. You may find it hard to accept compliments. You may shy away from some places or activities because you are afraid that you do not you look as good as other people there will.

Being attractive or slim is not necessarily an advantage. But not believing in yourself can certainly prove a handicap; if you do not believe in yourself, how will others be able to believe in you? Let us improve your self-image, to help you to see yourself as you truly are. You are going to learn how to accept that you already are an attractive, sensitive, intelligent person with a well-proportioned body and a self-assured, confident style.

You do not have to be ashamed of your body. You can and should be proud of your body, to accept yourself for the person you are.

I know you tend to compare yourself unfavorably to others. It can seem hard to accept your own body when all you see in the media are super-slim models and celebrities. You might think that this is the normal way to look. You have strived all of your life to attain similar physiques by dieting or extreme workouts.

But you do not see or feel how starved and image-obsessed celebrities often become.

Everything in their lives seems to revolve around their own self-image and how others perceive them and if they fail to live up to their self-imposed expectations this can often lead to disastrous consequences. They may feel under constant pressure to maintain unreasonable expectations and this can impact upon their personal life as they feel their privacy has been invaded. It is an ongoing cycle. Stress invariably begins to build up.

Others may be influenced by their images because they are bombarded with perfection with every magazine or popular film and that is all they tend to see. But the reality is that those celebrities often yearn for ordinary, normal lives like most of us enjoy.

You can set your own realistic standards without having to conform to other people's lofty expectations. You can concentrate on truly worthwhile achievements and becoming a contributing member of society. You can become a person who gives something back rather than who constantly seeks to bask in artificial adulation.

Focus on your positive qualities; things about you or your achievements that you are proud of, qualities which endear you to the people who matter most in your life. Focus on your eyes, the windows of your soul. Focus on your smile. Every smile is lovely, all eyes are truth and truth is beauty. Think about the new leanness of your torso after your fasting, diet, and exercise. Think about your new flexibility from the yoga practices you've been doing. Enjoy the new looseness you feel, the looks you've been getting from others. Do not be blind to them, do not turn away from happy happenstance. You deserve it and it will come to you. Do not ignore or deny it. Embrace it, embrace your eyes and your smile and your ever-improving body and mind. Embrace everything you have to offer, everything that you are.

Allow these to fill your mind as I'm quiet for a moment, and when you hear my voice again, your subconscious mind will be open and ready to embark on a short journey with me.

Now let's go for a walk along a path that represents your life. You will recognize some of the achievements you have accomplished. These could be described as quite small, such as learning to ride a bike, reading a book, and so forth. Others may be more important achievements, such as learning a language or getting a new job. It does not matter how small or large those achievements were, they are all there on your path of life.

When you are ready, we will begin at the very beginning of your beginning; your conception. The moment of conception, which has been caught on camera, is an explosion of sparks of light, like a tiny, natural fireworks display.

Even as a fetus, you achieved milestones as you reached crucial developmental stages until you were ready for birth. You are already on your own path of life where you continue to develop. As a baby, you mastered important skills like sitting up, crawling, feeding yourself, communicating. As a small child you had much to learn, yet you learned those new skills. See yourself, see that you have grown up and started at school. You made friends, you learned how to socialize; perhaps you met your first best friend or another person you played with at this time.

Walk along your path of life and note all which you have achieved. Acknowledge your attainments and successes, appreciate what a human being you already are. As you make your journey, note mirrors that reflect back all the positive contributions you have made throughout your life.

Catch a glimpse of yourself in the mirror. You may think: "Yes, that is me. That is what I did and I am proud of that accomplishment." You know and appreciate how there are many more important things than appearance, such as personality, kindness, respectfulness toward others.

You are also quite happy with the way that you look. You tell yourself, "I am great. I genuinely like myself. I love myself. I accept myself totally and unreservedly for the unique person I am." As you continue on the path you will see that there are some turning points on your path; major life changes.

See yourself walking this path, happy and calm. Note a bonfire a little bit. Tell me when you reach the bonfire.

You have travelled far and you still have a long way to go.

Give a little consideration to any negative comments or thoughts you have experienced or which you may have received about the way that you look. They may only have been words, and even though they lacked substance they were enough to make you emotionally upset.

It is time to reject those thoughts, feelings, emotions, and comments. Take each for what it is. Study it for a second or two to reassure yourself that it is not relevant to you and then toss it onto the bonfire. If anyone has ever put you down in any way, insulted you, or teasingly said something to upset you, examine those comments briefly before throwing them into the fire.

See your old hurts, sadness, insecurities, humiliation, anger, or embarrassment. Look at each one carefully before tossing them onto the bonfire and watch while they burn.

Remind yourself, "I am fine. I like myself. I love myself. I accept myself entirely for the unique person that I am." If there is anything else preventing you from loving and accepting yourself as the person you are, then get rid of it. It does not have any place in your life. All those harmful and negative emotions and feelings are gone. You truly and completely accept yourself for the unique individual that you are.

Acceptance does not mean you become complacent. You still strive to accomplish goals and satisfy desires, just like anybody does. But you are able to prioritize what is important to you and what is not.

As the negativities have all gone up in smoke, you note another mirror. Step over to the mirror and examine yourself from head to toe. See yourself standing tall, shoulders back, head held high and a confident smile on your face. And tell yourself, "I love myself, and I respect myself. I have a good body. I have a healthy body. I love my body. I accept my body. From now on, I recognize what is important to me and that is what matters.

Other people's opinions are just that; their opinions. If they are offensive or insulting, I can find it strangely amusing as it means that deep down, they are the insecure ones with problems about their body.

You accept these suggestions because you know they make sense. You know they are the truth, and truth is beauty. You love and respect your body. From now on you trust yourself. You trust your intuition, you trust your subconscious mind. You know that you are a good and worthwhile person who has achieved a lot in life. You are person who is admired by those around you. You are an example of personal excellence to others. You are secret desire of people and you do not even know it. You will likely never know it. But that is okay. Your confidence and best self will find what you need, who you need. You will no longer be distracted by what you imagine others may think of you either way. You are following your own path. You have your eye on a shining star over velvet-black sky. You reach for that star, you reach that star, you are that start. You will continue on your path without concern for what others think or say about you. We will talk more about it, I will make suggestions and these suggestions will be firmly embedded in your subconscious mind. They will grow stronger every day. They will become a part of your psyche, a part of your psychology. And in so being, they become a part of your mind-self and a part of your best self, body and mind. You will be open to the suggestions, mind and body both relaxed and alert. You are at the apex of your mind's powers and your body's strength.

In a moment, I will count the numbers from one to five and at the count of five, you will be fully refreshed and alert. You will be ready to allow these suggestions to work in your life. One … two … three, you're coming slowly back. Four … your eyelids are fluttering. Five … your eyes are open, you are wide awake, your mind and body are returning to normal.

Now let's relax and reflect. Do you feel better about your body? Do you feel more confident? Do you have more compassion for yourself, a greater appreciation of your own beauty, inward and outward? Do you feel that you can access that appreciation with greater ease? Have you gained a greater understanding of what people go through and suffer through in order to embrace that false sense of glamor and superiority?

All things in nature are beautiful. Beauty truly is in the eye of the beholder. Now your own eyes are open wider than they were, keener to observe the hidden beauty in all things, especially yourself. Hold onto that new perspective, using any of the techniques in the book to do so. Make it your mantra during meditation, envision it when you fast or diet. This is the idealized you that you're working toward, the better life and perfect future which is your goal, and to which you are more than entitled. Keep working, it is getting closer every day, in every way, and you're getting better and better.

Interrupted Sleep Relaxation

Ease your body and mind and relax. Leave your troubles behind you. You feel more at ease. It is okay if your mind wanders to pleasant but distracting thought. Your inner mind continues to listen. It enjoys the sense of harmony, peace, and tranquility that grows and develops inside you.

You know those feelings that you have when sleeping soundly, how you sometimes wish that you could just be left to sleep. Remember how you felt laying on a lawn or on a beach in the sun. You recall drifting in and out of sleep, yawning, and wanting nothing more than to stay just where you were.

Remember the comforting feeling of being a child, snug in your bed. You were safe, you were secure, you were looked after. Your childhood challenges may have seemed like a lot, but you can see them now for the mere trifles that they were. You were warm and comfortable and taken care of, a refuge that adult life rarely offers. You had no real responsibilities, as you do now. You faced no real risks, as you do now. Your life was simple, uncomplicated. Recall those warm, comforting feelings, of your mother's loving embrace and of a warm dinner in your belly. Sleep was a refuge then as it is today, necessary for body, mind, and soul. Sleep refreshes the mind as it give the body a chance to fast and to renew. Every morning you wake up, you are born anew.

Think about those rainy nights when you were a child, snuggled up warm. Reflect on those summer days when you could blissfully sleep in. Use your powerful subconscious mind to conjure the smells, the sights, your childhood bedroom. What was hanging on the walls? Were there pets in the room? Can you smell the cedar shavings of the hamster cage, or the briny scent of the fish food?

Relax and let your senses come alive. Be open and receptive, your mind ready to take you where you need and want to be. There's nothing stopping you, nothing threatening you. You are free. You are strong. You are in total control. You are in control of your body and mind. You are in control of your world, of all worlds.

You *are* all worlds.

You are free. You are free to travel where you wish, whenever you wish. You can travel to wherever you wish, to envision your ideal self in your ideal future. You can go to the past and forgive and let go, then release it forever. You can clean out the cupboards of your emotions, you can tell what is truth and what is a lie, an illusion meant to beguile. You cannot be fooled. You cannot be beguiled. You cannot be controlled. You cannot be contained. You cannot be constrained. You will not be controlled. You will not be contained. You will not be constrained.

I'm going to count slowly back from ten to zero and as I do, you find that you relax more and more with every number. You feel just now just as deeply relaxed as you did then.

Ten … feel yourself descending. Nine … you're drifting lazily. Eight … you're relaxing even more. Seven … you're going deeper. Six … deeper still. Five … you're halfway to total body relaxation. Four … that comfortable feeling is returning to your arms, legs, torso. Three, two … you're almost there. One … zero. Now you're looking up into a gorgeous night sky and that you can see a star in the distance. You can see one beautiful, solitary, silver star, shining down out of a velvety black night sky. That star is countless millions of miles away. You focus on that one solitary star. Note how it sparkles. You're even more relaxed now, more peaceful, calmer.

Envision yourself rising out of your body, drawn to that star. You move toward that star, through space and time and through the earth's stratosphere, passing planets and comets, passing through other galaxies, as you get closer to the star.

The nearer you get, the larger and brighter it is and the more comfortable and relaxed you are. Finally, you arrive at the star, it is right there in front of you … one solitary silver star. Now you are on the star, *in* the star … and the star is in you.

Now you *are* the star, the star is *you.*

Go deeper into a gentle hypnotic rest. Note the beautiful stairway in your star, with hundreds of sterling steps descending. You walk down the stairs, very nearly floating, your feet not touching the stairs at all. The word *relax* is written on each step. As you descend. you become even more comfortable, more at ease and relaxed. and at ease.

You're becoming sleepier, drifting deeper. From time to time, you may feel as if you are drifting off to sleep because you are so relaxed … so … relaxed.

For a while now, you know that you have been having trouble going back to sleep once you have been awakened and I know that you need to be fully alert once you awaken in order to deal with the situation in hand.

However, once you have dealt with the situation you have probably found that the harder you try to go back to sleep, the harder it is. This is known as *the law of reversed effect.* We are going to reverse that situation again by using a different technique.

Instead of trying to get back to sleep, you are going to learn how to put yourself into a hypnotic trance. And who knows? This may lead to sleep. But if it does not, you will still receive the same benefit as being asleep; because one hour of hypnosis is worth eight hours of quality sleep.

When your sleep is interrupted and it is time for you to go back to your bed, make yourself as comfortable as possible. Begin by imagining that you asked to perform a particularly unpleasant task. This chore is something you do not want to do, something you would go way out of your way to avoid doing, if possible. If you were asleep, you would not need to respond to the request. So pretend that you are asleep. Match the breathing pattern that you adapt when you are just falling asleep; slowly, rhythmically, deeply, evenly, breathing in slowly and holding that breath for a moment and then breathing out. Then again, breathing in slowly and holding before slowly releasing it. Go on with this this breathing technique for a minute or two.

As you breathe, feel your body starting to relax. Feel your body starting to feel heavy, starting to feel comfortable. That heaviness spreads up through your body, from the tips of your toes to the top of your head.

Take yourself back to the top of that beautiful staircase, noticing how safe and inviting it is as you descend … going down deeper … deeper with each step … relaxing more and then more still. You feel heavier and more comfortable than you ever thought possible.

Perhaps you can count those steps down, from twenty to zero, imagining yourself going deeper and deeper still, perhaps curious about what you will find at the bottom of those stairs.

Going down deeper, relaxing … easing … feeling oh so comfortable and so heavy and so relaxed. You do not care if you sleep, you enjoy this relaxation as you go deeper inside yourself.

The deeper you go the more comfortable and more relaxed you become, feeling heavy and detached, relaxed and happy and curious about what you will see at the bottom of your stairs.

The further down you go, the deeper into hypnosis you are. Perhaps you see the door at the bottom of the stairs, allow the door to formulate in your inner vision. Envision the door; the color, the size, the handle, what it is made out of.

Note your feelings. Are you intimidated by what may be behind that door? Are you afraid to walk through the door and face it? Or are you ready to open the door, eager to face whatever is on the other side. You know you have the power to control this world, that you are in the place of the mind-self. You are the master of this domain, and you are in complete control.

You are in complete control.

Open that door and walk through, closing it gently behind you. You will be in a place, having closed the door on any distractions.

Let the shadows rise to reveal that you're not in a room at all. The door has led to an outside realm, a beautiful and fanciful land of bright color and crisp beauty. Hear the birds tweeting, feel the breeze on your face. This is the place of your best self, the best place. Here, all is right and well. It is alive with activity, yet it is tranquil and languid, a place of perfect calm and relaxation.

Every time you go through this door you will discover something different, as you explore the beautiful realms of your subconscious mind. See the amazing misty colors swirling around, walk through a forest and note the fresh woodland smell and the leaves and patterns in the bark of the trees, where the branches intertwine with glimmers of sun shining through. Perhaps you will see a squirrel running up the tree and leaping among the branches before disappearing out of view.

The place is mercurial, changeable, adaptable, flexible. It contorts to your moods, it is the place where mind and body meet. And it is the gateway to all other places, all worlds. Because you are all worlds, and you are the mind-self of this space. From here, wherever you may be, you can open any door to any place or any time, far removed though it may be. You are at the central vortex of all space and time, of all worlds, of all the people you are or have been or could ever be.

Use this power. Use it at your will. It is a power that you and you alone can master for yourself. You can only transport yourself or help others to transport themselves, as I am doing for you now. But you alone hold the key to realizing your own inner vision. Only you can look into your own past. Only you know the pains of your past and the possibilities of your future. Only you can clear those emotional cupboards. Only you can open that door.

So go where only you can go, and do what only you can do. Visit exotic, faraway lands, take an ocean voyage or travel through time and space. Or you could visit a particularly happy memory from your past, or remember an event from your childhood that you had almost forgotten about.

Explore a tropical island out there in the sun and stroll along on the beach or splash in the warm water or relax and bask in the warmth of the summer sun. Go for a hike among the mighty redwoods of the Great

Northwest. Visit Stonehenge or London, hear Big Ben ring over the Thames. Compare it to Notre Dame, on the banks of the Seine. Climb Mt. Everest and make it back down; jump from the peak and fly down if you like, or just keep flying and never come down.

This is your special time. Utilize this experience and your creative imagination - to discover the journeys that lie inside you. You have the potential to go wherever you wish, knowing that when it is time to awaken you can do so, feeling calm and refreshed and ready to deal with anything.

Drift off to a place deep inside you, awakening at your regular time, alert and refreshed.

Remember that when your sleep has been interrupted for any reason that does not require your immediate attention, return to your bed or your couch or wherever you may be. Envision that you have been asked to perform a task that you'd rather not do. This could be something like going out in the wind and rain or sweeping leaves from outside your home. It is a task you would like to avoid at all costs, so you pretend to be asleep.

Mimic the actions and inactions of sleep by closing your eyes and breathing deeply and regularly as that warm heavy feeling spreads from the tips of your toes to the top of your head.

Take yourself to the top of that staircase as that heaviness increases and your tired body relaxes and drifts off to its own special place.

You are breathing slowly, rhythmically. As you descend the stairs and the heaviness and relaxation increases, a mist forms in your mind as faint images appear. Those images grow clearer as you embark on a different adventure before drifting back to sleep.

Feel that heaviness come over you, body and mind. Feel your body sink into the sheets, the mattress, the pillow. Feel the comforter wrap around you like your mother's loving embrace. Return to that time of peace in your life, when worry and responsibility were an illusion, where life was but a dream. There can be no distractions in that mindset, nothing will be able to pierce that comforting calm. You find yourself in a peaceful place, a peaceful space. There are no obstacles, nothing standing in the way of your restful repast. You will not toss and turn. You will not be hungry to distraction. Your body is perfectly comfortable, grateful to have this time to do what it needs to do, what it must do to create the best you, the best body for your best mind. This is what your want in body and mind, and what you deserve.

And you have it.

You find that sleep comes easily to you. When you return to bed after being interrupted, your body naturally resumes a comfortable position and you enjoy the rest of your rest.

I'm going to be quiet for a moment as you open that door and step through it to wherever it leads you.

These suggestions are deeply embedded in your subconscious mind. They grow stronger every day. They grow stronger by the day, stronger by the hour, stronger by the minute.

And while your strength increases, so does your power over the things which stood between you and a good night's sleep. The worries, the stresses, none can compete with your newly enlightened will. You will sleep through the night, because your mind will create a world where this happens. That world is your world. That world is you.

You can control your body, and only you can give it what it needs. It needs sleep. It wants sleep. Your mind needs sleep. Your mind wants sleep. And nothing in this world or any other can stop you, can interrupt you. No hunger pangs can get through that comfortable bed. No worries about self-image can violate the snug sanctity of your rest bed. Sleep is like a form of meditation. You focus on one thing, a good night's sleep. You focus on the dark of your closed eyes, the silence of the room around you. The world is sleeping, you too will sleep. Because there is nothing which can stand against your united mind and body, your best and strongest mind-self.

In a moment, I'm going to count you back up to normal conscious awareness. At the count of five you will be wide awake fully alert and refreshed and ready to allow these suggestions to work for you.

One … two … three … coming back slowly. Four … eyelids are fluttering. Five … your eyes are opening, you are wide awake, body mind and body are returning to normal.

Now let's relax and reflect. Where did you go with your special time? How did it feel to be there? What effects were there from your session? When descended into hypnotism, how did it feel? Was the sensation familiar? Did you feel the sensation of heaviness, calmness, ready for sleep? Was your mind peaceful, ready for rest? Do you feel more secure facing a night's sleep? Ae you looking forward to trying them just before bedtime? Are you confident or do you have trepidation? Either is normal, both are positive. They mean you're invested in you efforts, and they mean you have a good chance of success. The great thing is that you can always try again, with this or any of our specialized sessions. They'll become more familiar, easier to manage and more effective. If you made progress with this session, congratulations. If not, congratulations for trying. Even if you had success, try again anyway. That is what this book, what all of our books, are truly all about.

We have taken journeys to the limits of existence and then well beyond that. You now have the power and the experience to travel again, to make such travel a regular part of your life. You will find a richer world within and without. And what you learn will work with your other efforts toward total wellness. Congratulations on breaching that final frontier. You have worked hard and earned the value of the experiences you've had in the realm of the mind-self.

CONCLUSION

Congratulations! You started out this journey with a need, for change and for the knowledge of how to affect that change. Our promise was that if you retained just one significant lesson from this book, it could change your life. All of them could be a revolution for you and for everyone you know. But I'll bet you've picked up much more than that. So it's time for a personal review: Which lessons did you learn the most from? Which was the greater revelation, that cholesterol can be both good and bad, and that each comes from different types of foods? Did you realize how important hormones are to your overall wellness and good health? Did you ever realize you could manipulate your own hormone level and prevent hormonal imbalance? If you did know that, did you realize that some aspects of hormonal function are actually hereditary? Or was it the differences between the different kinds of fats? Was it the fasting? Which type did you try? If both, which worked best? Had you ever heard of autophagy before? How do people react when you explain it to them?

Had you ever practiced yoga before? If you read the book through a first time before applying any of it, are you looking forward to it? Or would meditation be a better place for you to start? At least you're thinking about these things, asking these questions, and that's the key to your ongoing success.

Keep asking these questions, because the nature of this book is to keep you interested and curious, to keep you learning more and teaching more about these things. You may have taken the journey from wanting better health to having it, from ignorance about the benefits and practices of yoga and meditation and exercise. But that journey doesn't really end. From the new perspective of your so-called destination, you can see that life itself is a journey and requires constant progress. As comprehensive as this book is, we acknowledge that it's just the first leg of your journey to wellness. There will be more scientific breakthrough and discoveries, and your journey calls upon you to be openminded to them. Keep abreast of the new studies, of the cutting edge tech. There are more exercises to learn, more complicated yoga classes, more intense meditative practices.

And when it comes to hypnosis, the sky is genuinely the limit. You've learned to let your mind control your body, but we've given you insight into ways to control your mind in a way you never thought possible. It's just another tool in your wellness toolbox, now it's one you can use.

You can always investigate new ways of thinking and being. You can and you must; you owe it to yourself and to those you love. And this book has shown you the way; it's up to you to make the most of it, to keep going on your journey. But take this book with you, as it has information you will go back to again and again. You may need refreshing as to all the complex facts and concepts. You may need a booster to your confidence. That's okay, everybody needs that from time to time.

But don't let this book be the only one you read. We offer other books on this subject, such as the one which focuses on women. Female bodies have particular needs and complexities which male bodies don't have. There will be some repeated information, but only what is required for complete understanding. There's more to learn, and we're dedicated to helping you through every new stage of your personal development.

Look our catalogue over and see if we don't have books for maladies you may not even know you suffer from. Open your mind and your heart to new avenues, new fields of study, new ways to make yourself a better person and your life a better experience. Helping yourself is a practice which transcends any single aspect of life. And, of course, every facet affects every other facet. These parts of our lives, of ourselves, are interlocked, each touching the other in critical and crucial ways. If this is the one lesson you took away from this book, then that alone is worth the price.

Still, you're now well-informed about dieting, nutrition, exercise, mental expansion, mental and physical unity. And you've seen not just how they work, but *that* they work. Since this is a book to be reread, to be used as a field guide for wellness, you may have read it once through just for a bedrock foundational understanding. You may not have tried any of the exercises yet, or the meditations. And that's excellent. Now you can go back with a sense of familiarity, with fewer questions and greater understanding. The dietary sections of the book aren't meant to be read once and memorized, but to be referred to often. So we encourage you to go back and read it again, to apply the exercises.

Or you might have dived right in and chosen a diet, engaged in some of these programs and exercises. That's great too! Neither approach is wrong if it's right for you. And if you did jump right in, now is the time to step back and reflect. How do you feel? How much better do you feel? How are our cholesterol levels? Did you lose weight? How much? It's probably something, and that's great. It may not be as much as you'd hoped. But guess what, that's great too! We agreed at the beginning that there were no magic bullets, no overnight miracles. Whatever progress you've made is proof positive that these exercises, diets, and other applications work. The more they are implemented, the more they will continue to work. Let your progress be your guide. Keep it up! You should have a new sense of empowerment and capability. You should have more energy and endurance to accomplish even more. Fast longer, exercise harder, be more mindful and more deliberate.

But remember or caveats: Good change is gradual change. Always transition into and out of any dietary or exercise application in the macro and the micro. Always consult a physician before starting a new dietary and/or exercise protocol. Keep in touch with your doctor too, to note any changes and make sure no damage is being done. Never overstress your body and mind; stress is good for your body, as it instigates change. Too much stress is harmful, as it can damage muscle, bone, and organ function. Remember that you're on a journey, and every so-called *destination* is just a waystation on the way to something bigger, someone better.

Keep up your journey, wherever it takes you. Every journey will be unique to the person taking it. Every discovery will reveal a new challenge, every destination points out the next road to travel. Along the way, you'll travel with more strength, more energy, more people following you. At the end, you'll find that idealized life and self you're working toward. Though chances are, once you've achieved that you'll only want to move forward still, improving things time and again. There's always room for improvement; and, as always, we'll be there with you every step of the way.

So let's keep going!

RESOURCES

https://getkion.com/blogs/all/intermittent-fasting-weight-loss
https://getkion.com/blogs/all/how-to-fast
https://getkion.com/blogs/all/breaking-a-fast-mindfully
https://intermittentdieter.com/best-foods-to-break-a-fast/
https://www.healthline.com/health/autophagy
https://www.medicalnewstoday.com/articles/autophagy#health-effects
https://www.whitneyerd.com/2020/01/the-truth-about-autophagy.html
https://paleoleap.com/long-fasts/
https://www.healthline.com/nutrition/6-ways-to-do-intermittent-fasting
https://www.jagranjosh.com/general-knowledge/list-of-important-hormones-and-their-functions-1516176713-1
https://www.hormone.org/your-health-and-hormones/glands-and-hormones-a-to-z
https://www.healthline.com/health/hormonal-imbalance#hair-loss
https://www.healthline.com/health/hormonal-imbalance#other-complications
https://www.ncbi.nlm.nih.gov/pmc/articles/PMC4445642/
https://www.arbor-health.com/blog/estrogen-dominance
https://www.uclahealth.org/endocrine-center/genetic-syndromes
https://health.clevelandclinic.org/are-you-planning-a-cleanse-or-detox-read-this-first/
https://www.healthline.com/nutrition/how-to-detox-your-body#The-Bottom-Line
https://skinkraft.com/blogs/articles/toxic-chemicals-in-cosmetics
https://thefoxandshe.com/skincare-ingredients-to-avoid/
https://experiencelife.lifetime.life/article/8-hidden-toxins-whats-lurking-in-your-cleaning-products/
https://www.lovense.com/bdsm-blog/enema-solutions
https://draxe.com/health/coffee-enema/
https://www.everydayhealth.com/diet-and-nutrition/diet/detox-cleanses-most-popular-types-what-know/
https://www.byrdie.com/best-juice-cleanses-4800007
https://www.cookinglight.com/eating-smart/clean-eating/3-cleanses-you-should-never-do-and-3-worth-trying
https://www.gaiam.com/blogs/discover/10-ways-to-detoxify-your-body
https://www.healthline.com/health/type-2-diabetes-ketogenic-diet
https://intermittentdieter.com/best-foods-to-break-a-fast/
https://www.mayoclinic.org/healthy-lifestyle/nutrition-and-healthy-eating/in-depth/paleo-diet/art-20111182
https://www.medicalnewstoday.com/articles/324405
https://www.webmd.com/diet/atkins-diet-what-you-can-eat#3
https://www.atkins.com/how-it-works/library/articles/7-day-keto-meal-plan
https://www.mayoclinic.org/diseases-conditions/diabetes/in-depth/diabetes-diet/art-20044295
https://www.marksdailyapple.com/how-to-exercise-while-fasting/
https://www.menshealth.com/fitness/a30300614/intermittent-fasting-working-out/
https://www.webmd.com/diet/a-z/hormone-diet
https://www.eatingwell.com/article/7805452/hormone-balancing-foods-how-diet-can-help/
https://www.health.harvard.edu/staying-healthy/the-truth-about-fats-bad-and-good
https://www.heart.org/en/healthy-living/healthy-eating/eat-smart/fats/dietary-fats
https://health.clevelandclinic.org/where-does-body-fat-go-when-you-lose-weight/

https://www.prevention.com/fitness/g20459708/best-workouts-to-target-belly-fat/
https://www.keckmedicine.org/what-is-the-difference-between-good-and-bad-cholesterol/
https://yogasynergy.com/article-on-fasting-and-yoga-by-john-mcwhorter/
https://dailycup.yoga/2019/11/10/why-you-should-consider-fasting-4-tips-to-prepare-for-your-first-fast/
https://www.chandriniyoga.com/blog/2018/4/29/the-practice-of-yoga-while-fasting
https://www.juruyoga.com/the-practice-of-yoga-while-fasting/
https://www.yogadownload.com/Utilities/ProgramDisplay/tabid/359/prodid/13004#.YH0Alz9lBPY
https://glennfay.medium.com/intermittent-fasting-and-meditation-remedies-for-weight-management-acdbf53ba76c
https://medium.com/the-ascent/meditation-intermittent-fasting-for-the-mind-7ab6a98cdb23
https://ourworldindata.org/obesity#what-are-the-drivers-of-obesity
https://www.ncbi.nlm.nih.gov/pmc/articles/PMC6347410/
https://www.healthline.com/nutrition/top-13-evidence-based-health-benefits-of-coffee#TOC_TITLE_HDR_5
https://courses.lumenlearning.com/introchem/chapter/hydrogenation/
https://booksy.com/blog/us/what-is-holistic-medicine-and-why-should-i-care/
https://www.nhs.uk/live-well/exercise/exercise-health-benefits/
https://www.hypno-fasting.com/faq
https://hypnotc.com/hypnotherapy-fasting-weight-loss/
https://www.verywellmind.com/best-hypnosis-apps-4800547
https://www.hypnotherapy-london.info/the-history-of-hypnosis/
https://www.spaceotechnologies.com/best-intermittent-fasting-apps/
https://www.tomsguide.com/best-picks/best-workout-apps
https://www.verywellfit.com/best-yoga-apps-4176689
https://www.nhs.uk/live-well/exercise/exercise-health-benefits/
https://www.hypnoticworld.com/hypnosis-scripts/
https://www.mayoclinic.org/healthy-lifestyle/nutrition-and-healthy-eating/in-depth/vegetarian-diet/art-20046446
https://www.tasteofhome.com/collection/vegetarian-meal-plan/

CPSIA information can be obtained
at www.ICGtesting.com
Printed in the USA
LVHW060025220521
688193LV00012B/753

9 781801 343183